D1524478

CONTENTS

INTRODUCTION 9

BREAKFAST RECIPES 13

1. Ham & Jicama Hash 13
2. Italian Breakfast Bake 13
3. Misto Quente 13
4. Zucchini Bread 13
5. Tortilla 13
6. Poached Eggs & Grits 14
7. Stuffed French Toast 14
8. Sunrise Smoothies 14
9. Strawberry & Ricotta Crepes 14
10. Apple Cinnamon Scones 14
11. Lemon Glazed Blueberry Bread 15
12. Simple Grain-free Biscuits 15
13. Strawberry Coconut Scones 15
14. Blueberry English Muffin Loaf 15
15. Cheese Spinach Waffles 16
16. Carrot And Oat Pancakes 16
17. Jicama Hash Browns 16
18. Spinach & Tomato Egg Muffins 16
19. Cinnamon Rolls 16
20. Strawberry Kiwi Smoothies 17
21. Hawaiian Breakfast Bake 17
22. Apple Topped French Toast 17
23. Pecan-oatmeal Pancakes 17
24. Pumpkin Spice French Toast 17
25. Tex Mex Breakfast Bake 18
26. Bagels 18
27. Cornbread 18
28. Ham & Broccoli Breakfast Bake 18
29. Muffins Sandwich 19
30. Cauliflower Potato Mash 19
31. Apple Cheddar Muffins 19
32. Mini Mushroom Egg Stacks 19
33. Savory Breakfast Egg Bites 19
34. Scallion Sandwich 20
35. Zucchini And Walnut Cake With Maple Flavor Icing 20
36. Easy Turkey Breakfast Patties 20
37. Sweet Nuts Butter 20
38. Apple Walnut Pancakes 20
39. Blueberry Muffins 21
40. Blueberry Buns 21
41. Cafe Mocha Smoothies 21
42. Baked Eggs 21
43. Blueberry Stuffed French Toast 21
44. Hot Maple Porridge 22

45. Cottage Cheese Pancakes 22
46. Scotch Eggs 22
47. Breakfast Pizza 22
48. French Toast In Sticks 22
49. Mango Strawberry Smoothies 23
50. Fried Egg 23
51. Tofu Scramble 23
52. Scrumptious Orange Muffins 23
53. Cauliflower Hash Browns 24
54. Grilled Sandwich With Three Types Of Cheese 24
55. Holiday Strata 24
56. Blueberry Cinnamon Muffins 24
57. Crab & Spinach Frittata 24
58. Apple Filled Swedish Pancake 25
59. Apple Cinnamon Muffins 25
60. Santa Fe Style Pizza 25
61. Brussels Sprout With Fried Eggs 25
62. Cauliflower Breakfast Hash 26
63. Peanut Butter And Berry Oatmeal 26
64. Quick Breakfast Yogurt Sundae 26
65. Olive & Mushroom Frittata 26
66. Pumpkin Muffins 26
67. Vanilla Mango Smoothies 27
68. Cheesy Spinach And Egg Casserole 27
69. Pumpkin Pie Smoothie 27
70. Berry Breakfast Bark 27
71. Lean Lamb And Turkey Meatballs With Yogurt 27
72. Cocotte Eggs 27
73. Cream Buns With Strawberries 28
74. Yogurt & Granola Breakfast Popsicles 28
75. Spinach Cheddar Squares 28
76. Peanut Butter Waffles 28
77. Bruschetta 29
78. Garlic Bread 29
79. Coconut Breakfast Porridge 29
80. Bacon Bbq 29

SNACK & DESSERTS RECIPES 30

81. Honeydew & Ginger Smoothies 30
82. Broiled Stone Fruit 30
83. Cheesy Onion Dip 30
84. Almond Coconut Biscotti 30
85. Margarita Chicken Dip 30
86. Parmesan Truffle Chips 30
87. Toffee Apple Mini Pies 31
88. Asian Chicken Wings 31
89. Apple Cinnamon Chimichanga 31

90. Lemon Biscuit 31
91. Cinnamon Apple Chips 32
92. Rustic Pear Pie With Nuts 32
93. Raspberry Peach Cobbler 32
94. Apricot Soufflé 32
95. Cinnamon Apple Popcorn 33
96. Blackberry Crostata 33
97. Chia And Raspberry Pudding 33
98. Palm Trees Holder 33
99. Almond Cheesecake Bites 33
100. Tortilla Chips 33
101. Blueberry Lemon "cup" Cakes 34
102. Hot & Spicy Mixed Nuts 34
103. Mozzarella Sticks 34
104. Café Mocha Torte 34
105. Candied Pecans 35
106. Baked Maple Custard 35
107. Buffalo Bites 35
108. Almond Flour Crackers 35
109. Cream Cheese Pound Cake 35
110. Oatmeal Peanut Butter Bars 36
111. Peach Custard Tart 36
112. Double Chocolate Biscotti 36
113. Apple Mini Cakes 36
114. Orange Oatmeal Cookies 37
115. Apple Pear & Pecan Dessert Squares 37
116. Mini Bread Puddings 37
117. Crab & Spinach Dip 37
118. Carrot Cupcakes 38
119. Sticky Ginger Cake 38
120. Cauliflower Hummus 38
121. Mini Apple Oat Muffins 38
122. Cappuccino Mousse 39
123. Cheesy Pita Crisps 39
124. Cranberry And Orange Muffins 39
125. Homemade Cheetos 39
126. Blt Stuffed Cucumbers 39
127. Espresso Chocolate Muffins 40
128. Coconutty Pudding Clouds 40
129. Freezer Fudge 40
130. Strawberry Sorbet 40
131. Italian Eggplant Rollups 40
132. Chocolate Chip Muffins 41
133. Banana Nut Cookies 41
134. Tropical Fruit Tart 41
135. Chocolate And Nut Cake 41
136. Pumpkin And Raspberry Muffins 42
137. Raspberry Lemon Cheesecake Squares 42
138. Raspberry Almond Clafoutis 42
139. Fried Zucchini 42
140. Fruity Coconut Energy Balls 43
141. Chewy Granola Bars 43
142. Blueberry No Bake Cheesecake 43
143. Honey Roasted Pumpkin Seeds 43
144. Fluffy Lemon Bars 44
145. Gingerbread Cookies 44
146. Mini Eggplant Pizzas 44
147. Peanut Butter Pie 44
148. Dark Chocolate Almond Yogurt Cups 44
149. Crispy Apple Chips 45
150. Zucchini Chips 45
151. Rum Spiced Nuts 45
152. Tiramisu 45
153. Raspberry Walnut Parfaits 45
154. Honey & Cinnamon Shortbread 45
155. Strawberry Cheesecake 46
156. Pistachio Cookies 46
157. Peach Ice Cream 46
158. Cheese Crisp Crackers 46
159. Chili Lime Tortilla Chips 47
160. Sangria Jello Cups 47
161. Mini Key Lime Tarts 47
162. Pumpkin Spice Snack Balls 47
163. Chocolate Cherry Cake Roll 47
164. Banana And Nut Bread 48
165. Soft Pretzel Bites 48
166. Apple Crisp 48
167. Strawberry Lime Pudding 48
168. Pineapple Frozen Yogurt 49
169. Cheesy Taco Chips 49
170. Tex Mex Popcorn 49
171. Pickled Cucumbers 49
172. Gingerbread Soufflés 49
173. Watermelon & Shrimp Ceviche 50
174. Chocolate Torte 50
175. Autumn Skillet Cake 50
176. German Chocolate Cake Bars 50
177. Watermelon Ice 51
178. Raspberry & Dark Chocolate Mini Soufflés 51
179. Chocolate Orange Bread Pudding 51
180. Fig Cookie Bars 51
181. Cranberry & Almond Granola Bars 52
182. Onion Rings 52
183. Coconut Milk Shakes 52
184. Coconut Macaroni 52
185. Crunchy Apple Fries 52
186. Whole-wheat Pumpkin Muffins 53
187. Caramel Pecan Pie 53

188. Light Cheese Cake With Strawberry Syrup..............53
189. Peanut Butter Banana "ice Cream"................................53
190. Pumpkin Ice Cream With Candied Pecans...........53
191. Chocolate Avocado Mousse..54
192. Dark Chocolate Coffee Cupcakes............................54
193. Easy Banana Mug Cake...54
194. Cinnamon Toasted Almonds.......................................54
195. Rosemary Potato Chips..54
196. Peanut Butter Oatmeal Cookies................................55
197. Moist Butter Cake...55
198. No Bake Lemon Tart...55
199. Coconut Cream Pie..55
200. Grain-free Berry Cobbler..56

BEEF, PORK & LAMB RECIPES................................. 57

201. Beef & Broccoli Skillet..57
202. Balsamic Chicken & Vegetable Skillet....................57
203. Russian Steaks With Nuts And Cheese....................57
204. Creamy Chicken Tenders...57
205. Tangy Balsamic Beef..57
206. Sirloin Strips & "rice"...58
207. Spicy Bbq Beef Brisket...58
208. Slow Cooker Lemon Chicken With Gravy................58
209. Ritzy Beef Stew..58
210. Pork Trinoza Wrapped In Ham....................................59
211. Mississippi Style Pot Roast...59
212. Spicy Grilled Turkey Breast...59
213. Stuffed Cabbage And Pork Loin Rolls......................59
214. Cheesy Chicken & Spinach..60
215. Bbq Chicken & Noodles...60
216. Homemade Flamingos...60
217. Pesto Chicken...60
218. Breaded Chicken With Seed Chips.............................60
219. Turkey Meatballs With Spaghetti Squash................60
220. Spicy Lettuce Wraps...61
221. Deconstructed Philly Cheesesteaks..........................61
222. Bbq Pork Tacos...61
223. Beef Picadillo..61
224. Citrus Pork Tenderloin...62
225. Beef Scallops...62
226. Chicken Pappardelle...62
227. One Pot Beef & Veggies...63
228. Zesty Chicken & Asparagus Pasta.............................63
229. Curried Chicken & Apples...63
230. Arroz Con Pollo...63
231. Tasty Harissa Chicken..64
232. Pork Souvlakia With Tzatziki Sauce...........................64
233. Salted Biscuit Pie Turkey Chops.................................64
234. Cheesy Beef & Noodles...64

235. Chicken's Liver...64
236. Chutney Turkey Burgers..65
237. Chicken Marsala..65
238. Poblano & Cheese Burgers..65
239. Ham And Cheese Stuffed Chicken Burgers.............65
240. Turkey Stuffed Peppers...66
241. Sausage & Spinach Frittata..66
242. Crust Less Pizza..66
243. Creamy Turkey & Peas With Noodles........................66
244. Classic Stroganoff...67
245. Ranch Chicken Casserole...67
246. Healthy Turkey Chili...67
247. Roasted Vegetable And Chicken Tortillas................67
248. Beer Braised Brisket..68
249. Beef With Sesame And Ginger.....................................68
250. Cheesy Beef Paseíllo...68
251. Pork Head Chops With Vegetables.............................68
252. Easy Lime Lamb Cutlets..68
253. Hot Chicken Salad Casserole..69
254. Horseradish Meatloaf...69
255. Beef Tenderloin With Roasted Vegetables...............69
256. Ginger Chili Broccoli...69
257. Fried Pork Chops...70
258. Southwest Turkey Lasagna..70
259. Stuffed Grilled Pork Tenderloin...................................70
260. Pasta Bolognese...70
261. Tasty Chicken Tenders..70
262. Creole Chicken...71
263. Potatoes With Loin And Cheese(1)...........................71
264. Kielbasa & Lamb Cassoulet..71
265. Crock Pot Carnitas...71
266. Zucchini Lasagna..71
267. Stuffed Flank Steak..72
268. Shepherd's Pie...72
269. Lemon Chicken With Basil..72
270. Turkey & Pepper Skillet...72
271. Taco Casserole...73
272. Spicy Grilled Flank Steak..73
273. Creamy And Aromatic Chicken....................................73
274. Orange Chicken..74
275. Cajun Chicken & Pasta...74
276. Breaded Chicken Fillets...74
277. Crunchy Grilled Chicken..74
278. Hawaiian Chicken...75
279. Lamb Ragu...75
280. Turkey Roulade...75
281. Jalapeno Turkey Burgers..75
282. Creamy Braised Oxtails..76
283. North Carolina Style Pork Chops.................................76

284. Seared Duck Breast With Red Wine & Figs 76
285. Alfredo Sausage & Vegetables 76
286. Cheesesteak Stuffed Peppers 77
287. Chicken Soup 77
288. French Onion Chicken & Vegetables 77
289. Pork On A Blanket 77
290. Chicken Thighs 77
291. Bacon & Cauliflower Casserole 78
292. Beef Tenderloin Steaks & Brandied Mushrooms ... 78
293. Turkey Stuffed Poblano Peppers 78
294. Hearty Beef Chili 78
295. Turkey Sloppy Joes 79
296. Chestnut Stuffed Pork Roast 79
297. Honey Bourbon Pork Chops 79
298. Pork Rind 79
299. Korean Chicken 80
300. Dry Rub Chicken Wings 80
301. Tandoori Lamb 80
302. Turkey & Mushroom Casserole 80
303. Meatloaf Reboot 81
304. Pork Loin With Onion Beer Sauce 81
305. Mediterranean Stuffed Chicken 81
306. Cajun Smothered Pork Chops 81
307. Pork Liver 81
308. French Onion Casserole 82
309. Cheesy Stuffed Chicken 82
310. Middle East Chicken Skewers 82
311. Chicken Tuscany 82
312. Ritzy Jerked Chicken Breasts 83
313. Lemon Chicken 83
314. Teriyaki Turkey Bowls 83
315. Garlic Honey Pork Chops 83
316. Chicken Stuffed With Mushrooms 84
317. Chicken Zucchini Patties With Salsa 84
318. Roast Turkey & Rosemary Gravy 84
319. Beef Goulash 84
320. Herbed Chicken And Artichoke Hearts 85
321. Mediterranean Lamb Meatballs 85
322. Italian Pork Medallions 85
323. Pork Diane 85
324. Turkey Noodle Casserole 86
325. Cheesy Chicken & "potato" Casserole 86
326. Beef & Veggie Quesadillas 86
327. Sumptuous Lamb And Pomegranate Salad 86
328. Mediterranean Grilled Chicken 87
329. Air Fried Meatloaf 87
330. Honey Garlic Chicken 87
331. Potatoes With Bacon, Onion And Cheese 87
332. Crock Pot Beef Roast With Gravy 88

333. Pork Paprika 88
334. Asian Roasted Duck Legs 88
335. Chicken & Spinach Pasta Skillet 88
336. Short Ribs 88
337. Turkey Meatball And Vegetable Kabobs 89
338. Roasted Duck Legs With Balsamic Mushrooms 89
339. South Of The Border Chicken Casserole 89
340. Swedish Beef Noodles 90
341. Grilled Cajun Beef Tenderloin 90
342. Cashew Chicken 90
343. Pork Chops With Creamy Marsala Sauce 90
344. Chicken Skewers With Yogurt 91
345. Provencal Ribs 91
346. Garlic Butter Steak 91
347. Blue Cheese Crusted Beef Tenderloin 91
348. Turkey Enchiladas 92
349. Easy Carbonara 92
350. Chicken Cordon Bleu 92
MEATLESS RECIPES **93**
351. Harvest Salad 93
352. Spicy Potatoes 93
353. Buffalo Cauliflower Wings 93
354. Asian Noodle Salad 93
355. Cheesy Mushroom And Pesto Flatbreads 94
356. Honey Roasted Carrots 94
357. Mushrooms Stuffed With Tomato 94
358. Cheesy Summer Squash And Quinoa Casserole 94
359. Eggplant Parmesan 94
360. Sweet Potato Salt And Pepper 95
361. Simple Sautéed Greens 95
362. Sweet Potato Chips 95
363. Chili Relleno Casserole 95
364. Cauliflower Rice 95
365. Autumn Slaw 96
366. Pizza Stuffed Portobello's 96
367. Cajun Style French Fries 96
368. Avocado & Citrus Shrimp Salad 96
369. Florentine Pizza 97
370. Vegetables In Air Fryer 97
371. Tofu Bento 97
372. Tofu In Peanut Sauce 97
373. Mexican Scrambled Eggs & Greens 97
374. Sweet Potato Cauliflower Patties 98
375. Healthy Taco Salad 98
376. Wilted Dandelion Greens With Sweet Onion 98
377. Asian Fried Eggplant 98
378. Chicken Guacamole Salad 99
379. Warm Portobello Salad 99

380. Layered Salad 99
381. Hassel Back Potatoes 99
382. Baked "potato" Salad 99
383. Butternut Noodles With Mushroom Sauce 100
384. Caprese Salad 100
385. Asparagus Avocado Soup 100
386. Roasted Broccoli With Garlic 100
387. Roasted Asparagus And Red Peppers 100
388. Chopped Veggie Salad 100
389. Zucchini Fritters 101
390. Egg Stuffed Zucchini Balls 101
391. Cauliflower "mac" And Cheese 101
392. Roasted Potatoes 101
393. Roasted Brussels Sprouts With Wild Rice Bowl 102
394. Garlicky Mushrooms 102
395. Tofu Salad Sandwiches 102
396. Roasted Tomato Brussels Sprouts 102
397. Butternut Fritters 102
398. Crock Pot Stroganoff 103
399. Lobster Roll Salad With Bacon Vinaigrette 103
400. Orange Tofu 103
401. Pomegranate & Brussels Sprouts Salad 103
402. Strawberry & Avocado Salad 104
403. Vegetables With Provolone 104
404. Potato Wedges 104
405. Crispy Tofu With Chili Garlic Noodles 104
406. Asian Style Slaw 104
407. Shrimp & Avocado Salad 105
408. Garden Vegetable Pasta 105
409. Teriyaki Tofu Burger 105
410. Tofu Curry 105
411. Faux Chow Mein 105
412. Roasted Tomato And Bell Pepper Soup 106
413. Festive Holiday Salad 106
414. Grilled Vegetable & Noodle Salad 106
415. Creamy Macaroni And Cheese 106
416. Creamy Pasta With Peas 107
417. Sesame Bok Choy With Almonds 107
418. Roasted Cauliflower With Tomatoes 107
419. Fried Avocado 107
420. French Toast 107
421. Butter-orange Yams 108
422. Grilled Portobello & Zucchini Burger 108
423. Tarragon Spring Peas 108
424. Potatoes With Provencal Herbs With Cheese 108
425. Spiced Potato Wedges 108
426. Roasted Delicata Squash With Thyme 109
427. Scrambled Eggs With Beans, Zucchini, Potatoes And Onions 109
428. Cantaloupe & Prosciutto Salad 109
429. Green Beans 109
430. Holiday Apple & Cranberry Salad 109
431. Asparagus & Bacon Salad 110
432. Eggplant-zucchini Parmesan 110
433. Southwest Chicken Salad 110
434. Tempeh Lettuce Wraps 110
435. Crispy Rye Bread Snacks With Guacamole 110
436. Lime Asparagus With Cashews 110
437. Cabbage Wedges 111
438. Broccoli & Bacon Salad 111
439. Black Pepper & Garlic Tofu 111
440. Watermelon & Arugula Salad 111
441. Broccoli & Mushroom Salad 112
442. Crust Less Broccoli Quiche 112
443. Zucchini "pasta" Salad 112
444. Homemade Vegetable Chili 112
445. Collard Greens With Tomato 113
446. Okra 113
447. Grilled Tofu & Veggie Skewers 113
448. Tex Mex Veggie Bake 113
449. Pad Thai 113
450. Pecan Pear Salad 114

OTHER FAVORITE RECIPES 115
451. Orange Marmalade 115
452. Homemade Pasta 115
453. Pizza Sauce 115
454. Beef Burgundy & Mushroom Stew 115
455. Kale Chips 116
456. Cucumber Ginger Detox 116
457. Spicy Tomato Chicken Soup 116
458. Chicken And Zoodle Soup 116
459. Beef And Mushroom Barley Soup 116
460. Cinnamon Blueberry Sauce 117
461. Bunless Sloppy Joes 117
462. Cilantro Lime Quinoa 117
463. Almond Vanilla Fruit Dip 117
464. Slow-cooked Simple Lamb And Vegetable Stew 117
465. Turkey, Barley And Vegetable Stock 118
466. Red Pepper, Goat Cheese, And Arugula Open-faced Grilled Sandwich 118
467. Roasted Salmon With Salsa Verde 118
468. Black Bean Enchilada Skillet Casserole 119
469. Pear & Poppy Jam 119
470. White Bean & Chicken Soup 119
471. Chocolate-zucchini Muffins 119
472. Slow Cooker Poblano Soup 120
473. Chicken & Pepper Stew 120

474. Lemon Garlic Green Beans................................120
475. "flour" Tortillas...120
476. African Christmas Stew 121
477. Cauliflower Pizza Crust.................................121
478. Crispy Cowboy Black Bean Fritters 121
479. Simple Deviled Eggs....................................121
480. Seafood, Mango, And Avocado Salad 121
481. Winter Chicken And Citrus Salad 122
482. Blueberry Orange Dessert Sauce.....................122
483. Homemade Turkey Breakfast Sausage 122
484. Almond Banana Smoothie..............................122
485. Roasted Mushroom & Cauliflower Soup 123
486. Spicy Sweet Dipping Sauce...........................123
487. Healthy Loaf Of Bread.................................123
488. Oat And Walnut Granola...............................123
489. Ginger-glazed Salmon And Broccoli 123
490. Tomato And Kale Soup.................................124
491. Blackened Tilapia With Mango Salsa.................124
492. Scallops And Asparagus Skillet......................124
493. Crab & Cauliflower Bisque............................124
494. Peanut Chicken Satay 125
495. Lamb Chops With Cherry Glaze 125
496. Garlic Dipping Sauce...................................125
497. Teriyaki Sauce...125
498. Clam & Bacon Soup.....................................126
499. Spinach, And Goat Cheese Breakfast Bake...........126
500. Pizza Crust..126
501. Cream Cheese Swirl Brownies 126
502. Citrus Vinaigrette.......................................127
503. Salmon Dill Soup..127
504. Smoky Pumpkin Soup..................................127
505. Sesame-ginger Chicken Soba.........................127
506. Apple Cider Vinaigrette................................127
507. Ginger Detox Twist......................................128
508. Cranberry Orange Compote...........................128
509. Crispy Parmesan Cups With Beans & Veggies......128
510. Saffron-spiced Chicken Breasts 128
511. Beef Vegetable Soup 128
512. Peaches And Cream Oatmeal Smoothie..............129
513. Roasted Tomato Salsa..................................129
514. Creamy Chicken & Cauliflower Rice Soup.............129
515. Italian Salad Dressing..................................129
516. Rainbow Black Bean Salad.............................129
517. Mango-glazed Pork Tenderloin Roast................130
518. Herb Vinaigrette..130
519. Low-carb No-cook Tomato Ketchup...................130
520. Sprig Of Parsley..130
521. Easy Thai Peanut Sauce................................130
522. Tomato Tuna Melts......................................130

523. Sweet Potato, Chickpea, And Kale Bowl With Creamy Tahini Sauce.......................................131
524. Spice-rubbed Crispy Roast Chicken 131
525. Cheesy Jalapeno Dip...................................131
526. Mashed Butternut Squash.............................131
527. Beef & Lentil Soup......................................131
528. Easy Coconut Chicken Tenders.......................132
529. Sweet Potato, Onion, And Turkey Sausage Hash.132
530. Greek Yogurt Sundae...................................132
531. Smoky Lentil & Leek Soup.............................132
532. "cornbread" Stuffing...................................132
533. Caramel Sauce..133
534. Chunky Chicken Noodle Soup.........................133
535. Light Beer Bread..133
536. Curried Carrot Soup....................................133
537. Marinara Sauce...133
538. Quick Coconut Flour Buns.............................134
539. Harvest Vegetable Soup...............................134
540. French Onion Soup.....................................134
541. Cheesy Vegetable And Hummus Pitas................134
542. Ginger-garlic Cod Cooked In Paper 135
543. Chipotle Chicken & Corn Soup........................135
544. Sautéed Spinach And Tomatoes......................135
545. Quick Tomato Marinara................................135
546. Baked Oysters..135
547. Macaroni And Vegetable Pie..........................136
548. South American Fish Stew..............................136
549. Oven-roasted Veggies..................................136
550. Pork Posole...136
551. Spaghetti Sauce..137
552. Dry Rub For Pork.......................................137
553. Mexican "rice"..137
554. Korean Beef Soup.......................................137
555. Beef & Sweet Potato Stew.............................137
556. Simple Buttercup Squash Soup........................138
557. Herbed Chicken Meatball Wraps......................138
558. Cheesy Broccoli Bites..................................138
559. Sausage & Pepper Soup...............................139
560. Walnut Vinaigrette.....................................139
561. Easy Chicken Cacciatore..............................139
562. Beet, Goat Cheese& Walnut Pesto With Zoodles139
563. Bacon Cheeseburger Dip..............................140
564. Spicy Asian Dipping Sauce............................140
565. Tuscan Sausage Soup..................................140
566. Blueberry & Chicken Salad On A Bed Of Greens.140
567. Grilled Tofu With Sesame Seeds......................140
568. Roasted Asparagus, Onions, And Red Peppers....141
569. Chinese Hot Mustard...................................141
570. Roasted Halibut WithGreen Beans, And Onions ..141

571. Comforting Squash Soup With Crispy Chickpeas 141
572. Beer Cheese & Chicken Soup 141
573. Curried Chicken Soup 142
574. Horseradish Mustard Sauce 142
575. Brown Rice With Carrot, And Scrambled Egg 142
576. Mozzarella & Artichoke Spaghetti Squash 142
577. Turkey Divan Casserole 143
578. Easy Italian Dressing 143
579. Coconut-berry Sunrise Smoothie 143
580. Tomato Soup With Seafood 143
581. Brown Rice & Lentil Salad 144
582. Vegetable Rice Pilaf 144
583. Turkey Chili 144
584. Tangy Asparagus Bisque 144
585. Wild Rice And Cranberries Salad 144

586. No Corn "cornbread" 145
587. Sugar Free Ketchup 145
588. Ritzy Calabaza Squash Soup 145
589. All Purpose Beef Marinade 145
590. Guinness Beef Stew With Cauliflower Mash 145
591. Maple Mustard Salad Dressing 146
592. Cauli-broccoli Tots 146
593. Basic Salsa 146
594. Cheesy Cauliflower Puree 146
595. Green Bean Casserole 146
596. Ceviche 147
597. Whole Veggie-stuffed Trout 147
598. Classic Texas Caviar 147
599. Avocado Cilantro Dressing 147
600. Green Protein Smoothie Recipe 148

INTRODUCTION

Eating and living healthy is not an option that you choose or refuse; it has become compulsory that we live healthy. For some of us, our definition of living healthy is simple and easy to follow. For others, especially those who suffer from Diabetes type 1 or type 2, eating healthy isn't so simple. It is tough and often requires the patient to careful concerning the amount of sugar taken while eating, and level of fat and calories and oil. Sometimes, trying to maintain a high level of carefulness can be really frustrating for the individual, especially when it seems like the condition of the diabetes isn't getting better.

However, it can be made less frustrating!
Meals are meant to be enjoyed not endured. You are not supposed to see meals as a nasty bit of chore that you have to do at a particular part of the day. They can be approached with delight and glee; hence, diabetes patients must live a full dietary life as much as they're staying healthy.I started becoming very concerned with the type of food that diabetic patients ate when someone I knew was diagnosed. The mood around the house the person stayed changed drastically. Although a friend tried to make light of the situation by saying *at least diabetes is not as bad as cancer,* people shushed him quickly. When the person's family and friends accepted that having diabetes was not a death sentence, we felt better. A few more visits to the doctor helped the patient's loved ones to see the light.

There was calm that followed when we learned that the diabetic patient we knew would not die soon. When that calm was present, we surged ahead with the action plan of creating a dietary plan for him. He could not eat the same way he used to as he had to change his diet to help him manage the sickness.At first, the diabetic patient didn't complain. It was okay to eat meals that were different from what the rest of the family. When we saw the dietary plan which contained the type of meals he had to eat, we knew it wasn't going to be an easy journey for him – and for all of us. If you have ever seen a dietary plan for diabetic patients, you would know it isn't really so nice. In the case of this friend of mine, he started to eat 'healthy' meals filled with loads of vegetables, fatty fish, fruits and whole grains. However, they tasted so bland and uninspiring that he avoided eating in the house during the first few weeks of the plan. In a tone that sounded funny but gloomy, he said he was being punished with the food.

It was a challenging experience for me too because watching my friend eat food he didn't feel satisfied with, was challenging. As a form of solidarity action, I adopted the dietary plan.It was hard for me at first, but like my friend, I got used to the meals and just accepted them. However, my curiosity got the better of me, and I started to crave for tastier, more pleasing meals for diabetics. I searched the internet for specific meals that were delicious and spicy. However, I did not see what I wanted, neither did they appeal to my sense of 'good and sumptuous dishes.'My frustration came to a tipping point and I decided it was best I created recipes to fit my need for delicious diabetes-healthy foods. *Afterall, who said eating healthy has to be tasteless?*The series of culinary experiments led me here. And it has been a wonderful journey so far, one I am grateful I embarked on.

The Meals Consideration For Diabetics

The types of food a diabetic patient should eat is not so different from what your doctor or dietician will prescribe as healthy foods. "There is no diabetic diet," says Erin Palinski Wade, RD, CDE. However, as a diabetic, you have to watch the type of food you eat and the nutrients quantities in those foods.When I was curating these recipes, there are some of foods I took into cognizance. These foods had rich and sumptuous blend of all the necessary dietary proportions. Let's examine them:

Veggies

There are no hard and fast rules to this: vegetables are a must-have for any dietary plan. As a diabetic, the one thing you should avoid is calories. Vegetables, especially leafy vegetables, are very low in calories and high in vitamin C.Research findings support the claims that people with diabetes have low levels of Vitamin C. Vegetables are rich in vitamin C; thus, they can help diabetics increase their Vitamin C levels. The antioxidant and anti-inflammatory qualities in Vitamin C are vital in healthy growth and living. The nutrients in vegetables are not only for reducing the amount of sugar in your body, there are other health benefits you get from leafy vegetables. When you take these leafy vegetables, the antioxidants vitamin C antioxidants help to protect your eyes from macular degeneration and cataracts, two common side effects of diabetes. Also, anti-inflammatory qualities reduce inflammation and cellular damage.

Fruits

Fruits are vital for everyone because they contain antioxidants and low levels of cholesterol. There are several fruits that you can take to help you increase the insulin sensitivity. Fruits like strawberries contain anthocyanins, an antioxidant that help reduce cholesterol and insulin levels.

What's more?

These fruits also contain polyphenols, which are great antioxidants. Also, some fruits contain high levels of fiber. Fibers are great for the body as they increase the Vitamin C levels and provide anti-inflammatory benefits that improve your immune system's overall functioning.

Whole Grains

Although whole grains are starchy, they are fibrous starch, and fibers are essential to healthy living. Grains such as brown rice, whole grain breads are some marvelous sources of whole grains. Whole grains are rich in fibers, and fibers are rich in antioxidants and reduce sugar levels.

Protein

The effects of healthy proteins can't be overemphasized. Proteins are healthy for diabetic patients as they help to balance blood sugar level.With proteins, you get high levels of Vitamin B and other useful minerals such as calcium, magnesium and potassium. Plus, did you know legumes such as beans are rich in fibers also? As a diabetic, it is vital that your glycaemic index shows a reduction. A glycaemic index is a tool used to calculate a person's sugar levels and a low glycaemic index shows good diabetic management.Beans are not just good because they help reduce glycaemic index, they are also useful in reducing your risk of cardiovascular diseases.

Greek Yoghurt

Diary is a great choice for diabetics. Various research shows that some dairy products are great for blood sugar management, which is vital in managing diabetes.The blood glucose and insulin levels are also greatly lowered, research has shown, when people take yogurts and some diary products. There are several researches that link reduced rate of type 1 diabetes progressing to type 2 with yogurt. Although some researches aren't altogether in support of this claim – yogurt linked with reduced diabetes – the link is still tangible, and more research is going on.A dietary plan with the right proportions also helps with weight reduction.

How?

A particular type of fat, the Conjugated linolic acid (CLA) found in yogurt, helps reduce your appetite, thereby making it easy for you to resist food.

Fatty Fish

For everyone who wants to live healthy, fatty fish is compulsory food. As a diabetic patient, you have an increased risk of heart disease. When you take fatty fishes such as salmon, sardines, the risk of you getting heart diseases is greatly reduced.The DHA and EPA in fatty fish help protect the cells that line your blood vessels, which improves the way your arteries function.Blood sugar regulation is another major benefit of fatty acids. And let's not forget the high-quality protein contained in fatty fishes. Protein helps stabilize blood sugar levels, which is what you need to be stabilized at all times.In this recipe book, I made sure that I combined these different food classes, in their right proportions, to help those suffering from diabetes to eat well, and eat healthy.

Some of the things I considered when curating these recipes are:

The Time It Takes to Cook These Meals

We all have several obligations, which are productive things that take our time. Many of us don't have the same work schedule. While some people have time to slow-cook their favorite Turkey sandwich on whole wheat with sliced veggies, some aren't so free. In this book, I categorized the recipes into 'quick meals' and 'slow-cooked meals'.Several recipes get cooked within the twinkle of an eye, while others need time and dedication to prepare them. Whether it is a meal that gets cooked in seven minutes, or those that need thirty minutes to cook, they are all healthy and tasty.Also, the recipes are specified into breakfast, lunch and dinner. I know there are people who are often at a crossroads on what to eat for the day, racking their brains nonstop, and feeling frustrated at their lack of food decisions. To help these type of people, I broke down the recipes into 'breakfast recipes for diabetics,' 'lunch recipes for diabetics,' and 'dinner recipes for diabetics'.

Easy stuff, right?

The Recipes Are Easy To Understand

As a person who wasn't particularly the 'cooking type', I always found recipe books filled with culinary jargon. While those jargons have somewhat become second nature to me, I don't think they should be used in a book for starter chefs and regular readers.The language was deliberately made simple and short so that everyone who picks up this book from the bookshelf in your local bookstore will read, understand and get cooking. When you get the book as a gift to the person, it will be easy to start cooking!It doesn't matter whether you are making fat-free cottage cheese with sliced peas or preparing tofu and veggie stir-fry over brown rice, you will easily understand the words. The procedures are easier, with a font that is beautiful and reader-friendly. The spacing was so you – the reader – don't feel overwhelmed by the clustered chunk of texts.Another wonderful benefit of this book is the pictures; they are crisp and clearly show how the already-prepared meal looks. And you can't help but savor the scintillating aroma of these meals wafting from the still pictures in the book.And if you aren't running to the kitchen to make your first salad (dark lettuce or leafy greens) topped with chicken breast and chickpeas with olive oil and vinegar dressing, then return the book to the bookstore.

The Foodstuffs Are Easy To Find

The early days of my friend's diabetic dietary plans had loved ones spending hours at the grocery store looking for foodstuffs to buy. It was a hellish experience for those loved ones because sometimes, they had to drive for almost an hour to get a foodstuff at another grocery store outside of town.The experience made me have a strong distaste for diabetic meals.

***Why would meal so bland require so much stress to buy?* I often asked myself.**

I ensured that the foodstuffs I picked are foodstuffs that you can find in every grocery store around you in this recipe book. Yes, there are some foodstuffs that you may not be familiar with. I wrote possible substitutes for these foodstuffs by the side if peradventure you are unable to get the first. I wouldn't want anyone else, especially beginners, to go through the stress of looking for foodstuffs for your meal.In conclusion, these recipes are the results of my years of experimenting with several recipes. It was no easy journey, but it was worth it!

BREAKFAST RECIPES

1. Ham & Jicama Hash

Servings: 4   Cooking Time: 15 Minutes

Ingredients:
- 6 eggs, beaten
- 2 cups jicama, grated
- 1 cup low fat cheddar cheese, grated
- 1 cup ham, diced
- What you'll need from store cupboard:
- Salt and pepper, to taste
- Nonstick cooking spray

Directions:
Spray a large nonstick skillet with cooking spray and place over medium-high heat. Add jicama and cook, stirring occasionally, until it starts to brown, about 5 minutes.   Add remaining Ingredients and reduce heat to medium. Cook about 3 minutes, then flip over and cook until eggs are set, about 3-5 minutes more. Season with salt and pepper and serve.

Nutrition Info: Calories 221 Total Carbs 8g Net Carbs 5g Protein 21g Fat 11g Sugar 2g Fiber 3g

2. Italian Breakfast Bake

Servings: 8   Cooking Time: 1 Hour

Ingredients:
- 19 oz. pkg. mild Italian sausages, remove casings
- 1 yellow onion, diced
- 8 eggs
- 2 cup half-and-half
- 2 cup reduced fat cheddar cheese, grated
- ¼ cup fresh parsley, diced
- 2 tbsp. butter, divided
- What you'll need from store cupboard:
- 1/2 loaf bread, (chapter 14), cut in cubes
- 1 tsp salt
- ¼ tsp pepper
- ¼ tsp red pepper flakes
- Nonstick cooking spray

Directions:
Spray a 9x13-inch baking dish with cooking spray. Melt 1 tablespoon butter in a skillet over medium heat. Add sausage and cook, breaking up with a spatula, until no longer pink. Transfer to a large bowl.   Add remaining tablespoon butter to the skillet with the onion and cook until soft, 3-5 minutes. Add to sausage with the cheese and bread cubes.   In a separate bowl, whisk together eggs, half-n-half, and seasonings. Pour over sausage mixture, tossing to mix all Ingredients. Pour into prepared baking dish, cover and chill 2 hours, or overnight.   Heat oven to 350 degrees. Remove cover and bake 50-60 minutes, or a knife inserted in center comes out clean. Serve immediately garnished with parsley.

Nutrition Info: Calories 300 Total Carbs 6g Net Carbs 5g Protein 22g Fat 20g Sugar 4g Fiber 1g

3. Misto Quente

Servings: 4   Cooking Time: 10 Minutes

Ingredients:

- 4 slices of bread without shell
- 4 slices of turkey breast
- 4 slices of cheese
- 2 tbsp. cream cheese
- 2 spoons of butter

Directions:
Preheat the air fryer. Set the timer of 5 minutes and the temperature to 200C.   Pass the butter on one side of the slice of bread, and on the other side of the slice, the cream cheese.   Mount the sandwiches placing two slices of turkey breast and two slices cheese between the breads, with the cream cheese inside and the side with butter.   Place the sandwiches in the basket of the air fryer. Set the timer of the air fryer for 5 minutes and press the power button.

Nutrition Info: Calories: 340 Fat: 15g Carbohydrates: 32g Protein: 15g Sugar: 0g Cholesterol: 0mg

4. Zucchini Bread

Servings: 8   Cooking Time: 40 Minutes

Ingredients:
- ¾ cup shredded zucchini
- 1/2 cup almond flour
- 1/4 teaspoon salt
- 1/4 cup cocoa powder, unsweetened
- 1/2 cup chocolate chips, unsweetened, divided
- 6 tablespoons erythritol sweetener
- 1/2 teaspoon baking soda
- 2 tablespoons olive oil
- 1/2 teaspoon vanilla extract, unsweetened
- 2 tablespoons butter, unsalted, melted
- 1 egg, pastured

Directions:
Switch on the air fryer, insert fryer basket, grease it with olive oil, then shut with its lid, set the fryer at 310 degrees F and preheat for 10 minutes.   Meanwhile, place flour in a bowl, add salt, cocoa powder and baking soda and stir until mixed.   Crack the eggs in another bowl, whisk in sweetener, egg, oil, butter, and vanilla until smooth and then slowly whisk in flour mixture until incorporated.   Add zucchini along with 1/3 cup chocolate chips and then fold until just mixed.   Take a mini loaf pan that fits into the air fryer, grease it with olive oil, then pour in the prepared batter and sprinkle remaining chocolate chips on top.   Open the fryer, place the loaf pan in it, close with its lid and cook for 30 minutes at the 310 degrees F until inserted toothpick into the bread slides out clean.   When air fryer beeps, open its lid, remove the loaf pan, then place it on a wire rack and let the bread cool in it for 20 minutes.   Take out the bread, let it cool completely, then cut it into slices and serve.

Nutrition Info: Calories: 356 Cal Carbs: 2 g Fat: 10 g Protein: 8 g Fiber: 2.5 g

5. Tortilla

Servings: Two   Cooking Time: 20 Minutes

Ingredients:
- 2 eggs

- 2 slices of ham, chopped
- 2 slices of chopped mozzarella
- 1 tbsp. chopped onion soup
- ½ cup chopped parsley and chives tea
- Salt, black pepper and oregano to taste
- Olive oil spread

Directions:
Preheat the air fryer for the time of 5 minutes and the temperature at 200C.   Spread a refractory that fits in the basket of the air fryer and has a high shelf and reserve. In a bowl, beat the eggs lightly with a fork. Add the fillings and spices. Place the refractory container in the basket of the air fryer and pour the beaten eggs being careful not to fall.   Set the time from 10 to 15 minutes and press the power button. The tortilla is ready when it is golden brown

Nutrition Info: Calories: 41 Fat: 1.01g Carbohydrates: 6.68g Protein: 1.08g Sugar: 0.25g Cholesterol: 0mg

6.   Poached Eggs & Grits

Servings: 4   Cooking Time: 10 Minutes

Ingredients:
- 4 eggs, poached
- 3 cups skim milk
- ¼ cup Colby cheese, grated
- What you'll need from store cupboard:
- 1 cup grits
- 2 tsp reduced fat parmesan cheese, grated

Directions:
In a large microwavable bowl, stir together the grits and most of the milk, save a little to stir in later. Cook 8-10 minutes, stirring every couple of minutes.   Meanwhile, poach the eggs in a large pot of boiling water.   When grits are done, stir in the cheese until melted and smooth. If they seem too stiff, add the remaining milk.   Ladle into 4 bowls and top each with a poached egg, serve.

Nutrition Info: Calories 180 Total Carbs 15g Net Carbs 14g Protein 13g Fat 6g Sugar 10g Fiber 1g

7.   Stuffed French Toast

Servings: 1   Cooking Time: 10 Minutes

Ingredients:
- 1 slice of brioche bread,
- 64 mm thick, preferably rancid
- 113g cream cheese
- 2 eggs
- 15 ml of milk
- 30 ml whipping cream
- 38g of sugar
- 3g cinnamon
- 2 ml vanilla extract
- Nonstick Spray Oil
- Pistachios chopped to cover
- Maple syrup, to serve

Directions:
Preheat the air fryer, set it to 175°C.   Cut a slit in the middle of the muffin.   Fill the inside of the slit with cream cheese. Leave aside.   Mix the eggs, milk, whipping cream, sugar, cinnamon, and vanilla extract. Moisten the stuffed French toast in the egg mixture for 10 seconds on each side.   Sprinkle each side of French

toast with oil spray.   Place the French toast in the preheated air fryer and cook for 10 minutes at 175°C Stir the French toast carefully with a spatula when you finish cooking.

Nutrition Info: Calories: 159Fat: 7.5g Carbohydrates: 25.2g Protein: 14g Sugar: 0g Cholesterol:90mg

8.   Sunrise Smoothies

Servings: 3   Cooking Time: 10 Minutes

Ingredients:
- 1 banana, frozen and sliced
- ¾ cup ruby red grapefruit juice
- ½ cup fresh pineapple, cubed
- ½ cup peach slices, unsweetened
- What you'll need from store cupboard:
- 4 ice cubes
- 1 tbsp. Splenda

Directions:
Combine all Ingredients in a blender. Process until smooth. Pour into chilled glasses and serve.

Nutrition Info: Calories 97 Total Carbs 24g Net Carbs 22g Protein 1g Fat 0g Sugar 18g Fiber 2g

9.   Strawberry & Ricotta Crepes

Servings: 4   Cooking Time: 15 Minutes

Ingredients:
- 8 eggs
- 1 cup strawberries, sliced
- 1 cup low-fat ricotta cheese
- What you'll need from store cupboard:
- 2 tsp Splenda
- 2 tsp vanilla
- Nonstick cooking spray

Directions:
In a small bowl, place strawberries and sprinkle with 1 teaspoon Splenda, set aside.   In a large mixing bowl, whisk ½ cup ricotta cheese with remaining Ingredients. Spray a small nonstick skillet with cooking spray and heat over medium heat.   Pour ¼ cup batter at a time into hot pan, swirling the pan to cover the bottom. Cook until bottom is brown, about 1-2 minutes. Flip over and cook 1 minute more.   To serve, spread each crepe with 2 tablespoons ricotta cheese and fold over. Top with strawberries.

Nutrition Info: Calories 230 Total Carbs 10g Net Carbs 8g Protein 17g Fat 14g Sugar 9g Fiber 2g

10.   Apple Cinnamon Scones

Servings: 16   Cooking Time: 25 Minutes

Ingredients:
- 2 large eggs
- 1 apple, diced
- ¼ cup + ½ tbsp. margarine, melted and divided
- 1 tbsp. half-n-half
- What you'll need from store cupboard:
- 3 cups almond flour
- 1/3 cup + 2 tsp Splenda
- 2 tsp baking powder
- 2 tsp cinnamon
- 1 tsp vanilla
- ¼ tsp salt

14

Directions:
Heat oven to 325 degrees. Line a large baking sheet with parchment paper.   In a large bowl, whisk flour, 1/3 cup Splenda, baking powder, 1 ½ teaspoons cinnamon, and salt together. Stir in apple.   Add the eggs, ¼ cup melted margarine, cream, and vanilla. Stir until the mixture forms a soft dough.   Divide the dough in half and pat into 2 circles, about 1-inch thick, and 7-8 inches around.   In a small bowl, stir together remaining 2 teaspoons Splenda, and ½ teaspoon cinnamon. Brush the ½ tablespoon melted margarine over dough and sprinkle with cinnamon mixture. Cut each into 8 equal pieces and place on prepared baking sheet. Bake 20-25 minutes, or until golden brown and firm to the touch.
Nutrition Info: Calories 176 Total Carbs 12g Net Carbs 9g Protein 5g Fat 12g Sugar 8g Fiber 3g

11. Lemon Glazed Blueberry Bread

Servings: 12   Cooking Time: 50 Minutes
Ingredients:
- 5 eggs
- ½ cup blueberries
- 5 tbsp. half-n-half, divided
- 3 tbsp. butter, soft
- What you'll need from store cupboard:
- 2 cup almond flour, sifted
- ½ cup Splenda
- 2 tbsp. coconut flour
- 2 tbsp. Swerve confectioners
- 1 ½ tsp baking powder
- 1 tsp vanilla
- Butter flavored cooking spray

Directions:
Heat oven to 350 degrees. Spray an 8.5-inch loaf pan with cooking spray.   In a large bowl, beat the eggs, ½ cup Splenda, and vanilla 2-3 minutes or until the eggs look frothy. Add 3 tablespoons half-n-half and mix again. In a separate bowl, combine flours and baking powder. Add to egg mixture and beat to combine. Beat in the butter then fold in berries.   Transfer to prepared pan and bake 45-50 minutes or it passes the toothpick test. Let cool 10 minutes in the pan, then invert onto serving plate.   In a small bowl, whisk together remaining 2 tablespoons half-n-half, powdered Splenda and lemon juice. When bread has cooled drizzle glaze over top, letting it drip down the sides. Slice and serve.
Nutrition Info: Calories 185 Total Carbs 14g Net Carbs 11g Protein 5g Fat 12g Sugar 10g Fiber 3g

12. Simple Grain-free Biscuits

Servings: 4   Cooking Time: 15 Minutes
Ingredients:
- 2 tablespoons unsalted butter
- ¼ cup plain low-fat Greek yogurt
- Pinch salt
- 1½ cups finely ground almond flour

Directions:
Preheat the oven to 375ºF (190ºC). Line a baking sheet with parchment paper and set aside.   Place the butter in a microwave-safe bowl and microwave for 15 to 20 seconds, or until it is just enough to soften.   Add the yogurt and salt to the bowl of butter and blend well. Slowly pour in the almond flour and keep stirring until the mixture just comes together into a slightly sticky, shaggy dough.   Use a ¼-cup measuring cup to mound balls of dough onto the parchment-lined baking sheet and flatten each into a rounded biscuit shape, about 1 inch thick.   Bake in the preheated oven for 13 to 15 minutes, or until the biscuits are lightly golden brown. Let the biscuits cool for 5 minutes before serving.
Nutrition Info:calories: 309   fat: 28.1g   protein: 9.9g   carbs: 8.7g   fiber: 5.1g   sugar: 2.0g   sodium: 31mg

13. Strawberry Coconut Scones

Servings: 8   Cooking Time: 40 Minutes
Ingredients:
- 1 ½ cup strawberries, chopped
- 1 large egg
- What you'll need from store cupboard:
- 1 ½ cups almond flour
- ¼ cup coconut oil, melted
- ¼ cup Splenda
- ¼ cup unsweetened coconut, grated
- 2 tbsp. cornstarch
- 1 tsp vanilla
- 1 tsp baking powder

Directions:
Heat oven to 350 degrees. Line a 9-inch round baking dish with parchment paper.   In a large bowl, beat egg, oil, Splenda, and vanilla until smooth. Scrape sides as needed.   Turn mixer to low, and add flour, cornstarch, coconut, and baking powder until incorporated.   Fold in strawberries. Spread batter evenly in prepared pan. Bake 35-40 minutes.   Let cool 15 minutes before removing from pan. Slice into 8 pieces.
Nutrition Info: Calories 225 Total Carbs 14g Net Carbs 11g Protein 5g Fat 17g Sugar 8g Fiber 3g

14. Blueberry English Muffin Loaf

Servings: 12   Cooking Time: 1 Hour
Ingredients:
- 6 eggs beaten
- ½ cup almond milk, unsweetened
- ½ cup blueberries
- What you'll need from store cupboard:
- ½ cup cashew butter
- ½ cup almond flour
- ¼ cup coconut oil
- 2 tsp baking powder
- ½ tsp salt
- Nonstick cooking spray

Directions:
Heat oven to 350 degrees. Line a loaf pan with parchment paper and spray lightly with cooking spray. In a small glass bowl, melt cashew butter and oil together in the microwave for 30 seconds. Stir until well combined.   In a large bowl, stir together the dry Ingredients. Add cashew butter mixture and stir well. In a separate bowl, whisk the milk and eggs together. Add to flour mixture and stir well. Fold in blueberries.

Pour into the prepared pan and bake 45 minutes, or until it passes the toothpick test. Cook 30 minutes, remove from pan and slice.

Nutrition Info: Calories 162 Total Carbs 5g Net Carbs 4g Protein 6g Fat 14g Sugar 1g Fiber 1g

15. Cheese Spinach Waffles

Servings: 4   Cooking Time: 20 Minutes
Ingredients:
- 2 strips of bacon, cooked and crumbled
- 2 eggs, lightly beaten
- ½ cup cauliflower, grated
- ½ cup frozen spinach, chopped (squeeze water out first)
- ½ cup low fat mozzarella cheese, grated
- ½ cup low fat cheddar cheese, grated
- 1 tbsp. margarine, melted
- What you'll need from store cupboard:
- ¼ cup reduced fat Parmesan cheese, grated
- 1 tsp onion powder
- 1 tsp garlic powder
- Nonstick cooking spray

Directions:
Thaw spinach and squeeze out as much of the water as you, place in a large bowl. Heat your waffle iron and spray with cooking spray. Add remaining Ingredients to the spinach and mix well. Pour small amounts on the waffle iron and cook like you would for regular waffles. Serve warm.

Nutrition Info: Calories 186 Total Carbs 2g Protein 14g Fat 14g Sugar 1g Fiber 0g

16. Carrot And Oat Pancakes

Servings: 4   Cooking Time: 8 Minutes
Ingredients:
- ¼ cup plain Greek yogurt
- 1 tablespoon pure maple syrup
- 1 cup rolled oats
- 1 cup low-fat cottage cheese
- 1 cup shredded carrots
- ½ cup unsweetened plain almond milk
- 2 eggs
- 1 teaspoon baking powder
- 2 tablespoons ground flaxseed
- ½ teaspoon ground cinnamon
- 2 teaspoons canola oil, divided

Directions:
Stir together the yogurt and maple syrup in a small bowl and set aside. Grind the oats in a blender, or until they are ground into a flour-like consistency. Make the batter: Add the cheese, carrots, almond milk, eggs, baking powder, flaxseed, and cinnamon to the blender, and process until fully mixed and smooth. Heat 1 teaspoon of canola oil in a large skillet over medium heat. Make the pancakes: Pour ¼ cup of batter into the skillet and swirl the pan so the batter covers the bottom evenly. Cook for 1 to 2 minutes until bubbles form on the surface. Gently flip the pancake with a spatula and cook for 1 to 2 minutes more, or until the pancake turns golden brown around the edges. Repeat with the remaining canola oil

and batter. Top the pancakes with the maple yogurt and serve warm.

Nutrition Info: calories: 227   fat: 8.1g   protein: 14.9g   carbs: 24.2g   fiber: 4.0g   sugar: 7.0g   sodium: 403mg

17. Jicama Hash Browns

Servings: 2   Cooking Time: 20 Minutes
Ingredients:
- 2 cups jicama, peeled and grated
- ½ small onion, diced
- What you'll need from the store cupboard
- 1 tbsp. vegetable oil
- A pinch of salt to taste
- A pinch of pepper to taste

Directions:
Add the oil to a large skillet and heat over med-high heat. Add the onion and cook until translucent. Add the jicama and salt and pepper to taste. Cook until nicely browned on both sides. Serve immediately.

Nutrition Info: Calories 113 Total Carbs 12g Net Carbs 6g Protein 1g Fat 7g Sugar 3g Fiber 6g

18. Spinach & Tomato Egg Muffins

Servings: 6   Cooking Time: 25 Minutes
Ingredients:
- 6 eggs
- 2 green onions, sliced
- 1 avocado, sliced
- ½ cup fresh spinach, diced
- 1/3 cup tomatoes, diced
- 1/3 cup reduced-fat cheddar cheese, grated
- ¼ cup almond milk, unsweetened
- What you'll need from the store cupboard:
- Salt and pepper
- Nonstick cooking spray

Directions:
Heat oven to 350 degrees. Spray a muffin pan with cooking spray. In a large bowl, beat together eggs, milk, and salt and pepper to taste. Add remaining Ingredients and mix well. Divide evenly between 6 muffin cups. Bake 20-25 minutes or until egg is set in the middle. Remove from oven let cool 5 minutes. Serve topped with sliced avocado.

Nutrition Info: Calories 176 Total Carbs 5g Net Carbs 2g Protein 8g Fat 15g Sugar 1g Fiber 3g

19. Cinnamon Rolls

Servings: 6   Cooking Time: 20 Minutes
Ingredients:
- 4 eggs
- 1 ripe banana
- What you'll need from store cupboard:
- 2/3 cup coconut flour
- 6 tbsp. honey, divided
- 6 tbsp. coconut oil, soft, divided
- 1 tsp vanilla
- 1 tsp baking soda
- ½ tsp salt
- 1 tbsp. + ½ tsp cinnamon

Directions:

Heat oven to 350 degrees. Line a cookie sheet with parchment paper.   In a medium bowl, lightly beat eggs. Beat in the banana. Add 2 tablespoons honey, 2 tablespoons melted coconut oil, and vanilla and mix to combine.   Mix in flour, salt, baking soda, and ½ teaspoon cinnamon until thoroughly combined. If dough is too sticky add more flour, a little at a time.   Line a work surface with parchment paper and place dough on top. Place another sheet of parchment paper on top and roll out into a large rectangle.   In a small bowl, combine 2 tablespoons honey, 2 tablespoons coconut oil, and 1 tablespoons of cinnamon and spread on dough. Roll up and cut into 6 equal pieces. Place on prepared pan and bake 15-30 minutes, or until golden brown. Let cool 10 minutes. Stir together the remaining 2 tablespoons of honey and coconut oil and spread over warm rolls. Serve.

Nutrition Info: Calories 247 Total Carbs 23g Protein 4g Fat 17g Sugar 20g Fiber 1g

20. Strawberry Kiwi Smoothies

Servings: 4   Cooking Time: 3 Minutes
Ingredients:
- 2 kiwi, peel & quarter
- 6 oz. strawberry yogurt
- 1 cup strawberries, frozen
- ½ cup skim milk
- What you'll need from store cupboard:
- 2 tbsp. honey

Directions:
Place all Ingredients in a blender and process until smooth.   Pour into glasses and serve immediately.

Nutrition Info: Calories 120 Total Carbs 26g Net Carbs 24g Protein 3g Fat 1g Sugar 23g Fiber 2g

21. Hawaiian Breakfast Bake

Servings: 6   Cooking Time: 20 Minutes
Ingredients:
- 6 slice ham, sliced thin
- 6 eggs
- ¼ cup reduced fat cheddar cheese, grated
- What you'll need from store cupboard:
- 6 pineapple slices
- 2 tbsp. salsa
- ½ tsp seasoning blend, salt-free

Directions:
Heat oven to 350 degrees.   Line 6 muffin cups, or ramekins with sliced ham. Layer with cheese, salsa, and pineapple.   Crack one egg into each cup, sprinkle with seasoning blend.   If using ramekins place them on a baking sheet, bake 20-25 minutes or until egg whites are completely set but yolks are still soft. Serve immediately.

Nutrition Info: Calories 135 Total Carbs 5g Net Carbs 4g Protein 12g Fat 8g Sugar 3g Fiber 1g

22. Apple Topped French Toast

Servings: 2   Cooking Time: 10 Minutes
Ingredients:
- 1 apple, peel and slice thin
- 1 egg
- ¼ cup skim milk
- 2 tbsp. margarine, divided
- What you'll need from store cupboard:
- 4 slices Healthy Loaf Bread, (chapter 14)
- 1 tbsp. Splenda brown sugar
- 1 tsp vanilla
- ¼ tsp cinnamon

Directions:
Melt 1 tablespoon margarine in a large skillet over med-high heat. Add apples, Splenda, and cinnamon and cook, stirring frequently, until apples are tender.   In a shallow dish, whisk together egg, milk, and vanilla. Melt the remaining margarine in a separate skillet over med-high heat. Dip each slice of bread in the egg mixture and cook until golden brown on both sides.   Place two slices of French toast on plates, and top with apples. Serve immediately.

Nutrition Info: Calories 394 Total Carbs 27g Net Carbs 22g Protein 10g Fat 23g Sugar 19g Fiber 5g

23. Pecan-oatmeal Pancakes

Servings: 6   Cooking Time: 15 Minutes
Ingredients:
- 1 cup quick-cooking oats
- 1½ teaspoons baking powder
- 2 eggs
- ⅓ cup mashed banana (about ½ medium banana)
- ⅓ cup skim milk
- ½ teaspoon vanilla extract
- 2 tablespoons chopped pecans
- 1 tablespoon canola oil

Directions:
Pulse the oats in a food processor until they are ground into a powder-like consistency.   Transfer the ground oats to a small bowl, along with the baking powder. Mix well.   Whisk together the eggs, mashed banana, skim milk, and vanilla in another bowl. Pour into the bowl of dry ingredients and stir with a spatula just until well incorporated. Add the chopped pecans and mix well. In a large nonstick skillet, heat the canola oil over medium heat.   Spoon ¼ cup of batter for each pancake onto the hot skillet, swirling the pan so the batter covers the bottom evenly. Cook for 1 to 2 minutes until bubbles form on top of the pancake. Flip the pancake and cook for an additional 1 to 2 minutes, or until the pancake is browned and cooked through. Repeat with the remaining batter.   Remove from the heat and serve on a plate.

Nutrition Info:(1 Pancake)calories: 131   fat: 6.9g protein: 5.2g carbs: 13.1g fiber: 2.0g sugar: 2.9g sodium: 120mg

24. Pumpkin Spice French Toast

Servings: 4   Cooking Time: 20 Minutes
Ingredients:
- 6 eggs
- 1 ½ cup skim milk
- What you'll need from store cupboard:
- 8 slices Healthy Loaf Bread, (chapter 15)
- ¼ cup pumpkin
- 1 tsp salt

- 1 tsp pumpkin pie spice
- 1 tsp vanilla
- Butter flavored cooking spray

Directions:

In a large bowl, whisk together all Ingredients, except bread, until combined. Add the bread slices and toss to coat.   Spray a large, nonstick skillet with cooking spray and place over medium heat. Add bread, two slices, or what fits in the pan, at a time and cook 2-3 minutes per side. Serve as is, or with sugar-free maple syrup.

Nutrition Info: Calories 295 Total Carbs 10g net Carbs 8g Protein 17g Fat 20g Sugar 5g Fiber 2g

25. Tex Mex Breakfast Bake

Servings: 9   Cooking Time: 40 Minutes

Ingredients:
- 2 cups egg substitute
- 4 scallions, sliced
- 1 cup reduced-fat Monterey Jack cheese, grated and divided
- ¾ cup bell pepper, diced
- ½ cup fat-free milk
- ½ cup salsa, (chapter 16)
- What you'll need from the store cupboard
- 10 slices light whole-grain bread, cut into 1-inch pieces
- 1 (4-ounce) can green chilies, diced and drained
- ½ tsp chili powder
- ½ tsp garlic powder
- ¼ tsp black pepper
- Nonstick cooking spray

Directions:

Spray a 9x13-inch baking dish with cooking spray. Place bread evenly on the bottom.   Spray a small skillet with cooking spray and place over medium heat. Add bell pepper and cook until tender, about 5 minutes.   In a medium bowl, whisk together remaining Ingredients, reserving ½ cup cheese.   Place the cooked peppers over the bread, then pour in the egg mixture. Cover and chill at least 2 hours or overnight.   Heat oven to 350 degrees. Sprinkle the reserved ½ cheese over the top of casserole and bake, covered, 20 minutes. Remove the cover and bake 15 – 20 minutes more, or until the eggs are firm in the center.   Serve immediately topped salsa.

Nutrition Info: Calories 197 Total Carbs 25g Net Carbs 19g Protein 16g Fat 4g Sugar 9g Fiber 6g

26. Bagels

Servings: 6   Cooking Time: 20 Minutes

Ingredients:
- 2 cups almond flour
- 2 cups shredded mozzarella cheese, low-fat
- 2 tablespoons butter, unsalted
- 1 1/2 teaspoon baking powder
- 1-teaspoon apple cider vinegar
- 1 egg, pastured
- For Egg Wash:
- 1 egg, pastured
- 1-teaspoon butter, unsalted, melted

Directions:

Place flour in a heatproof bowl, add cheese and butter, then stir well and microwave for 90 seconds until butter and cheese has melted.   Then stir the mixture until well combined, let it cool for 5 minutes and whisk in the egg, baking powder, and vinegar until incorporated and dough comes together.   Let the dough cool for 10 minutes, then divide the dough into six sections, shape each section into a bagel and let the bagels rest for 5 minutes.   Prepare the egg wash and for this, place the melted butter in a bowl, whisk in the egg until blended and then brush the mixture generously on top of each bagel.   Take a fryer basket, line it with parchment paper and then place prepared bagels in it in a single layer.   Switch on the air fryer, insert fryer, then shut with its lid, set the fryer at 350 degrees F and cook for 10 minutes at the 350 degrees F until bagels are nicely golden and thoroughly cooked, turning the bagels halfway through the frying.   When air fryer beeps, open its lid, transfer bagels to a serving plate and cook the remaining bagels in the same manner.

Nutrition Info: Calories: 408.7 Cal Carbs: 8.3 g Fat: 33.5 g Protein: 20.3 g Fiber: 4 g

27. Cornbread

Servings: 8   Cooking Time: 25 Minutes

Ingredients:
- 3/4 cup almond flour
- 1-cup white cornmeal
- 1-tablespoon erythritol sweetener
- 1 1/2 teaspoons baking powder
- 1/4 teaspoon salt
- 1/2 teaspoon baking soda
- 6 tablespoons butter, unsalted; melted
- 2 eggs; beaten
- 1 1/2 cups buttermilk, low fat

Directions:

Switch on the air fryer, insert fryer pan, grease it with olive oil, then shut with its lid, set the fryer at 360 degrees F and preheat for 5 minutes.   Meanwhile, crack the egg in a bowl and then whisk in butter and milk until blended. Place flour in another bowl, add remaining ingredients, stir until well mixed and then stir in egg mixture until incorporated.   Open the fryer, pour the batter into the fryer pan, close with its lid and cook for 25 minutes at the 360 degrees F until nicely golden and crispy, shaking halfway through the frying.   When air fryer beeps, open its lid, take out the fryer pan, and then transfer the bread onto a serving plate.   Cut the bread into pieces and serve.

Nutrition Info: Calories: 138 Cal Carbs: 2 g Fat:3 g Protein: 5 g Fiber: 2 g

28. Ham & Broccoli Breakfast Bake

Servings: 8   Cooking Time: 35-40 Minutes

Ingredients:
- 8-10 eggs, beaten
- 4-6 cup small broccoli florets, blanch for 2 minutes, then drain well
- 1-2 cup ham, diced
- 1 cup mozzarella cheese, grated
- 1/3 cup green onion, sliced thin

- What you'll need from store cupboard:
- 1 tsp all-purpose seasoning
- Fresh-ground black pepper, to taste
- Nonstick cooking spray

Directions:
Heat oven to 375. Spray a 9x12-inch baking dish with cooking spray. Layer broccoli, ham, cheese and onions in the dish. Sprinkle with seasoning and pepper. Pour eggs over everything. Using a fork, stir the mixture to make sure everything is coated with the egg. Bake 35-40 minutes, or until eggs are set and top is starting to brown. Serve immediately.
Nutrition Info: Calories 159 Total Carbs 7g Net Carbs 5g Protein 15g Fat 9g Sugar 2g Fiber 2g

29. Muffins Sandwich

Servings: 1   Cooking Time: 10 Minutes
Ingredients:
- Nonstick Spray Oil
- 1 slice of white cheddar cheese
- 1 slice of Canadian bacon
- 1 English muffin, divided
- 15 ml hot water
- 1 large egg
- Salt and pepper to taste

Directions:
Spray the inside of an 85g mold with oil spray and place it in the air fryer. Preheat the air fryer, set it to 160ºC. Add the Canadian cheese and bacon in the preheated air fryer. Pour the hot water and the egg into the hot pan and season with salt and pepper. Select Bread, set to 10 minutes. Take out the English muffins after 7 minutes, leaving the egg for the full time. Build your sandwich by placing the cooked egg on top of the English muffing and serve
Nutrition Info: Calories 400 Fat 26g, Carbohydrates 26g, Sugar 15 g, Protein 3 g, Cholesterol 155 mg

30. Cauliflower Potato Mash

Servings: 4   Cooking Time: 30 Minutes
Ingredients:
- 2 cups potatoes, peeled and cubed
- 2 tbsp. butter
- ¼ cup milk
- 10 oz. cauliflower florets
- ¾ tsp. salt

Directions:
Add water to the saucepan and bring to boil. Reduce heat and simmer for 10 minutes. Drain vegetables well. Transfer vegetables, butter, milk, and salt in a blender and blend until smooth.
Nutrition Info: Calories 128 Fat 6.2 g, Carbohydrates 16.3 g, Sugar 3.3 g, Protein 3.2 g, Cholesterol 17 mg

31. Apple Cheddar Muffins

Servings: 12   Cooking Time: 20 Minutes
Ingredients:
- 1 egg
- ¾ cup tart apple, peel & chop
- 2/3 cup reduced fat cheddar cheese, grated
- 2/3 cup skim milk

- What you'll need from store cupboard:
- 2 cup low carb baking mix
- 2 tbsp. vegetable oil
- 1 tsp cinnamon.

Directions:
Heat oven to 400 degrees F. Line a 12 cup muffin pan with paper liners. In a medium bowl, lightly beat the egg. Stir in remaining Ingredients just until moistened. Divide evenly between prepared muffin cups. Bake 17-20 minutes or until golden brown. Serve warm.
Nutrition Info: Calories 162 Total Carbs 17g Net Carbs 13g Protein 10g Fat 5g Sugar 8g Fiber 4g

32. Mini Mushroom Egg Stacks

Servings: 3   Cooking Time: 25 Minutes
Ingredients:
- 6 mini Portobello mushrooms, rinse and remove stems
- 4 cup of mixed baby kale
- 4 eggs, beaten
- 3 green onions, diced
- 3 slices bacon, cooked crisp and crumbled
- ½ red pepper, diced
- 6 tbsp. low fat cheddar cheese, grated
- What you'll need from store cupboard:
- 3 tbsp. olive oil, divided
- Salt and pepper

Directions:
Heat oven to 350 degrees. Lay mushrooms on baking sheet and brush with 1 tablespoon oil. Sprinkle with salt and pepper and bake 10-15 minutes, or until tender but firm enough to hold their shape. Heat 1 tablespoon oil in a large skillet over med-high heat. Add vegetables and salt and pepper to taste. Cook, stirring frequently until kale has wilted and peppers are tender. Transfer to a bowl. Wipe skillet clean and heat remaining tablespoon oil. Add eggs and scramble to desired doneness. To assemble, top each mushroom with the kale mixture, then eggs. Sprinkle one tablespoon cheese on top then the bacon. One serving is 2 mushroom stacks.
Nutrition Info: Calories 256 Total Carbs 10g Net Carbs 8g Protein 21g Fat 15g Sugar 2g Fiber 2g

33. Savory Breakfast Egg Bites

Servings: 8   Cooking Time: 20 To 25 Minutes
Ingredients:
- 6 eggs, beaten
- ¼ cup unsweetened plain almond milk
- ¼ cup crumbled goat cheese
- ½ cup sliced brown mushrooms
- 1 cup chopped spinach
- ¼ cup sliced sun-dried tomatoes
- 1 red bell pepper, diced
- Salt and freshly ground black pepper, to taste
- Nonstick cooking spray

- Special Equipment:
- An 8-cup muffin tin

Directions:
Preheat the oven to 350ºF (180ºC). Grease an 8-cup muffin tin with nonstick cooking spray. Make the egg bites: Mix together the beaten eggs, almond milk, cheese,

mushroom, spinach, tomatoes, bell pepper, salt, and pepper in a large bowl, and whisk to combine. Spoon the mixture into the prepared muffin cups, filling each about three-quarters full. Bake in the preheated oven for 20 to 25 minutes, or until the top is golden brown and a fork comes out clean. Let the egg bites sit for 5 minutes until slightly cooled. Remove from the muffin tin and serve warm.

Nutrition Info:(1 Egg Bite)calories: 68 fat: 4.1g protein: 6.2g carbs: 2.9g fiber: 1.1g sugar: 2.0g sodium: 126mg

34. Scallion Sandwich

Servings: 1   Cooking Time: 10 Minutes

Ingredients:
- 2 slices wheat bread
- 2 teaspoons butter, low fat
- 2 scallions, sliced thinly
- 1 tablespoon of parmesan cheese, grated
- 3/4 cup of cheddar cheese, reduced fat, grated

Directions:
Preheat the Air fryer to 356 degrees. Spread butter on a slice of bread. Place inside the cooking basket with the butter side facing down. Place cheese and scallions on top. Spread the rest of the butter on the other slice of bread Put it on top of the sandwich and sprinkle with parmesan cheese. Cook for 10 minutes.

Nutrition Info: Calorie: 154Carbohydrate: 9g Fat: 2.5g Protein: 8.6g Fiber: 2.4g

35. Zucchini And Walnut Cake With Maple Flavor Icing

Servings: 5   Cooking Time: 35 Minutes

Ingredients:
- 1 9-ounce package of yellow cake mix
- 1 egg
- ⅓ cup of water
- ½ cup grated zucchini
- ¼ cup chopped walnuts
- ¾ tsp. of cinnamon
- ¼ tsp. nutmeg
- ¼ tsp. ground ginger
- Maple Flavor Glaze

Directions:
Preheat the fryer to a temperature of 350°F. Prepare an 8 x 3⅞ inch loaf pan. Prepare the cake dough according to package directions, using ⅓ cup of water instead of ½ cup. Add zucchini, nuts, cinnamon, nutmeg, and ginger. Pour the dough into the prepared mold and put it inside the basket. Bake until a toothpick inserted in the middle of the cake is clean when removed for 32 to 34 minutes. Remove the cake from the fryer and let it cool on a grill for 10 minutes. Then, remove the cake and place it on a serving plate. Stop cooling just warm. Spray it with maple flavor glaze.

Nutrition Info: Calories: 196 Carbohydrates: 27gFat: 11g Protein: 1g Sugar: 7g Cholesterol: 0mg

36. Easy Turkey Breakfast Patties

Servings: 8   Cooking Time: 10 Minutes

Ingredients:
- 1 pound (454 g) lean ground turkey
- ½ teaspoon dried thyme
- ½ teaspoon dried sage
- ½ teaspoon salt
- ½ teaspoon freshly ground black pepper
- ¼ teaspoon ground fennel seeds
- 1 teaspoon extra-virgin olive oil

Directions:
Mix the ground turkey, thyme, sage, salt, pepper, and fennel in a large bowl, and stir until well combined. Form the turkey mixture into 8 equal-sized patties with your hands. In a skillet, heat the olive oil over medium-high heat. Cook the patties for 3 to 4 minutes per side until cooked through. Transfer the patties to a plate and serve hot.

Nutrition Info:(1 Patty)calories: 91 fat: 4.8g protein: 11.2g carbs: 0.1g fiber: 0.1g sugar: 0g sodium: 155mg

37. Sweet Nuts Butter

Servings: 5   Cooking Time: 25 Minutes

Ingredients:
- 1½ pounds sweet potatoes, peeled and cut into ½ inch pieces (2 medium)
- ½ tbsp. olive oil
- 1 tbsp. melted butter
- 1 tbsp. finely chopped walnuts
- ½ tsp. grated one orange
- ⅛ tsp. nutmeg
- ⅛ tsp. ground cinnamon

Directions:
Put sweet potatoes in a small bowl and sprinkle with oil. Stir until covered and then pour into the basket, ensuring that they are in a single layer. Cook at a temperature of 350°F for 20 to 25 minutes, stirring or turning halfway through cooking. Remove them to the serving plate. Combine the butter, nuts, orange zest, nutmeg, and cinnamon in a small bowl and pour the mixture over the sweet potatoes.

Nutrition Info: Calories: 141 Fat: 1.01g Carbohydrates: 6.68g Protein: 1.08g Sugar: 0.25g Cholesterol: 7mg

38. Apple Walnut Pancakes

Servings: 18   Cooking Time: 30 Minutes

Ingredients:
- 1 apple, peeled and diced
- 2 cup skim milk
- 2 egg whites
- 1 egg, beaten
- What you'll need from store cupboard:
- 1 cup flour
- 1 cup whole wheat flour
- ½ cup walnuts, chopped
- 2 tbsp. sunflower oil
- 1 tbsp. Splenda brown sugar
- 2 tsp baking powder
- 1 tsp salt
- Nonstick cooking spray

Directions:

In a large bowl, combine dry Ingredients. In a separate bowl, combine egg whites, egg, milk, and oil and add to dry Ingredients. Stir just until moistened. Fold in apple and walnuts. Spray a large griddle with cooking spray and heat. Pour batter, ¼ cup on to hot griddle. Flip when bubbles form on top. Cook until second side is golden brown. Serve with sugar free syrup.

Nutrition Info: Calories 120 Total Carbs 15g Net Carbs 13g Protein 4g Fat 5g Sugar 3g Fiber 2g

39. Blueberry Muffins

Servings: 14   Cooking Time: 30 Minutes

Ingredients:
- 1-cup almond flour
- 1 cup frozen blueberries
- 2 teaspoons baking powder
- 1/3 cup erythritol sweetener
- 1 teaspoon vanilla extract, unsweetened
- ½-teaspoon salt
- ¼ cup melted coconut oil
- 1 egg, pastured
- ¼ cup applesauce, unsweetened
- ¼ cup almond milk, unsweetened

Directions:
Switch on the air fryer, insert fryer basket, grease it with olive oil, then shut with its lid, set the fryer at 360 degrees F and preheat for 10 minutes. Meanwhile, place flour in a large bowl, add berries, salt, sweetener, and baking powder and stir until well combined. Crack the eggs in another bowl, whisk in vanilla, milk, and applesauce until combined and then slowly whisk in flour mixture until incorporated. Take fourteen silicone muffin cups, grease them with oil, and then evenly fill them with the prepared batter. Open the fryer; stack muffin cups in it, close with its lid and cook for 10 minutes until muffins are nicely golden brown and set. When air fryer beeps, open its lid, transfer muffins onto a serving plate and then remaining muffins in the same manner.

Nutrition Info: Calories: 201 Cal Carbs: 27.3 g Fat: 8.8 g Protein: 3 g

40. Blueberry Buns

Servings: 6   Cooking Time: 12 Minutes

Ingredients:
- 240g all-purpose flour
- 50g granulated sugar
- 8g baking powder
- 2g of salt
- 85g chopped cold butter
- 85g of fresh blueberries
- 3g grated fresh ginger
- 113 ml whipping cream
- 2 large eggs
- 4 ml vanilla extract
- 5 ml of water

Directions:
Put sugar, flour, baking powder and salt in a large bowl. Put the butter with the flour using a blender or your hands until the mixture resembles thick crumbs. Mix the blueberries and ginger in the flour mixture and set aside Mix the whipping cream, 1 egg and the vanilla

extract in a different container. Put the cream mixture with the flour mixture until combined. Shape the dough until it reaches a thickness of approximately 38 mm and cut it into eighths. Spread the buns with a combination of egg and water. Set aside Preheat the air fryer set it to 180°C. Place baking paper in the preheated inner basket and place the buns on top of the paper. Cook for 12 minutes at 180°C, until golden brown

Nutrition Info: Calories: 105 Fat: 1.64g Carbohydrates: 20.09g Protein: 2.43g Sugar: 2.1g Cholesterol: 0mg

41. Cafe Mocha Smoothies

Servings: 3   Cooking Time: 5 Minutes

Ingredients:
- 1 avocado, remove pit and cut in half
- 1 ½ cup almond milk, unsweetened
- ½ cup canned coconut milk
- What you'll need from store cupboard:
- 3 tbsp. Splenda
- 3 tbsp. unsweetened cocoa powder
- 2 tsp instant coffee
- 1 tsp vanilla

Directions:
Place everything but the avocado in the blender. Process until smooth. Add the avocado and blend until smooth and no chunks remain. Pour into glasses and serve.

Nutrition Info: Calories 109 Total Carbs 15g Protein 6g Fat 1g Sugar 13g Fiber 0g

42. Baked Eggs

Servings: 2   Cooking Time: 17 Minutes

Ingredients:
- 2 tablespoons frozen spinach, thawed
- ½-teaspoon salt
- ¼-teaspoon ground black pepper
- 2 eggs, pastured
- 3 teaspoons grated parmesan cheese, reduced-fat
- 2 tablespoons milk, unsweetened, reduced-fat

Directions:
Switch on the air fryer, insert fryer basket, grease it with olive oil, then shut with its lid, set the fryer at 330 degrees F and preheat for 5 minutes. Meanwhile, take two silicon muffin cups, grease them with oil, then crack an egg into each cup and evenly add cheese, spinach, and milk. Season the egg with salt and black pepper and gently stir the ingredients, without breaking the egg yolk. Open the fryer, add muffin cups in it, close with its lid and cook for 8 to 12 minutes until eggs have cooked to desired doneness. When air fryer beeps, open its lid, take out the muffin cups and serve.

Nutrition Info: Calories: 161 Cal Carbs: 3 g Fat: 11.4 g Protein: 12.1 g Fiber: 1.1

43. Blueberry Stuffed French Toast

Servings: 8   Cooking Time: 20 Minutes

Ingredients:
- 4 eggs
- 1 ½ cup blueberries
- ½ cup orange juice

- 1 tsp orange zest
- What you'll need from store cupboard:
- 16 slices bread, (chapter 14)
- 3 tbsp. Splenda, divided
- 1/8 tsp salt
- Blueberry Orange Dessert Sauce, (chapter 15)
- Nonstick cooking spray

Directions:
Heat oven to 400 degrees. Spray a large baking sheet with cooking spray. In a small bowl, combine berries with 2 tablespoons of Splenda. Lay 8 slices of bread on work surface. Top with about 3 tablespoons of berries and place second slice of bread on top. Flatten slightly. In a shallow dish, whisk remaining Ingredients together. Carefully dip both sides of bread in egg mixture and place on prepared pan. Bake 7-12 minutes per side, or until lightly browned. Heat up dessert sauce until warm. Plate the French toast and top with 1-2 tablespoons of the sauce. Serve.

Nutrition Info: Calories 208 Total Carbs 20g Net Carbs 18g Protein 7g Fat 10g Sugar 14g Fiber 2g

44. Hot Maple Porridge

Servings: 1   Cooking Time: 1 Minute

Ingredients:
- 1 tsp margarine
- What you'll need from store cupboard:
- 1/2 cup water
- 2 tbsp. flax meal
- 1 tbsp. almond flour
- 1 tbsp. coconut flour
- 1 tsp Splenda
- ¼ tsp maple extract
- Pinch salt

Directions:
In a microwave safe bowl, combine all Ingredients, except margarine, and mix thoroughly. Microwave on high for one minute. Stir in margarine and serve.

Nutrition Info: Calories 143 Total Carbs 9g Net Carbs 2g Protein 5g Fat 1g Sugar 0g Fiber 7g

45. Cottage Cheese Pancakes

Servings: 2   Cooking Time: 5 Minutes

Ingredients:
- 1 cup low-fat cottage cheese
- 4 egg whites
- What you'll need from the store cupboard
- ½ cup oats
- 1 tbsp. Stevia, raw, optional
- 1 tsp vanilla
- Nonstick cooking spray

Directions:
Place all Ingredients into a blender and process until smooth. Spray a medium skillet with cooking spray and heat over medium heat. Pour about ¼ cup batter into hot pan and cook until golden brown on both sides. Serve with sugar-free syrup, fresh berries, or topping of your choice.

Nutrition Info: Calories 250 Total carbs 25g Net Carbs 23g Protein 25g Fat 4g Sugar 7g Fiber 2g

46. Scotch Eggs

Servings: 4   Cooking Time: 15 Minutes

Ingredients:
- 1-pound pork sausage, pastured
- 2 tablespoons chopped parsley
- 1/8 teaspoon salt
- 1/8 teaspoon grated nutmeg
- 1 tablespoon chopped chives
- 1/8 teaspoon ground black pepper
- 2 teaspoons ground mustard and more as needed
- 4 eggs, hard-boiled, shell peeled
- 1 cup shredded parmesan cheese, low-fat

Directions:
Switch on the air fryer, insert fryer basket, grease it with olive oil, then shut with its lid, set the fryer at 400 degrees F and preheat for 10 minutes. Meanwhile, place sausage in a bowl, add salt, black pepper, parsley, chives, nutmeg, and mustard, then stir until well mixed and shape the mixture into four patties. Peel each boiled egg, then place an egg on a patty and shape the meat around it until the egg has evenly covered. Place cheese in a shallow dish, and then roll the egg in the cheese until covered completely with cheese; prepare remaining eggs in the same manner. Then open the fryer, add eggs in it close with its lid and cook for 15 minutes at the 400 degrees F until nicely golden and crispy, turning the eggs and spraying with oil halfway through the frying. When air fryer beeps, open its lid, transfer eggs onto a serving plate and serve with mustard.

Nutrition Info: Calories: 533 Cal Carbs: 0.6 g Fat: 7 g Protein: 6.3 g Fiber: 0 g

47. Breakfast Pizza

Servings: 8   Cooking Time: 30 Minutes

Ingredients:
- 12 eggs
- ½ lb. breakfast sausage
- 1 cup bell pepper, sliced
- 1 cup red pepper, sliced
- 1 cup cheddar cheese, grated
- ½ cup half-n-half
- What you'll need from store cupboard:
- ½ tsp salt
- ¼ tsp pepper

Directions:
Heat oven to 350 degrees. In a large cast iron skillet, brown sausage. Transfer to bowl. Add peppers and cook 3-5 minutes or until they begin to soften. Transfer to a bowl. In a small bowl, whisk together the eggs, cream, salt and pepper. Pour into skillet. Cook 5 minutes or until the sides start to set. Bake 15 minutes. Remove from oven and set it to broil. Top "crust" with sausage, peppers, and cheese. Broil 3 minutes, or until cheese is melted and starts to brown. Let rest 5 minutes before slicing and serving.

Nutrition Info: Calories 230 Total Carbs 4g Protein 16g Fat 17g Sugar 2g Fiber 0g

48. French Toast In Sticks

Servings: 4   Cooking Time: 10 Minutes

Ingredients:
- 4 slices of white bread, 38 mm thick, preferably hard
- 2 eggs
- 60 ml of milk
- 15 ml maple sauce
- 2 ml vanilla extract
- Nonstick Spray Oil
- 38g of sugar
- 3ground cinnamon
- Maple syrup, to serve
- Sugar to sprinkle

Directions:
Cut each slice of bread into thirds making 12 pieces. Place sideways   Beat the eggs, milk, maple syrup and vanilla. Preheat the air fryer, set it to 175°C.   Dip the sliced bread in the egg mixture and place it in the preheated air fryer. Sprinkle French toast generously with oil spray. Cook French toast for 10 minutes at 175°C. Turn the toast halfway through cooking.   Mix the sugar and cinnamon in a bowl.   Cover the French toast with the sugar and cinnamon mixture when you have finished cooking.

Nutrition Info: Calories 128 Fat 6.2 g, Carbohydrates 16.3 g, Sugar 3.3 g, Protein 3.2 g, Cholesterol 17 mg

49.   Mango Strawberry Smoothies

Servings: 2   Cooking Time: 10 Minutes
Ingredients:
- ½ mango, peeled and diced
- ¾ cup strawberries, halved
- ½ cup skim milk
- ¼ cup vanilla yogurt
- What you'll need from store cupboard:
- 3 ice cubes
- 2 tsp Splenda

Directions:
Combine all Ingredients in a blender. Process until smooth. Pour into chilled glasses and serve immediately.

Nutrition Info: Calories 132 Total Carbs 26g Net Carbs 24g Protein 5g Fat 1g Sugar 23g Fiber 2g

50.   Fried Egg

Servings: 1   Cooking Time: 4 Minutes
Ingredients:
- 1 egg, pastured
- 1/8 teaspoon salt
- 1/8 teaspoon cracked black pepper

Directions:
Take the fryer pan, grease it with olive oil and then crack the egg in it.   Switch on the air fryer, insert fryer pan, then shut with its lid, and set the fryer at 370 degrees F. Set the frying time to 3 minutes, then when the air fryer beep, open its lid and check the egg; if egg needs more cooking, then air fryer it for another minute.   Transfer the egg to a serving plate, season with salt and black pepper and serve.

Nutrition Info: Calories: 90 Cal Carbs: 0.6 g Fat: 7 g Protein: 6.3 g Fiber: 0 g

51.   Tofu Scramble

Servings: 3   Cooking Time: 18 Minutes
Ingredients:
- 12 ounces tofu, extra-firm, drained, ½-inch cubed
- 1 teaspoon garlic powder
- 1 teaspoon onion powder
- 1 teaspoon paprika
- 1/2 teaspoon ground black pepper
- 1/2 teaspoon salt
- 1 tablespoon olive oil
- 2 teaspoon xanthan gum

Directions:
Switch on the air fryer, insert fryer basket, grease it with olive oil, then shut with its lid, set the fryer at 220 degrees F and preheat for 5 minutes.   Meanwhile, place tofu pieces in a bowl, drizzle with oil, and sprinkle with xanthan gum and toss until well coated.   Add remaining ingredients to the tofu and then toss until well coated.   Open the fryer, add tofu in it, close with its lid and cook for 13 minutes until nicely golden and crispy, shaking the basket every 5 minutes.   When air fryer beeps, open its lid, transfer tofu onto a serving plate and serve.

Nutrition Info: Calories: 94 Cal Carbs: 5 g Fat: 5 g Protein: 6 g Fiber: 0 g

52.   Scrumptious Orange Muffins

Servings: 8   Cooking Time: 15 Minutes
Ingredients:
- Dry Ingredients
- 2½ cups finely ground almond flour
- ½ teaspoon baking powder
- ½ teaspoon ground cardamom
- ¾ teaspoon ground cinnamon
- ¼ teaspoon salt
- Wet Ingredients
- 2 large eggs
- 4 tablespoons avocado or coconut oil
- 1 tablespoon raw honey
- ¼ teaspoon vanilla extract
- Grated zest and juice of 1 medium orange
- Special Equipment:
- An 8-cup muffin tin

Directions:
Preheat the oven to 375°F (190°C) and line an 8-cup muffin tin with paper liners.   Stir together the almond flour, baking powder, cardamon, cinnamon, and salt in a large bowl. Set aside.   Whisk together the eggs, oil, honey, vanilla, zest and juice in a medium bowl. Pour the mixture into the bowl of dry ingredients and stir with a spatula just until incorporated.   Pour the batter into the prepared muffin cups, filling each about three-quarters full.   Bake in the preheated oven for 15 minutes, or until the tops are golden and a toothpick inserted in the center comes out clean.   Let the muffins cool for 10 minutes before serving.

Nutrition Info:calories: 287   fat: 23.5g   protein: 7.9g   carbs: 15.8g   fiber: 3.8g   sugar: 9.8g   sodium: 96mg

53. Cauliflower Hash Browns

Servings: 6   Cooking Time: 25 Minutes
Ingredients:
- 1/4 cup chickpea flour
- 4 cups cauliflower rice
- 1/2 medium white onion, peeled and chopped
- 1/2 teaspoon garlic powder
- 1-tablespoon xanthan gum
- 1/2 teaspoon salt
- 1-tablespoon nutritional yeast flakes
- 1-teaspoon ground paprika

Directions:
Switch on the air fryer, insert fryer basket, grease it with olive oil, then shut with its lid, set the fryer at 375 degrees F and preheat for 10 minutes.   Meanwhile, place all the ingredients in a bowl, stir until well mixed and then shape the mixture into six rectangular disks, each about ½-inch thick.   Open the fryer, add hash browns in it in a single layer, close with its lid and cook for 25 minutes at the 375 degrees F until nicely golden and crispy, turning halfway through the frying.   When air fryer beeps, open its lid, transfer hash browns to a serving plate and serve.

Nutrition Info: Calories: 115.2 Cal Carbs: 6.2 g Fat: 7.3 g Protein: 7.4 g Fiber: 2.2 g

54. Grilled Sandwich With Three Types Of Cheese

Servings: Two   Cooking Time: 8 Minutes
Ingredients:
- 2 tbsp. mayonnaise
- ⅛ tsp. dried basil
- ⅛ tsp. dried oregano
- 4 slices of whole wheat bread
- 2 slices of ½ to 1-ounce cheddar cheese
- 2 slices of Monterey Jack cheese
- ½ to 1 ounce
- 2 thin slices of tomato
- 2 slices of ½ to 1 oz. provolone cheese Soft butter

Directions:
Mix mayonnaise with basil and oregano in a small bowl and then spread the mixture on each side of the slice. Cover each slice with a slice of each cheese and tomato, and then the other slice of bread.   Lightly brush each side of the sandwich and put the sandwiches in the basket. Cook at a temperature of 400°F for 8 minutes, turning halfway through cooking.

Nutrition Info: Calories: 141 Fat: 1.01g Carbohydrates: 68g Protein: 1.08g Sugar: 0.25g Cholesterol: 33mg

55. Holiday Strata

Servings: 8   Cooking Time: 1 Hour
Ingredients:
- 8 eggs
- 6 slices bacon, diced
- 4 breakfast sausages, casings removed and meat crumbled
- 1 onion, diced fine
- 1 pint cherry tomatoes
- 4 cup spinach
- 3 cup skim milk
- 1 cup reduced fat cheddar cheese, grated
- What you'll need from store cupboard:
- ½ loaf Italian bread, cut in 2-inch cubes
- 2 tsp Dijon mustard
- 1 tsp salt
- ¼ tsp pepper
- Butter flavored cooking spray

Directions:
Spray a 13x9-inch baking dish with cooking spray. Heat a large non-stick skillet over medium heat. Add bacon and sausage and cook until bacon is crisp, and sausage is cooked through, about 5-7 minutes. Transfer to paper towel lined plate. Drain all but 1 tablespoon of fat from the pan.   Add onion and cook until soft and golden brown, about 6 minutes.   Add tomatoes and spinach and cook until tomatoes start to soften and spinach wilts, about 2 minutes. Remove from heat and set aside to cool.   In a large bowl, beat eggs with milk, Dijon, salt and pepper. Mix in cheese, bread, bacon, sausage, and spinach mixture. Pour into prepared pan and cover with plastic wrap.   Refrigerate for two hours or overnight.   Heat oven to 359 degrees. Uncover and bake 1 hour, or until set in the center. Cool slightly before serving.

Nutrition Info: Calories 343 Total Carbs 24g Net Carbs 22g Protein 25g Fat 16g Sugar 7g Fiber 2g

56. Blueberry Cinnamon Muffins

Servings: 10   Cooking Time: 30 Minutes
Ingredients:
- 3 eggs
- 1 cup blueberries
- 1/3 cup half-n-half
- ¼ cup margarine, melted
- What you'll need from store cupboard:
- 1½ cup almond flour
- ⅓ cup Splenda
- 1 tsp baking powder
- 1 tsp cinnamon

Directions:
Heat oven to 350 degrees. Line 10 muffin cups with paper liners.   In a large mixing bowl, combine dry Ingredients.   Stir in wet Ingredients and mix well. Fold in the blueberries and spoon evenly into lined muffin pan.   Bake 25-30 minutes or they pass the toothpick test.

Nutrition Info: Calories 194 Total Carbs 12g Net Carbs 10g Protein 5g Fat 14g Sugar 9g Fiber 2g

57. Crab & Spinach Frittata

Servings: 10   Cooking Time: 30 Minutes
Ingredients:
- ¾ lb. crabmeat
- 8 eggs
- 10 oz. spinach, frozen and thawed, squeeze dry
- 2 stalks celery, diced
- 2 cup half-n-half
- 1 cup Swiss cheese

- ½ cup onion, diced
- ½ cup red pepper, diced
- ¼ cup mushrooms, diced
- 2 tbsp. margarine
- What you'll need from store cupboard:
- 1 cup bread crumbs
- ½ tsp salt
- ¼ tsp pepper
- ¼ tsp nutmeg
- Nonstick cooking spray

Directions:
Heat oven to 375 degrees. Spray a large casserole, or baking dish with cooking spray.   In a large bowl, beat eggs and half-n-half. Stir in crab, spinach, bread crumbs, cheese, and seasonings.   Melt butter in a large skillet over medium heat. Add celery, onion, rep pepper, and mushrooms. Cook, stirring occasionally, until vegetables are tender, about 5 minutes. Add to egg mixture.   Pour mixture into prepared baking dish and bake 30-35 minutes, or until eggs are set and top is light brown. Cool 10 minutes before serving.
Nutrition Info: Calories 261 Total Carbs 18g Net Carbs 16g Protein 14g Fat 15g Sugar 4g Fiber 2g

58. Apple Filled Swedish Pancake

Servings: 6   Cooking Time: 20 Minutes
Ingredients:
- 2 apples, cored and sliced thin
- ¾ cup egg substitute
- ½ cup fat-free milk
- ½ cup sugar-free caramel sauce
- 1 tbsp. reduced calorie margarine
- What you'll need from the store cupboard
- ½ cup flour
- 1`1/2 tbsp. brown sugar substitute
- 2 tsp water
- ¼ tsp cinnamon
- 1/8 tsp cloves
- 1/8 tsp salt
- Nonstick cooking spray

Directions:
Heat oven to 400 degrees. Place margarine in cast iron, or ovenproof, skillet and place in oven until margarine is melted.   In a medium bowl, whisk together flour, milk, egg substitute, cinnamon, cloves and salt until smooth. Pour batter in hot skillet and bake 20 – 25 minutes until puffed and golden brown.   Spray a medium saucepan with cooking spray. Heat over medium heat.   Add apples, brown sugar and water. Cook, stirring occasionally, until apples are tender and golden brown, about 4 – 6 minutes.   Pour the caramel sauce into a microwave-proof measuring glass and heat 30 – 45 seconds, or until warmed through.   To serve, spoon apples into pancake and drizzle with caramel. Cut into wedges.
Nutrition Info: Calories 193 Total Carbs 25g Net Carbs 23g Protein 6g Fat 2g Sugar 12g Fiber 2g

59. Apple Cinnamon Muffins

Servings: 12   Cooking Time: 25 Minutes
Ingredients:

- 1 cup apple, diced fine
- 2/3 cup skim milk
- ¼ cup reduced-calorie margarine, melted
- 1 egg, lightly beaten
- What you'll need from the store cupboard
- 1 2/3 cups flour
- 1 tbsp. Stevia
- 2 ½ tsp baking powder
- 1 tsp cinnamon
- ½ tsp sea salt
- ¼ tsp nutmeg
- Nonstick cooking spray

Directions:
Heat oven to 400 degrees F. Spray a 12-cup muffin pan with cooking spray.   In a large bowl, combine dry Ingredients and stir to mix.   In another bowl, beat milk, margarine, and egg to combine.   Pour wet Ingredients into dry Ingredients and stir just until moistened. Gently fold in apples.   Spoon into prepared muffin pan. Bake 25 minutes, or until tops are lightly browned.
Nutrition Info: Calories 119 Total Carbs 17g Net Carbs 16g Protein 3g Fat 4g Sugar 3g Fiber 1g

60. Santa Fe Style Pizza

Servings: Two   Cooking Time: 10 Minutes
Ingredients:
- 1 tsp. vegetable oil
- ½ tsp. ground cumin
- 2 tortillas 7 to 8 inches in diameter
- ¼ cup black bean sauce prepared
- 4 ounces cooked chicken, in strips or grated
- 1 tbsp. taco seasonings
- 2 tbsp. prepared chipotle sauce, or preferred sauce
- ¼ cup plus 2 tbsp. corn kernels, fresh or frozen (thawed)
- 1 tbsp. sliced scallions
- 1 tsp. chopped cilantro
- ⅔ cup grated pepper jack cheese

Directions:
Put the oil with the cumin in a small bowl; spread the mixture on both tortillas. Then spread the black bean sauce evenly over both tortillas. Put the chicken pieces and taco seasonings in medium bowl; Stir until chicken is covered. Add the sauce and mix it with the covered chicken.   Remove half of the chicken and place it over the bean sauce in one of the tortillas. Put half the corn, chives, and cilantro over the tortilla and then cover with half the cheese. Put the pizza inside the basket and cook it at a temperature of 400°F for 10 minutes. Prepare the other tortilla and cook it after removing the first one.
Nutrition Info: Calories: 41 Fat: 1.01g Carbohydrates: 6.68g Protein: 1.08g Sugar: 0.25g Cholesterol: 0mg

61. Brussels Sprout With Fried Eggs

Servings: 4   Cooking Time: 15 Minutes
Ingredients:
- 3 teaspoons extra-virgin olive oil, divided
- 1 pound (454 g) Brussels sprouts, sliced
- 2 garlic cloves, thinly sliced
- ¼ teaspoon salt
- Juice of 1 lemon

- 4 eggs

Directions:

Heat 1½ teaspoons of olive oil in a large skillet over medium heat.   Add the Brussels sprouts and sauté for 6 to 8 minutes until crispy and tender, stirring frequently. Stir in the garlic and cook for about 1 minute until fragrant. Sprinkle with the salt and lemon juice. Remove from the skillet to a plate and set aside.   Heat the remaining oil in the skillet over medium-high heat. Crack the eggs one at a time into the skillet and fry for about 3 minutes. Flip the eggs and continue cooking, or until the egg whites are set and the yolks are cooked to your liking.   Serve the fried eggs over the crispy Brussels sprouts.

Nutrition Info:calories: 157   fat: 8.9g   protein: 10.1g   carbs: 11.8g   fiber: 4.1g   sugar: 4.0g   sodium: 233mg

62. Cauliflower Breakfast Hash

Servings: 2   Cooking Time: 20 Minutes

Ingredients:
- 4 cups cauliflower, grated
- 1 cup mushrooms, diced
- ¾ cup onion, diced
- 3 slices bacon
- ¼ cup sharp cheddar cheese, grated

Directions:

In a medium skillet, over med-high heat, fry bacon, set aside.   Add vegetables to the skillet and cook, stirring occasionally, until golden brown.   Cut bacon into pieces and return to skillet.   Top with cheese and allow it to melt. Serve immediately.

Nutrition Info: Calories 155 Total Carbs 16g Net Carbs 10g Protein 10g Fat 7g Sugar 7g Fiber 6g

63. Peanut Butter And Berry Oatmeal

Servings: 2   Cooking Time: 15 Minutes

Ingredients:
- 1½ cups unsweetened vanilla almond milk
- ¾ cup rolled oats
- 1 tablespoon chia seeds
- 2 tablespoons natural peanut butter
- ¼ cup fresh berries, divided (optional)
- 2 tablespoons walnut pieces, divided (optional)

Directions:

Add the almond milk, oats, and chia seeds to a small saucepan and bring to a boil.   Cover and continue cooking for about 10 minutes, stirring often, or until the oats have absorbed the milk.   Add the peanut butter and keep stirring until the oats are thick and creamy. Divide the oatmeal into two serving bowls. Serve topped with the berries and walnut pieces, if desired.

Nutrition Info:calories: 260   fat: 13.9g   protein: 10.1g   carbs: 26.9g   fiber: 7.1g   sugar: 1.0g   sodium: 130mg

64. Quick Breakfast Yogurt Sundae

Servings: 1   Cooking Time: 0 Minutes

Ingredients:
- ¾ cup plain Greek yogurt

- ¼ cup mixed berries (blueberries, strawberries, blackberries)
- 2 tablespoons cashew, walnut, or almond pieces
- 1 tablespoon ground flaxseed
- 2 fresh mint leaves, shredded

Directions:

Pour the yogurt into a tall parfait glass and scatter the top with the berries, cashew pieces, and flaxseed.   Sprinkle the mint leaves on top for garnish and serve chilled.

Nutrition Info:calories: 238   fat: 11.2g   protein: 20.9g   carbs: 15.8g   fiber: 4.1g   sugar: 8.9g   sodium: 63mg

65. Olive & Mushroom Frittata

Servings: 4   Cooking Time: 20 Minutes

Ingredients:
- 2 cups fresh spinach, chopped
- 1 cup cremini mushrooms, sliced
- 4 eggs
- 2 egg whites
- 1/3 cup reduced-fat Parmesan cheese, grated
- ¼ cup Kalamata olives, pitted and sliced thin
- 1 large shallot, sliced thin
- What you'll need from the store cupboard
- 1 tbsp. olive oil
- ½ tsp rosemary
- ¼ tsp black pepper
- 1/8 tsp salt

Directions:

Preheat broiler.   In a nonstick, broiler proof skillet, heat oil over medium heat. Add mushrooms and cook 3 minutes, stirring occasionally. Add spinach and shallot and cook until mushrooms and spinach are tender, about 5 minutes.   In a medium bowl, whisk together eggs and seasonings. Pour egg mixture into skillet. Cook, as it cooks, use a spatula around the edge of skillet, lifting the frittata so uncooked eggs flow underneath. Cook until eggs are almost set.   Sprinkle the olives and cheese over the top. Broil 4-inches from heat until top is lightly browned, about 2 minutes. Let stand 5 minutes before cutting into 4 wedges to serve.

Nutrition Info: Calories 146 Total Carbs 3g Protein 10g Fat 11g Sugar 0g Fiber 0g

66. Pumpkin Muffins

Servings: 10   Cooking Time: 20 Minutes

Ingredients:
- 2 eggs
- ¼ cup butter, melted
- What you'll need from store cupboard:
- 2 cup almond flour
- ¾ cup pumpkin
- ⅓ cup Splenda
- 2 tbsp. pumpkin seeds
- 2 tsp baking powder
- 1 tsp cinnamon
- 1 tsp vanilla
- ½ tsp salt

Directions:

Heat oven to 400 degrees. Line a muffin pan with paper liners.   In a large bowl, combine butter, pumpkin, eggs

and vanilla. Whisk until smooth. In another bowl, combine flour, Splenda, baking powder, cinnamon and salt. Add to pumpkin mixture and stir to combine. Divide evenly between muffin cups. Sprinkle the pumpkin seeds on the top and bake 20 minutes, or they pass the toothpick test. Let cool 10 minutes before serving.
Nutrition Info: Calories 212 Total Carbs 13g Net Carbs 10g Protein 6g Fat 16g Sugar 8g Fiber 3g

67. Vanilla Mango Smoothies

Servings: 3   Cooking Time: 5 Minutes
Ingredients:
- 1 cup mango, frozen chunks
- 6 oz. vanilla yogurt
- ½ cup orange juice, unsweetened
- What you'll need from store cupboard:
- 1 tbsp. honey

Directions:
Place all Ingredients in a blender. Process until smooth. Pour into chilled glasses and serve.
Nutrition Info: Calories 112 Total Carbs 22g Net Carbs 21g Protein 4g Fat 1g Sugar 21g Fiber 1g

68. Cheesy Spinach And Egg Casserole

Servings: 8   Cooking Time: 35 Minutes
Ingredients:
- 1 (10-ounce / 284-g) package frozen spinach, thawed and drained
- 1 (14-ounce / 397-g) can artichoke hearts, drained
- ¼ cup finely chopped red bell pepper
- 8 eggs, lightly beaten
- ¼ cup unsweetened plain almond milk
- 2 garlic cloves, minced
- ½ teaspoon salt
- ½ teaspoon freshly ground black pepper
- ½ cup crumbled goat cheese
- Nonstick cooking spray

Directions:
Preheat the oven to 375ºF (190ºC). Spray a baking dish with nonstick cooking spray and set aside. Mix the spinach, artichoke hearts, bell peppers, beaten eggs, almond milk, garlic, salt, and pepper in a large bowl, and stir to incorporate. Pour the mixture into the greased baking dish and scatter the goat cheese on top. Bake in the preheated oven for 35 minutes, or until the top is lightly golden around the edges and eggs are set. Remove from the oven and serve warm.
Nutrition Info:calories: 105   fat: 4.8g   protein: 8.9g   carbs: 6.1g   fiber: 1.7g   sugar: 1.0g   sodium: 486mg

69. Pumpkin Pie Smoothie

Servings: 2   Cooking Time: 5 Minutes
Ingredients:
- 1 ½ cup almond milk, unsweetened
- 4 oz. reduced fat cream cheese, soft
- ½ cup Greek yogurt
- What you'll need from store cupboard:
- ¼ cup pumpkin puree
- 2 tbsp. Splenda
- 1/8 tsp cinnamon
- Pinch ginger

Directions:
Place all Ingredients in a blender. Process until smooth and everything is combined. Pour into two glasses and garnish with the pinch of ginger on top.
Nutrition Info: Calories 220 Total Carbs 27g Net Carbs 25g Protein 13g Fat 5g Sugar 15g Fiber 2g

70. Berry Breakfast Bark

Servings: 6   Cooking Time: 2 Hours
Ingredients:
- 3-4 strawberries, sliced
- 1 ½ cup plain Greek yogurt
- ½ cup blueberries
- What you'll need from store cupboard:
- ½ cup low fat granola
- 3 tbsp. sugar free maple syrup

Directions:
Line a baking sheet with parchment paper. In a medium bowl, mix yogurt and syrup until combined. Pour into prepared pan and spread in a thin even layer. Top with remaining Ingredients. Cover with foil and freeze two hours or overnight. To serve: slice into squares and serve immediately. If bark thaws too much it will lose its shape. Store any remaining bark in an airtight container in the freezer.
Nutrition Info: Calories 69 Total Carbs 18g Net Carbs 16g Protein 7g Fat 6g Sugar 7g Fiber 2g

71. Lean Lamb And Turkey Meatballs With Yogurt

Servings: 4   Cooking Time: 10 Minutes
Ingredients:
- 1 egg white
- 4 ounces ground lean turkey
- 1 pound of ground lean lamb
- 1 teaspoon each of cayenne pepper, ground coriander, red chili paste, salt, and ground cumin
- 2 garlic cloves, minced
- 1 ½ tablespoons parsley, chopped
- 1 tablespoon mint, chopped
- 1/4 cup of olive oil
- For the yogurt
- 2 tablespoons of buttermilk
- 1 garlic clove, minced
- 1/4 cup mint, chopped
- 1/2 cup of Greek yogurt, non-fat
- Salt to taste

Directions:
Set the Air Fryer to 390 degrees. Mix all the ingredients for the meatballs in a bowl. Roll and mold them into golf-size round pieces. Arrange in the cooking basket. Cook for 8 minutes. While waiting, combine all the ingredients for the mint yogurt in a bowl. Mix well.
Nutrition Info: Calorie: 154 Carbohydrate: 9g Fat: 2.5g Protein: 8.6g Fiber: 2.4g

72. Cocotte Eggs

Servings: 1   Cooking Time: 15 Minutes
Ingredients:
- 1 tbsp. olive oil soup

- 2 tbsp. crumbly ricotta
- 1 tbsp. parmesan cheese soup
- 1 slice of gorgonzola cheese
- 1 slice of Brie cheese
- 1 tbsp. cream soup
- 1 egg
- Nutmeg and salt to taste
- Butternut to taste

Directions:
Spread with olive oil in the bottom of a small glass refractory. Place the cheese in the bottom and season with nutmeg and salt. Add the cream.   Break the egg into a cup and gently add it to the refractory mixture. Preheat the air fryer for the time of 5 minutes and the temperature at 200C. Put the refractory in the basket of the air fryer, set the time to 10 minutes, and press the power button. Remove and serve still hot.
Nutrition Info: Calories: 138 Cal Carbs: 3 g Fat: 33 g Protein: 7.4 g Fiber: 2.2 g

73. Cream Buns With Strawberries

Servings: 6   Cooking Time: 12 Minutes
Ingredients:
- 240g all-purpose flour
- 50g granulated sugar
- 8g baking powder
- 1g of salt
- 85g chopped cold butter
- 84g chopped fresh strawberries
- 120 ml whipping cream
- 2 large eggs
- 10 ml vanilla extract
- 5 ml of water

Directions:
Sift flour, sugar, baking powder and salt in a large bowl. Put the butter with the flour using a blender or your hands until the mixture resembles thick crumbs.   Mix the strawberries in the flour mixture. Set aside for the mixture to stand. Beat the whipping cream, 1 egg and the vanilla extract in a separate bowl.   Put the cream mixture in the flour mixture until they are homogeneous, then spread the mixture to a thickness of 38 mm.   Use a round cookie cutter to cut the buns. Spread the buns with a combination of egg and water. Set aside Preheat the air fryer, set it to 180°C.   Place baking paper in the preheated inner basket.   Place the buns on top of the baking paper and cook for 12 minutes at 180°C, until golden brown.
Nutrition Info: Calories: 150Fat: 14g Carbohydrates: 3g Protein: 11g Sugar: 8g Cholesterol: 0mg

74. Yogurt & Granola Breakfast Popsicles

Servings: 6   Cooking Time: 8 Hours
Ingredients:
- 1 ½ cups fresh berries, chopped
- 1 ¼ cups plain low-fat yogurt
- What you'll need from the store cupboard
- 6 tbsp. granola, crumbled
- 4 tsp sugar free maple syrup, divided
- 1 tsp vanilla
- 6 3-oz Popsicle molds

Directions:
In a medium bowl, stir together yogurt, berries, 2 teaspoons maple syrup, and vanilla together.   Pour evenly into Popsicle molds.   In a small bowl, stir together remaining syrup and granola together. Top each Popsicle with 1 tablespoon of the granola mixture. Insert sticks and freeze 8 hours, or overnight. Popsicles can be stored in the freezer up to 1 week.
Nutrition Info: Calories 73 Total Carbs 20g Net Carbs 18g Protein 5g Fat 4g Sugar 7g Fiber 2g

75. Spinach Cheddar Squares

Servings: 4   Cooking Time: 40 Minutes
Ingredients:
- 10 oz. spinach, frozen, thaw and squeeze dry
- 1 ½ cup egg substitute
- ¾ cup skim milk
- ¾ cup reduced fat cheddar cheese, grated
- ¼ cup red pepper, diced
- What you'll need from store cupboard:
- 2 tbsp. reduced fat parmesan cheese
- 1 tbsp. bread crumbs
- ½ tsp minced onion, dried
- ½ tsp salt
- ¼ tsp garlic powder
- ¼ tsp pepper
- Nonstick cooking spray

Directions:
Heat oven to 350 degrees. Spray an 8-inch square baking dish with cooking spray.   Sprinkle bread crumbs over the bottom of prepared dish. Top with ½ cup cheese, spinach, and red pepper.   In a small bowl, whisk together remaining Ingredients. Pour over vegetables. Bake 35 minutes. Sprinkle with remaining cheese and bake 2-3 minutes more, or until cheese is melted and a knife inserted in the center comes out clean.   Let cool 15 minutes before cutting and serving.
Nutrition Info: Calories 159 Total Carbs 7g Net Carbs 5g Protein 22g Fat 5g Sugar 4g Fiber 2g

76. Peanut Butter Waffles

Servings: 4   Cooking Time: 10 Minutes
Ingredients:
- 4 eggs
- ½ cup low fat cream cheese
- ½ cup half-n-half
- 2 tbsp. margarine
- What you'll need from store cupboard:
- 2/3 cup low fat peanut butter
- 2 tsp Splenda
- 1 tsp baking powder
- Nonstick cooking spray

Directions:
Lightly spray waffle iron with cooking spray and preheat. In a medium glass bowl, place peanut butter, margarine, and cream cheese. Microwave 30 seconds and stir to combine.   Stir in the cream, baking powder, and Splenda and mix until all the Ingredients are combined. Stir in eggs and mix well.   Ladle into waffle iron and cook until golden brown and crisp on the outside. Serve.

Nutrition Info: Calories 214 Total Carbs 9g Net Carbs 8g Protein 9g Fat 15g Sugar 2g Fiber 1g

77. Bruschetta

Servings: 2   Cooking Time: 10 Minutes

Ingredients:
- 4 slices of Italian bread
- 1 cup chopped tomato tea
- 1 cup grated mozzarella tea
- Olive oil
- Oregano, salt, and pepper
- 4 fresh basil leaves

Directions:
Preheat the air fryer. Set the timer of 5 minutes and the temperature to 2000C.   Sprinkle the slices of Italian bread with olive oil. Divide the chopped tomatoes and mozzarella between the slices. Season with salt, pepper, and oregano.   Put oil in the filling. Place a basil leaf on top of each slice.   Put the bruschetta in the basket of the air fryer being careful not to spill the filling. Set the timer of 5 minutes, set the temperature to 180C, and press the power button.   Transfer the bruschetta to a plate and serve.

Nutrition Info: Calories: 434 Fat: 14g Carbohydrates: 63g Protein: 11g Sugar: 8g Cholesterol: 0mg

78. Garlic Bread

Servings: 4-5   Cooking Time: 15 Minutes

Ingredients:
- 2 stale French rolls
- 4 tbsp. crushed or crumpled garlic
- 1 cup of mayonnaise
- Powdered grated Parmesan
- 1 tbsp. olive oil

Directions:
Preheat the air fryer. Set the time of 5 minutes and the temperature to 2000C.   Mix mayonnaise with garlic and set aside.   Cut the baguettes into slices, but without separating them completely.   Fill the cavities of equals. Brush with olive oil and sprinkle with grated cheese.   Place in the basket of the air fryer. Set the

timer to 10 minutes, adjust the temperature to 1800C and press the power button.

Nutrition Info: Calories: 340 Fat: 15g Carbohydrates: 32g Protein: 15g Sugar: 0g Cholesterol: 0mg

79. Coconut Breakfast Porridge

Servings: 4   Cooking Time: 10 Minutes

Ingredients:
- 4 cup vanilla almond milk, unsweetened
- What you'll need from store cupboard:
- 1 cup unsweetened coconut, grated
- 8 tsp coconut flour

Directions:
Add coconut to a saucepan and cook over med-high heat until it is lightly toasted. Be careful not to let it burn. Add milk and bring to a boil. While stirring, slowly add flour, cook and stir until mixture starts to thicken, about 5 minutes.   Remove from heat, mixture will thicken more as it cools. Ladle into bowls, add blueberries, or drizzle with a little honey if desired.

Nutrition Info: Calories 231 Total Carbs 21g Net Carbs 8g Protein 6g Fat 14g Sugar 4g Fiber 13g

80. Bacon Bbq

Servings: 2   Cooking Time: 8 Minutes

Ingredients:
- 13g dark brown sugar
- 5g chili powder
- 1g ground cumin
- 1g cayenne pepper
- 4 slices of bacon, cut in half

Directions:
Mix seasonings until well combined.   Dip the bacon in the dressing until it is completely covered. Leave aside. Preheat the air fryer, set it to 160°C.   Place the bacon in the preheated air fryer   Select Bacon and press Start/Pause.

Nutrition Info: Calories: 1124 Fat: 72g Carbohydrates: 59g Protein: 49g Sugar: 11g Cholesterol: 77mg

Snack & Desserts Recipes

81. Honeydew & Ginger Smoothies

Servings: 3   Cooking Time: 3 Minutes
Ingredients:
- 1 ½ cup honeydew melon, cubed
- ½ cup banana
- ½ cup nonfat vanilla yogurt
- ¼ tsp fresh ginger, grated
- What you'll need from store cupboard:
- ½ cup ice cubes

Directions:
Place all Ingredients in a blender and pulse until smooth. Pour into glasses and serve immediately.

Nutrition Info: Calories 68 Total Carbs 16g Net Carbs 15g Protein 2g Fat 0g Sugar 12g Fiber 1g

82. Broiled Stone Fruit

Servings: 2   Cooking Time: 5 Minutes
Ingredients:
- 1 peach
- 1 nectarine
- 2 tbsp. sugar free whipped topping
- What you'll need from store cupboard:
- 1 tbsp. Splenda brown sugar
- Nonstick cooking spray

Directions:
Heat oven to broil. Line a shallow baking dish with foil and spray with cooking spray.   Cut the peach and nectarine in half and remove pits. Place cut side down in prepared dish. Broil 3 minutes.   Turn fruit over and sprinkle with Splenda brown sugar. Broil another 2-3 minutes.   Transfer 1 of each fruit to a dessert bowl and top with 1 tablespoon of whipped topping. Serve.

Nutrition Info: Calories 101 Total Carbs 22g Net Carbs 20g Protein 1g Fat 1g Sugar 19g Fiber 2g

83. Cheesy Onion Dip

Servings: 8   Cooking Time: 5 Minutes
Ingredients:
- 8 oz. low fat cream cheese, soft
- 1 cup onions, grated
- 1 cup low fat Swiss cheese, grated
- What you'll need from store cupboard:
- 1 cup lite mayonnaise

Directions:
Heat oven to broil.   Combine all Ingredients in a small casserole dish. Microwave on high, stirring every 30 seconds, until cheese is melted and Ingredients are combined.   Place under the broiler for 1-2 minutes until the top is nicely browned. Serve warm with vegetables for dipping.

Nutrition Info: Calories 158 Total Carbs 5g Protein 9g Fat 11g Sugar 1g Fiber 0g

84. Almond Coconut Biscotti

Servings: 16   Cooking Time: 50 Minutes
Ingredients:
- 1 egg, room temperature
- 1 egg white, room temperature
- ½ cup margarine, melted
- What you'll need from store cupboard:
- 2 ½ cup flour
- 1 1/3 cup unsweetened coconut, grated
- ¾ cup almonds, sliced
- 2/3 cup Splenda
- 2 tsp baking powder
- 1 tsp vanilla
- ½ tsp salt

Directions:
Heat oven to 350 degrees.   Line a baking sheet with parchment paper.   In a large bowl, combine dry Ingredients.   In a separate mixing bowl, beat other Ingredients together. Add to dry Ingredients and mix until thoroughly combined.   Divide dough in half. Shape each half into a loaf measuring 8x2 ¾-inches. Place loaves on pan 3 inches apart.   Bake 25-30 minutes or until set and golden brown. Cool on wire rack 10 minutes.   With a serrated knife, cut loaf diagonally into ½-inch slices. Place the cookies, cut side down, back on the pan and bake another 20 minutes, or until firm and nicely browned. Store in airtight container. Serving size is 2 cookies.

Nutrition Info: Calories 234 Total Carbs 13g Net Carbs 10g Protein 5g Fat 18g Sugar 9g Fiber 3g

85. Margarita Chicken Dip

Servings: 12   Cooking Time: 1 Hour
Ingredients:
- 2 ½ cup Monterrey jack cheese, grated
- 1 ½ cup chicken, cooked and shredded
- 1 ½ blocks cream cheese, soft, cut into cubes
- ¼ cup fresh lime juice
- 2 tbsp. fresh orange juice
- 2 tbsp. Pico de Gallo
- 1 tbsp. lime zest
- What you'll need from store cupboard:
- ¼ cup tequila
- 2 cloves garlic, diced fine
- 1 tsp cumin
- 1 tsp salt

Directions:
Place the cream cheese on bottom of crock pot. Top with chicken, then grated cheese. Add remaining Ingredients, except the Pico de Gallo.   Cover and cook on low 60 minutes. Stir the dip occasionally to combine Ingredients. When dip is done transfer to serving bowl. Top with Pico de Gallo and serve with tortilla chips.

Nutrition Info: Calories 169 Total Carbs 5g Protein 14g Fat 8g Sugar 1g Fiber 0g

86. Parmesan Truffle Chips

Servings: 4   Cooking Time: 20 Minutes
Ingredients:
- 4 egg whites
- ½ tsp fresh parsley, diced fine
- What you'll need from store cupboard:
- 3 tbsp. reduced fat parmesan cheese, divided
- 2 tsp water

- ½ tsp salt
- Truffle oil to taste
- Nonstick cooking spray

Directions:
Heat oven to 400 degrees. Spray two muffin pans with cooking spray. In a small bowl, whisk together egg whites, water, and salt until combined. Spoon just enough egg white mixture into each muffin cup to barely cover the bottom. Sprinkle a small pinch of parmesan on each egg white. Bake 10-15 minutes or until the edges are dark brown, be careful not to burn them. Let cool in the pans 3-4 minutes then transfer to a small bowl and drizzle lightly with truffle oil. Add parsley and ½ tablespoon parmesan and toss to coat. Serve.
Nutrition Info: Calories 47 Total Carbs 0g Protein 4g Fat 3g Sugar 0g Fiber 0g

87. Toffee Apple Mini Pies

Servings: 12   Cooking Time: 25 Minutes
Ingredients:
- 2 9-inch pie crusts, soft
- 2 cup Gala apples, diced fine
- 1 egg, beaten
- 1 tbsp. butter, cut in 12 cubes
- 1 ½ tsp fresh lemon juice
- What you'll need from store cupboard:
- 2 tbsp. toffee bits
- 1 tbsp. Splenda
- ½ tsp cinnamon
- Nonstick cooking spray

Directions:
Heat oven to 375 degrees. Spray a cookie sheet with cooking spray. In a medium bowl, stir together apples, toffee, Splenda, lemon juice, and cinnamon. Roll pie crusts, one at a time, out on a lightly floured surface. Use a 3-inch round cookie cutter to cut 12 circles from each crust. Place 12 on prepared pan. Brush the dough with half the egg. Spoon 1 tablespoon of the apple mixture on each round, leaving ½- inch edge. Top with pat of butter. Place second dough round on top and seal edges closed with a fork. Brush with remaining egg. Bake 25 minutes, or until golden brown. Serve warm.
Nutrition Info: Calories 154 Total Carbs 17g Net Carbs 16g Protein 1g Fat 9g Sugar 6g Fiber 1g

88. Asian Chicken Wings

Servings: 3   Cooking Time: 30 Minutes
Ingredients:
- 24 chicken wings
- What you'll need from store cupboard:
- 6 tbsp. soy sauce
- 6 tbsp. Chinese 5 spice
- Salt & pepper
- Nonstick cooking spray

Directions:
Heat oven to 350 degrees. Spray a baking sheet with cooking spray. Combine the soy sauce, 5 spice, salt, and pepper in a large bowl. Add the wings and toss to coat. Pour the wings onto the prepared pan. Bake 15 minutes. Turn chicken over and cook another 15 minutes

until chicken is cooked through. Serve with your favorite low carb dipping sauce (see chapter 15).
Nutrition Info: Calories 178 Total Carbs 8g Protein 12g Fat 11g Sugar 1g Fiber 0g

89. Apple Cinnamon Chimichanga

Servings: 4   Cooking Time: 15 Minutes
Ingredients:
- 2 apple, cored and chopped
- 3 tablespoons splenda, divided
- ¼ cup water
- ½ teaspoon ground cinnamon
- 4 (8-inch) whole-wheat flour tortillas
- Nonstick cooking spray
- Special Equipment:
- 4 toothpicks, soaked in water for at least 30 minutes

Directions:
Preheat the oven to 400°F (205°C). Line a baking sheet with parchment paper and set aside. Make the apple filling: Add the apples, 2 tablespoons of splenda, water, and cinnamon to a medium saucepan over medium heat. Stir to combine and allow the mixture to boil for 5 minutes, or until the apples are fork-tender, but not mushy. Remove the apple filling from the heat and let it cool to room temperature. Make the chimichangas: Place the tortillas on a lightly floured surface. Spoon 2 teaspoons of prepared apple filling onto each tortilla and fold the tortilla over to enclose the filling. Roll each tortilla up and run the toothpicks through to secure. Spritz the tortillas lightly with nonstick cooking spray. Arrange the tortillas on the prepared baking sheet, seam-side down. Scatter the remaining splenda all over the tortillas. Bake in the preheated oven for 10 minutes, flipping the tortillas halfway through, or until they are crispy and golden brown on each side. Remove from the oven to four plates and serve while warm.
Nutrition Info:(1 Chimichanga)calories: 201   fat: 6.2g   protein: 3.9g   carbs: 32.8g   fiber: 5.0g   sugar: 7.9g   sodium: 241mg

90. Lemon Biscuit

Servings: 1   Cooking Time: 30 Minutes
Ingredients:
- 120g all-purpose flour
- 4g baking powder
- A pinch of salt
- 84g unsalted butter, softened
- 130g granulated sugar
- 1 large egg
- 15g of fresh lemon juice
- 1 lemon, lemon zest
- 56g whey

Directions:
Mix the flour, baking powder and salt in a bowl. Set aside. Add the softened butter to an electric mixer and beat until soft and fluffy. Approximately 3 minutes Beat the sugar in the butter for 1 minute. Beat the flour mixture in the butter until it is completely united, for about 1 minute. Add the egg, lemon juice and lemon zest. Mix until everything is completely united. Slowly pour the whey

while mixing at medium speed. Add the mixture to a tray of greased mini loaves on top.   Preheat the air fryer set the temperature to 160°C.   Place the cake in the preheated air fryer. Set the time to 30 minutes at 160°C.
Nutrition Info: Calories: 420 Fat: 0g Carbohydrates: 0g Protein: 0g Sugar: 0gCholesterol: 0mg

91. Cinnamon Apple Chips

Servings: 2   Cooking Time: 10 Minutes
Ingredients:
- 1 medium apple, sliced thin
- What you'll need from store cupboard:
- ¼ tsp cinnamon
- ¼ tsp nutmeg
- Nonstick cooking spray

Directions:
Heat oven to 375. Spray a baking sheet with cooking spray.   Place apples in a mixing bowl and add spices. Toss to coat.   Arrange apples, in a single layer, on prepared pan. Bake 4 minutes, turn apples over and bake 4 minutes more.   Serve immediately or store in airtight container.
Nutrition Info: Calories 58 Total Carbs 15g Protein 0g Fat 0g Sugar 11g Fiber 3g

92. Rustic Pear Pie With Nuts

Servings: 4   Cooking Time: 45 Minutes
Ingredients:
- Cake
- 100g all-purpose flour
- 1g of salt
- 12g granulated sugar
- 84g unsalted butter, cold, cut into 13 mm pieces
- 30 ml of water, frozen
- 1 egg, beaten
- 12g turbinated sugar
- Nonstick Spray Oil
- 20g of honey
- 5 ml of water
- Roasted nuts, chopped, to decorate
- Filling:
- 1 large pear, peeled, finely sliced
- 5g cornstarch
- 24g brown sugar
- 1g ground cinnamon
- A pinch salt

Directions:
Mix 90 g of flour, salt, and granulated sugar in a large bowl until well combined. Join the butter in the mixture using a pastry mixer or food processor until thick crumbs form. Add cold water and mix until it joins. Shape the dough into a bowl, cover with plastic and let cool in the refrigerator for 1 hour.   Mix the stuffing ingredients in a bowl until they are combined. Roll a roll through your cooled dough until it is 216 mm in diameter. Add 10 g of flour on top of the dough leaving 38 mm without flour. Place the pear slices in decorative circles superimposed on the floured part of the crust. Remove any remaining pear juice on the slices. Fold the edge over the filling. Cover the edges with beaten eggs and sprinkle the sugar over the whole cake. Set aside   Preheat the air fryer set

the temperature to 160°C. Spray the preheated air fryer with oil spray and place the cake inside. Set the time to 45 minutes at 1600C. Mix the honey and water and pass the mixture through the cake when you finish cooking. Garnish with toasted chopped nuts.
Nutrition Info: Calories: 20 Fat: 0g Carbohydrates: 0g Protein: 0g Sugar: 0gCholesterol: 0mg

93. Raspberry Peach Cobbler

Servings: 8   Cooking Time: 40 Minutes
Ingredients:
- 1 ¼ lbs. peaches, peeled and sliced
- 2 cups fresh raspberries
- ½ cup low-fat buttermilk
- 2 tbsp. cold margarine, cut into pieces
- 1 tsp lemon zest
- What you'll need from store cupboard:
- ¾ cup + 2 tbsp. flour, divided
- 4 tbsp. + 2 tsp Splenda, divided
- ½ tsp baking powder
- ½ tsp baking soda
- 1/8 tsp salt
- Nonstick cooking spray

Directions:
Heat oven to 425 degrees. Spray an 11×7-inch baking dish with cooking spray.   In a large bowl, stir together 2 tablespoons Splenda and 2 tablespoons flour. Add the fruit and zest and toss to coat. Pour into prepared baking dish. Bake 15 minutes, or until fruit is bubbling around the edges.   In a medium bowl, combine remaining flour, 2 tablespoons Splenda, baking powder, baking soda, and salt. Cut in margarine with pastry cutter until it resembles coarse crumbs. Stir in the buttermilk just until moistened.   Remove the fruit from the oven and top with dollops of buttermilk mixture. Sprinkle the remaining 2 teaspoons of Splenda over the top and bake 18-20 minutes or top is lightly browned. Serve warm.
Nutrition Info: Calories 130 Total Carbs 22g Net Carbs 19g Protein 2g Fat 3g Sugar 10g Fiber 3g

94. Apricot Soufflé

Servings: 6   Cooking Time: 30 Minutes
Ingredients:
- 4 egg whites
- 3 egg yolks, beaten
- 3 tbsp. margarine
- What you'll need from store cupboard
- ¾ cup sugar free apricot fruit spread
- 1/3 cup dried apricots, diced fine
- ¼ cup warm water
- 2 tbsp. flour
- ¼ tsp cream of tartar
- 1/8 tsp salt

Directions:
Heat oven to 325 degrees.   In a medium saucepan, over medium heat, melt margarine. Stir in flour and cook, stirring, until bubbly.   Stir together the fruit spread and water in a small bowl and add it to the saucepan with the apricots. Cook, stirring, 3 minutes or until mixture thickens.   Remove from heat and whisk in egg yolks. Let cool to room temperature, stirring occasionally.   In

a medium bowl, beat egg whites, salt, and cream of tartar on high speed until stiff peaks form. Gently fold into cooled apricot mixture.   Spoon into a 1 1/2 –quart soufflé dish. Bake 30 minutes, or until puffed and golden brown. Serve immediately.

Nutrition Info: Calories 116 Total Carbs 7g Protein 4g Fat 8g Sugar 1g Fiber 0g

95. Cinnamon Apple Popcorn

Servings: 11   Cooking Time: 50 Minutes

Ingredients:
- 4 tbsp. margarine, melted
- What you'll need from store cupboard
- 10 cup plain popcorn
- 2 cup dried apple rings, unsweetened and chopped
- ½ cup walnuts, chopped
- 2 tbsp. Splenda brown sugar
- 1 tsp cinnamon
- ½ tsp vanilla

Directions:
Heat oven to 250 degrees.   Place chopped apples in a 9x13-inch baking dish and bake 20 minutes. Remove from oven and stir in popcorn and nuts.   In a small bowl, whisk together margarine, vanilla, Splenda, and cinnamon. Drizzle evenly over popcorn and toss to coat. Bake 30 minutes, stirring quickly every 10 minutes. If apples start to turn a dark brown, remove immediately. Pout onto waxed paper to cool at least 30 minutes. Store in an airtight container. Serving size is 1 cup.

Nutrition Info: Calories 133 Total Carbs 14g Net Carbs 11g Protein 3g Fat 8g Sugar 7g Fiber 3g

96. Blackberry Crostata

Servings: 6   Cooking Time: 20 Minutes

Ingredients:
- 1 9-inch pie crust, unbaked
- 2 cup fresh blackberries
- Juice and zest of 1 lemon
- 2 tbsp. butter, soft
- What you'll need from store cupboard:
- 3 tbsp. Splenda, divided
- 2 tbsp. cornstarch

Directions:
Heat oven to 425 degrees. Line a large baking sheet with parchment paper and unroll pie crust in pan.   In a medium bowl, combine blackberries, 2 tablespoons Splenda, lemon juice and zest, and cornstarch. Spoon onto crust leaving a 2-inch edge. Fold and crimp the edges.   Dot the berries with 1 tablespoon butter. Brush the crust edge with remaining butter and sprinkle crust and fruit with remaining Splenda.   Bake 20-22 minutes or until golden brown. Cool before cutting and serving.

Nutrition Info: Calories 206 Total Carbs 24g Net Carbs 21g Protein 2g Fat 11g Sugar 9g Fiber 3g

97. Chia And Raspberry Pudding

Servings: 4   Cooking Time: 0 Minutes

Ingredients:
- 1 cup unsweetened vanilla almond milk
- 2 cup plus ½ cup raspberries, divided
- ¼ cup chia seeds
- 1½ teaspoons lemon juice
- ½ teaspoon lemon zest
- 1 tablespoon honey

Directions:
Stir together the almond milk, 2 cups of raspberries, chia seeds, lemon juice, lemon zest, and honey in a small bowl. Transfer the bowl to the fridge to thicken for at least 1 hour, or until a pudding-like texture is achieved. When the pudding is ready, give it a good stir. Scatter with the remaining ½ cup raspberries and serve immediately.

Nutrition Info:calories: 122   fat: 5.2g   protein: 3.1g carbs: 17.9g   fiber: 9.0g   sugar: 6.8g   sodium: 51mg

98. Palm Trees Holder

Servings: 2   Cooking Time: 15 Minutes

Ingredients:
- 1 Sheet of puff pastry
- Sugar

Directions:
Stretch the puff pastry sheet.   Pour the sugar over and fold the puff pastry sheet in half.   Put a thin layer of sugar on top and fold the puff pastry in half again.   Roll the puff pastry sheet from both ends towards the center (creating the shape of the palm tree).   Cut into sheets 5-8 mm thick.   Preheat the air fryer to 1800C and put the palm trees in the basket.   Set the timer about 10 minutes at 1800C.

Nutrition Info: Calories: 108 Fat: 12g Carbohydrates: 29g Protein: 4g Sugar: 100g Cholesterol: 56g

99. Almond Cheesecake Bites

Servings: 6   Cooking Time: 30 Minutes

Ingredients:
- ½ cup reduced-fat cream cheese, soft
- What you'll need from store cupboard:
- ½ cup almonds, ground fine
- ¼ cup almond butter
- 2 drops liquid stevia

Directions:
In a large bowl, beat cream cheese, almond butter and stevia on high speed until mixture is smooth and creamy. Cover and chill 30 minutes.   Use your hands to shape the mixture into 12 balls.   Place the ground almonds in a shallow plate. Roll the balls in the nuts completely covering all sides. Store in an airtight container in the refrigerator.

Nutrition Info: Calories 68 Total Carbs 3g Net Carbs 2 Protein 5g Fat 5g Sugar 0g Fiber 1g

100. Tortilla Chips

Servings: 4   Cooking Time: 10 Minutes

Ingredients:
- 2 cup part-skim grated mozzarella cheese, grated
- What you'll need from store cupboard:
- ¾ cup super fine almond flour
- ½ tsp salt
- ½ tsp chili powder

Directions:

Heat oven to 375 degrees.   Prepare a double boiler. Over high heat, bring the water in the pot to a simmer, then turn heat to low. Add all the Ingredients to the top of the double boiler and stir constantly until cheese melts and mixture holds together in a ball. Turn out onto a large piece of parchment paper and let cool 5 minutes. Knead the dough to thoroughly combine all the Ingredients. Separate into 2 equal portions. Working with one portion at a time, roll dough out between two pieces of parchment paper into 9x15-inch rectangle. Remove top piece of parchment and with a pizza cutter, or sharp knife, cut rectangle into squares or triangles. Slide the parchment paper onto a cookie sheet and arrange dough shapes so they have ½-inch space between them. Repeat with second dough portion. Bake 5-8 minutes, or until centers are golden brown. Remove from oven and transfer to wire rack to cool. Chips will crisp up as they cool. Store in an airtight container.

Nutrition Info: Calories 95 Total Carbs 3g Net Carbs 2g Protein 5g Fat 8g Sugar 0g Fiber 1g

101. Blueberry Lemon "cup" Cakes

Servings: 5   Cooking Time: 10 Minutes
Ingredients:
- 4 eggs
- ½ cup coconut milk
- ½ cup blueberries
- 2 tbsp. lemon zest
- What you'll need from store cupboard
- ½ cup + 1 tsp coconut flour
- ¼ cup Splenda
- ¼ cup coconut oil, melted
- 1 tsp baking soda
- ½ tsp lemon extract
- ¼ tsp stevia extract
- Pinch salt

Directions:
In a small bowl, toss berries in the 1 teaspoon of flour. In a large bowl, stir together remaining flour, Splenda, baking soda, salt, and zest.   Add the remaining Ingredients and mix well. Fold in the blueberries. Divide batter evenly into 5 coffee cups. Microwave, one at a time, for 90 seconds, or until they pass the toothpick test.

Nutrition Info:al Facts Per ServingCalories 263 Total Carbs 14g Net Carbs 12g Protein 5g Fat 20g Sugar 12g Fiber 2g

102. Hot & Spicy Mixed Nuts

Servings: 6   Cooking Time: 10 Minutes
Ingredients:
- What you'll need from store cupboard:
- ½ cup whole almonds
- ½ cup pecan halves
- ½ cup walnut halves
- 1 tsp sunflower oil
- ½ tsp cumin
- ½ tsp curry powder
- 1/8 tsp cayenne pepper
- Dash of white pepper

Directions:
Heat oven to 350 degrees.   Place the nuts in a large bowl. Add the oil and toss to coat.   Stir the spices together in a small bowl. Add to nuts and toss to coat. Spread nuts on a large baking sheet in a single layer. Bake 10 minutes.   Remove from oven and let cool. Store in airtight container. Serving size is ¼ cup.

Nutrition Info: Calories 257 Total Carbs 5g Net Carbs 1g Protein 6g Fat 25g Sugar 1g Fiber 4g

103. Mozzarella Sticks

Servings: 4   Cooking Time: 30 Minutes
Ingredients:
- 8 string cheese sticks, halved
- 2 eggs, beaten
- What you'll need from store cupboard:
- 1 cup reduced fat parmesan cheese
- ½ cup sunflower oil
- 1 tbsp. Italian seasoning
- 1 clove garlic, diced fine

Directions:
Heat oil in a pot over med-high heat.   In a medium bowl, combine parmesan cheese, Italian seasoning and garlic.   In a small bowl, beat the eggs.   Dip string cheese in eggs then in parmesan mixture to coat, pressing coating into cheese.   Place in hot oil and cook until golden brown. Transfer to paper towel lined plate. Serve warm with marinara sauce, (chapter 16).

Nutrition Info: Calories 290 Total Carbs 3g Protein 24g Fat 20g Sugar 0g Fiber 0g

104. Café Mocha Torte

Servings: 14   Cooking Time: 25 Minutes
Ingredients:
- 8 eggs
- 1 cup margarine, cut into cubes
- What you'll need from store cupboard:
- 1 lb. bittersweet chocolate, chopped
- ¼ cup brewed coffee, room temperature
- Nonstick cooking spray

Directions:
Heat oven to 325 degrees. Spray an 8-inch springform pan with cooking spray. Line bottom of sides with parchment paper and spray again. Wrap the outside with a double layer of foil and place in 9x13-inch baking dish. Put a small saucepan of water on to boil.   In a large bowl, beat the eggs on med speed until doubled in volume, about 5 minutes.   Place the chocolate, margarine and coffee into microwave safe bowl and microwave on high, until chocolate is melted and mixture is smooth, stir every 30 seconds.   Fold 1/3 of the eggs into chocolate mixture until almost combined. Add the remaining eggs, 1/3 at a time and fold until combined.   Pour into prepared pan. Pour boiling water around the springform pan until it reaches halfway up the sides. Bake 22-25 minutes, or until cake has risen slightly and edges are just beginning to set.   Remove from water bath and let cool completely. Cover with plastic wrap and chill 6 hours or overnight. About 30 minutes before serving, run a knife around the edges and remove the side of the pan. Slice and serve.

Nutrition Info: Calories 260 Total Carbs 12g Net Carbs 11g Protein 5g Fat 21g Sugar 11g Fiber 1g

105. Candied Pecans

Servings: 6   Cooking Time: 10 Minutes
Ingredients:
- 1 ½ tsp butter
- What you'll need from store cupboard:
- 1 ½ cup pecan halves
- 2 ½ tbsp. Splenda, divided
- 1 tsp cinnamon
- ¼ tsp ginger
- 1/8 tsp cardamom
- 1/8 tsp salt

Directions:
In a small bowl, stir together 1 1/2 teaspoons Splenda, cinnamon, ginger, cardamom and salt. Set aside.   Melt butter in a medium skillet over med-low heat. Add pecans, and two tablespoons Splenda. Reduce heat to low and cook, stirring occasionally, until sweetener melts, about 5 to 8 minutes.   Add spice mixture to the skillet and stir to coat pecans. Spread mixture to parchment paper and let cool for 10-15 minutes. Store in an airtight container. Serving size is ¼ cup.

Nutrition Info: Calories 173 Total Carbs 8g Net Carbs 6g Protein 2g Fat 16g Sugar 6g Fiber 2g

106. Baked Maple Custard

Servings: 6   Cooking Time: 1 Hour 15 Minutes
Ingredients:
- 2 ½ cup half-and-half
- ½ cup egg substitute
- What you'll need from store cupboard
- 3 cup boiling water
- ¼ cup Splenda
- 2 tbsp. sugar free maple syrup
- 2 tsp vanilla
- Dash nutmeg
- Nonstick cooking spray

Directions:
Heat oven to 325°degrees. Lightly spray 6 custard cups or ramekins with cooking spray.   In a large bowl, whisk together half-n-half, egg substitute, Splenda, vanilla, and nutmeg. Pour evenly into prepared custard cups. Place cups in a 13x9-inch baking dish.   Pour boiling water around, being careful not to splash it into, the cups. Bake 1 hour 15 minutes, centers will not be completely set.   Remove cups from pan and cool completely. Cover and chill overnight.   Just before serving, drizzle with the maple syrup.

Nutrition Info: Calories 190 Total Carbs 15g Protein 5g Fat 12g Sugar 8g Fiber 0g

107. Buffalo Bites

Servings: 4   Cooking Time: 10 Minutes
Ingredients:
- 1 egg
- ½ head of cauliflower, separated into florets
- What you'll need from store cupboard:
- 1 cup panko bread crumbs
- 1 cup low-fat ranch dressing
- ½ cup hot sauce
- ½ tsp salt
- ½ tsp garlic powder
- Black pepper
- Nonstick cooking spray

Directions:
Heat oven to 400 degrees. Spray a baking sheet with cooking spray.   Place the egg in a medium bowl and mix in the salt, pepper and garlic. Place the panko crumbs into a small bowl.   Dip the florets first in the egg then into the panko crumbs. Place in a single layer on prepared pan.   Bake 8-10 minutes, stirring halfway through, until cauliflower is golden brown and crisp on the outside.   In a small bowl stir the dressing and hot sauce together. Use for dipping.

Nutrition Info: Calories 132 Total Carbs 15g Net Carbs 14g Protein 6g Fat 5g Sugar 4g Fiber 1g

108. Almond Flour Crackers

Servings: 8   Cooking Time: 15 Minutes
Ingredients:
- ½ cup coconut oil, melted
- What you'll need from the store cupboard
- 1 ½ cups almond flour
- ¼ cup Stevia

Directions:
Heat oven to 350 degrees. Line a cookie sheet with parchment paper.   In a mixing bowl, combine all Ingredients and mix well.   Spread dough onto prepared cookie sheet, ¼-inch thick. Use a paring knife to score into 24 crackers.   Bake 10 – 15 minutes or until golden brown.   Separate and store in air-tight container.

Nutrition Info: Calories 281 Total Carbs 16g Net Carbs 14g Protein 4g Fat 23g Sugar 13g Fiber 2g

109. Cream Cheese Pound Cake

Servings: 14   Cooking Time: 35 Minutes
Ingredients:
- 4 eggs
- 3 ½ oz. cream cheese, soft
- 4 tbsp. butter, soft
- What you'll need from store cupboard:
- 1 ¼ cup almond flour
- ¾ cup Splenda
- 1 tsp baking powder
- 1 tsp of vanilla
- ¼ tsp of salt
- Butter flavored cooking spray

Directions:
Heat oven to 350 degrees. Spray an 8-inch loaf pan with cooking spray.   In a medium bowl, combine flour, baking powder, and salt.   In a large bowl, beat butter and Splenda until light and fluffy. And cream cheese and vanilla and beat well.   Add the eggs, one at a time, beating after each one. Stir in the dry Ingredients until thoroughly combined.   Pour into prepared pan and bake 30-40 minutes or cake passes the toothpick test. Let cool 10 minutes in the pan, then invert onto serving plate. Slice and serve.

Nutrition Info: Calories 202 Total Carbs 15g Net Carbs 14g Protein 5g Fat 13g Sugar 13g Fiber 1g

110. Oatmeal Peanut Butter Bars

Servings: 10   Cooking Time: 10 Minutes
Ingredients:
- ½ cup almond milk, unsweetened
- What you'll need from store cupboard:
- 1 cup oats
- ¼ cup agave syrup
- 6tbsp. raw peanut butter
- 2 tbsp. peanuts, chopped
- 1 tsp pure vanilla

Directions:
Heat oven to 325 degrees. Line a cookie sheet with parchment paper.   Place all Ingredients, except the peanuts, into a food processor. Process until you have a sticky dough. Use your hands to mix in the peanuts. Separate the dough into 10 equal balls on the prepared cookie sheet. Shape into squares or bars. Press the bars flat to ¼-inch thickness.   Bake 8-12 minutes, or until the tops are nicely browned. Remove from oven and cool completely. The bars will be soft at first but will stiffen as they cool.
Nutrition Info: Calories 125 Total Carbs 14g Net Carbs 12g Protein 4g Fat 6g Sugar 1g Fiber 2g

111. Peach Custard Tart

Servings: 8   Cooking Time: 40 Minutes
Ingredients:
- 12 oz. frozen unsweetened peach slices, thaw and drain
- 2 eggs, separated
- 1 cup skim milk
- 4 tbsp. cold margarine, cut into pieces
- What you'll need from store cupboard:
- 1 cup flour
- 3 tbsp. Splenda
- 2-3 tbsp. cold water
- 1 tsp vanilla
- ¼ tsp + 1/8 tsp salt, divided
- ¼ tsp nutmeg

Directions:
Heat oven to 400 degrees.   In a medium bowl, stir together flour and ¼ teaspoon salt. With a pastry blender, cut in margarine until mixture resembles coarse crumbs. Stir in cold water, a tablespoon at a time, just until moistened. Shape into a disc.   On a lightly floured surface, roll out dough to an 11-inch circle. Place in bottom of a 9-inch tart pan with a removable bottom. Turn the edge under and pierce the sides and bottom with a fork.   In a small bowl, beat 1 egg white with a fork, discard the other or save for another use. Lightly brush crust with egg. Place the tart pan on a baking sheet and bake 10 minutes. Cool.   In a large bowl, whisk together egg yolks, Splenda, vanilla, nutmeg, and 1/8 teaspoon salt until combined.   Pour milk in a glass measuring cup and microwave on high for 1 minute. Do not boil. Whisk milk into egg mixture until blended. Arrange peaches on the bottom of the crust and pour egg mixture over the top. Bake 25-30 minutes, or until set.

Cool to room temperature. Cover and chill at least 2 hours before serving.
Nutrition Info:al Facts Per ServingCalories 180 Total Carbs 22g Net Carbs 21g Protein 5g Fat 7g Sugar 9g Fiber 1g

112. Double Chocolate Biscotti

Servings: 27   Cooking Time: 30 Minutes
Ingredients:
- 3 egg whites, divided
- 2 eggs
- 1 tbsp. orange zest
- What you'll need from store cupboard:
- 2 cup flour
- ½ cup Splenda
- ½ cup almonds, toasted and chopped
- 1/3 cup cocoa, unsweetened
- ¼ cup mini chocolate chips
- 1 tsp vanilla
- 1 tsp instant coffee granules
- 1 tsp water
- ½ tsp salt
- ½ tsp baking soda
- Nonstick cooking spray

Directions:
Heat oven to 350 degrees. Spray a large baking sheet with cooking spray.   In a large bowl, combine flour, Splenda, cocoa, salt, and baking soda.   In a small bowl, whisk the eggs, 2 egg whites, vanilla, and coffee. Let rest 3-4 minutes to dissolve the coffee.   Stir in the orange zest and add to dry Ingredients, stir to thoroughly combine. Fold in the nuts and chocolate chips.   Divide dough in half and place on prepared pan. Shape each half into 14x1 ¾-inch rectangle.   Stir water and remaining egg white together. Brush over the top of the dough. Bake 20-25 minutes, or until firm to the touch. Cool on wire racks 5 minutes.   Transfer biscotti to a cutting board. Use a serrated knife to cut diagonally into ½-inch slice. Place cut side down on baking sheet and bake 5-7 minutes per side. Store in airtight container. Serving size is 2 pieces.
Nutrition Info: Calories 86 Total Carbs 13g Net Carbs 12g Protein 3g Fat 3g Sugar 5g Fiber 1g

113. Apple Mini Cakes

Servings: 2   Cooking Time: 10 Minutes
Ingredients:
- 1 medium apple, peeled and diced, into bite-sized pieces
- 18g granulated sugar
- 18g unsalted butter
- 2g ground cinnamon
- 1g ground nutmeg
- 1g ground allspice
- 1 sheet prefabricated cake dough
- 1 beaten egg
- 5 ml of milk

Directions:
Put diced apples, granulated sugar, butter, cinnamon, nutmeg, and allspice in a medium saucepan or in a skillet over medium-low heat.   Simmer for 2 minutes and

remove from heat. Allow the apples to cool, discovered at room temperature for 30 minutes. Cut the cake dough into circles of 127 mm. Add the filling to the center of each circle and use your finger to apply water to the outer ends. Some filler will be left unused. Close the cake cut a small opening at the top. Preheat the air fryer for a few minutes and set the temperature to 175°C. Mix the eggs and milk and spread the mixture on each foot. Place the cakes in the preheated air fryer and cook at 175°C for 10 minutes until the cakes are golden brown.

Nutrition Info:(Nutrition per Serving)Calories: 185 Fat: 11Carbohydrates: 38g Protein: 5g Sugar: 20gCholesterol: 11mg

114. Orange Oatmeal Cookies

Servings: 18 (2 Cookies Per Serving)   Cooking Time: 10 Minutes

Ingredients:
- 1 orange, zested and juiced
- ½ cup margarine
- 1 egg white
- 1 tbsp. orange juice
- What you'll need from the store cupboard
- 1 cup whole wheat pastry flour
- 1 cup oats
- ¼ cup stevia
- ¼ cup dark brown sugar substitute
- ¼ cup applesauce, unsweetened
- 1/3 cup wheat bran
- ½ tsp baking soda
- ½ tsp cream of tartar
- ¼ tsp cinnamon

Directions:
Heat oven to 350 degrees. Line two cookie sheets with parchment paper. In a medium mixing bowl, cream butter. Gradually add the sugars and beat 2 -3 minutes. Add egg white and applesauce and beat just to combine. Sift the dry Ingredients together in a large mixing bowl. Add the wet Ingredients, the orange juice, and the zest. Drop the dough by tablespoons onto the prepared cookie sheets. Bake 10 minutes, or until the bottoms are brown. Cool on wire rack. Store in an airtight container.

Nutrition Info: Calories 129 Total Carbs 17g Net Carbs 16g Protein 2g Fat 6g Sugar 8g Fiber 1g

115. Apple Pear & Pecan Dessert Squares

Servings: 24   Cooking Time: 25 Minutes

Ingredients:
- 1 Granny Smith apple, sliced, leave peel on
- 1 Red Delicious apple, sliced, leave peel on
- 1 ripe pear, sliced, leave peel on
- 3 eggs
- ½ cup plain fat-free yogurt
- 1 tbsp. lemon juice
- 1 tbsp. margarine
- What you'll need from store cupboard:
- 1 package spice cake mix
- 1 ¼ cup water, divided
- ½ cup pecan pieces
- 1 tbsp. Splenda

- 1 tsp cinnamon
- ½ tsp vanilla
- ¼ tsp nutmeg
- Nonstick cooking spray

Directions:
Heat oven to 350°F. Spray jelly-roll pan with nonstick cooking spray. In a large bowl, beat cake mix, 1 cup water, eggs and yogurt until smooth. Pour into prepared pan and bake 20 minutes or it passes the toothpick test. Cool completely. In a large nonstick skillet, over med-high heat, toast the pecans, stirring, about 2 minutes or until lightly browned. Remove to a plate. Add the remaining ¼ cup water, sliced fruit, juice and spices to the skillet. Bring to a boil. Reduce heat to medium and cook 3 minutes or until fruit is tender crisp. Remove from heat and stir in Splenda, margarine, vanilla, and pecans. Spoon evenly over cooled cake. Slice into 24 squares and serve.

Nutrition Info: Calories 130 Total Carbs 20g Net Carbs 19g Protein 2g Fat 5g Sugar 10g Fiber 1g

116. Mini Bread Puddings

Servings: 12   Cooking Time: 35 Minutes

Ingredients:
- 6 slices cinnamon bread, cut into cubes
- 1 ¼ cup skim milk
- ½ cup egg substitute
- 1 tbsp. margarine, melted
- What you'll need from store cupboard
- 1/3 cup Splenda
- 1 tsp vanilla
- 1/8 tsp salt
- 1/8 tsp nutmeg

Directions:
Heat oven to 350°F. Line 12 medium-size muffin cups with paper baking cups. In a large bowl, stir together milk, egg substitute, Splenda, vanilla, salt and nutmeg until combined. Add bread cubes and stir until moistened. Let rest 15 minutes. Spoon evenly into prepared baking cups. Drizzle margarine evenly over the tops. Bake 30-35 minutes or until puffed and golden brown. Remove from oven and let cool completely.

Nutrition Info: Calories 105 Total Carbs 16 Net Carbs 15g Protein 4g Fat 2g Sugar 9g Fiber 1g

117. Crab & Spinach Dip

Servings: 10   Cooking Time: 2 Hours

Ingredients:
- 1 pkg. frozen chopped spinach, thawed and squeezed nearly dry
- 8 oz. reduced-fat cream cheese
- What you'll need from store cupboard:
- 6 ½ oz. can crabmeat, drained and shredded
- 6 oz.jar marinated artichoke hearts, drained and diced fine
- ¼ tsp hot pepper sauce
- Melba toast or whole grain crackers (optional)

Directions:
Remove any shells or cartilage from crab. Place all Ingredients in a small crock pot. Cover and cook on high 1 ½ - 2 hours, or until heated through and cream cheese

is melted. Stir after 1 hour.   Serve with Melba toast or whole grain crackers. Serving size is ¼ cup.
Nutrition Info: Calories 106 Total Carbs 7g Net Carbs 6g Protein 5g Fat 8g Sugar 3g Fiber 1g

118. Carrot Cupcakes

Servings: 12   Cooking Time: 35 Minutes
Ingredients:
- 2 cup carrots, grated
- 1 cup low fat cream cheese, soft
- 2 eggs
- 1-2 tsp skim milk
- What you'll need from store cupboard:
- ½ cup coconut oil, melted
- ¼ cup coconut flour
- ¼ cup Splenda
- ¼ cup honey
- 2 tsp vanilla, divided
- 1 tsp baking powder
- 1 tsp cinnamon
- Nonstick cooking spray

Directions:
Heat oven to 350 degrees. Lightly spray a muffin pan with cooking spray, or use paper liners.   In a large bowl, stir together the flour, baking powder, and cinnamon. Add the carrots, eggs, oil, Splenda, and vanilla to a food processor. Process until Ingredients are combined but carrots still have some large chunks remaining. Add to dry Ingredients and stir to combine.   Pour evenly into prepared pan, filling cups 2/3 full. Bake 30-35 minutes, or until cupcakes pass the toothpick test. Remove from oven and let cool.   In a medium bowl, beat cream cheese, honey, and vanilla on high speed until smooth. Add milk, one teaspoon at a time, beating after each addition, until frosting is creamy enough to spread easily. Once cupcakes have cooled, spread each one with about 2 tablespoons of frosting. Chill until ready to serve.
Nutrition Info:al Facts Per ServingCalories 160 Total Carbs 13g Net Carbs 12g Protein 4g Fat 10g Sugar 11g Fiber 1g

119. Sticky Ginger Cake

Servings: 16   Cooking Time: 30 Minutes
Ingredients:
- 2 eggs, beaten
- 1 cup buttermilk
- 2 tbsp. butter
- 2 tsp fresh ginger, grated
- What you'll need from store cupboard:
- 1 cup flour
- ¼ cup + 1 tbsp. honey
- ¼ cup + 1 tbsp. molasses
- ¼ cup Splenda brown sugar
- 1 tbsp. water
- 1 tsp baking soda
- 1 tsp ginger
- 1 tsp cinnamon
- ½ tsp allspice
- ¼ tsp salt
- Nonstick cooking spray
- Swerve confections sugar, for dusting

Directions:
Heat oven to 400 degrees. Spray an 8-inch square pan with cooking spray.   In a saucepan over medium heat, stir together ¼ honey, ¼ cup molasses, Splenda, butter and grated ginger until butter is melted. Remove from heat and let cool 5 minutes.   In a medium bowl, stir together the dry Ingredients.   In a small bowl, beat the eggs and buttermilk together. Whisk into the molasses mixture until combined. Add to dry Ingredients and mix well. Pour into prepared pan.   Bake 25 minutes. Use a skewer to poke holes every inch across the top of the cake. In a small bowl mix remaining honey, molasses and water together. Brush over hot cake. Cool completely and dust lightly with confectioner's sugar before serving.
Nutrition Info: Calories 102 Total Carbs 18g Protein 2g Fat 2g Sugar 11g Fiber 0g

120. Cauliflower Hummus

Servings: 6   Cooking Time: 15 Minutes
Ingredients:
- 3 cup cauliflower florets
- 3 tbsp. fresh lemon juice
- What you'll need from store cupboard:
- 5 cloves garlic, divided
- 5 tbsp. olive oil, divided
- 2 tbsp. water
- 1 ½ tbsp. Tahini paste
- 1 ¼ tsp salt, divided
- Smoked paprika and extra olive oil for serving

Directions:
In a microwave safe bowl, combine cauliflower, water, 2 tablespoons oil, ½ teaspoon salt, and 3 whole cloves garlic. Microwave on high 15 minutes, or until cauliflower is soft and darkened.   Transfer mixture to a food processor or blender and process until almost smooth. Add tahini paste, lemon juice, remaining garlic cloves, remaining oil, and salt. Blend until almost smooth.   Place the hummus in a bowl and drizzle lightly with olive oil and a sprinkle or two of paprika. Serve with your favorite raw vegetables.
Nutrition Info: Calories 107 Total Carbs 5g Net Carbs 3g Protein 2g Fat 10g Sugar 1g Fiber 2g

121. Mini Apple Oat Muffins

Servings: 24   Cooking Time: 25 Minutes
Ingredients:
- 1 ½ cups old-fashioned oats
- 1-teaspoon baking powder
- ½-teaspoon ground cinnamon
- ¼-teaspoon baking soda
- ¼-teaspoon salt
- ½ cup unsweetened applesauce
- ¼-cup light brown sugar
- 3 tablespoons canola oil
- 3 tablespoons water
- 1-teaspoon vanilla extract
- ½ cup slivered almonds

Directions:
Preheat the oven to 350°F and grease a mini muffin pan. Place the oats in a food processor and pulse into a fine flour.   Add the baking powder, cinnamon, baking soda,

38

and salt.   Pulse until well combined then add the applesauce, brown sugar, canola oil, water, and vanilla then blend smooth.   Fold in the almonds and spoon the mixture into the muffin pan.   Bake for 22 to 25 minutes until a knife inserted in the center comes out clean.   Cool the muffins for 5 minutes then turn out onto a wire rack.

Nutrition Info: Calories 70Total Fat 0.7g, Saturated Fat 0.1g, Total Carbs 14.7g, Net Carbs 12.2g, Protein 2.1g, Sugar 2.2g, Fiber 2.5g, Sodium 1mg

122. Cappuccino Mousse

Servings: 8   Cooking Time: 1 Hour
Ingredients:
- 2 cup low fat cream cheese, soft
- 1 cup half-n-half
- ½ cup almond milk, unsweetened
- 1/4 cup strong brewed coffee, cooled completely
- What you'll need from store cupboard:
- 1-2 tsp coffee extract
- 1 tsp vanilla liquid sweetener
- Whole coffee beans for garnish

Directions:
In a large bowl, beat cream cheese and coffee on high speed until smooth. Add milk, 1 teaspoon coffee extract and liquid sweetener. Beat until smooth and thoroughly combined.   Pour in half-n-half and continue beating until mixture resembles the texture of mousse.   Spoon into dessert glasses or ramekins, cover and chill at least 1 hour before serving. Garnish with a coffee bean and serve.

Nutrition Info:al Facts Per ServingCalories 98 Total Carbs 5g Protein 9g Fat 5g Sugar 0g Fiber 0g

123. Cheesy Pita Crisps

Servings: 8   Cooking Time: 15 Minutes
Ingredients:
- ½ cup mozzarella cheese
- ¼ cup margarine, melted
- What you'll need from store cupboard:
- 4 whole-wheat pita pocket halves
- 3 tbsp. reduced fat parmesan
- ½ tsp garlic powder
- ½ tsp onion powder
- ¼ tsp salt
- ¼ tsp pepper
- Nonstick cooking spray

Directions:
Heat oven to 400 degrees. Spray a baking sheet with cooking spray.   Cut each pita pocket in half. Cut each half into 2 triangles. Place, rough side up, on prepared pan.   In a small bowl, whisk together margarine, parmesan and seasonings. Spread each triangle with margarine mixture. Sprinkle mozzarella over top. Bake 12-15 minutes or until golden brown.

Nutrition Info: Calories 131 Total Carbs 14g Net Carbs 12g Protein 4g Fat 7g Sugar 1g Fiber 2g

124. Cranberry And Orange Muffins

Servings: 6-8   Cooking Time: 15 Minutes
Ingredients:
- 120g all-purpose flour
- 66g of sugar
- 4g baking powder
- 2g of baking soda
- A pinch salt
- 100g of blueberries
- 1 egg
- 80 ml of orange juice
- 60 ml of vegetable oil
- 1 orange, zest
- Nonstick Spray Oil

Directions:
Mix the flour, baking powder, baking soda, salt, and blueberries in a large bowl.   Beat the egg, orange juice, oil, and orange zest in a separate bowl.   Mix the wet and dry ingredients until well combined.   Grease the muffin pans with oil spray and pour the mixture until they are filled to ¾.   Preheat the air fryer for a few minutes and set the temperature to 150°C.   Place the muffin molds carefully in the preheated air fryer. You may have to work in parts. Set the time to 15 minutes at 150°C.

Nutrition Info: Calories: 215 Fat: 0g Carbohydrates: 0g Protein: 0g Sugar: 0gCholesterol: 17.1mg

125. Homemade Cheetos

Servings: 6   Cooking Time: 30 Minutes
Ingredients:
- 3 egg whites
- ½ cup cheddar cheese, grated and frozen
- What you'll need from store cupboard:
- ¼ cup reduced fat parmesan cheese
- 1/8 tsp cream of tartar

Directions:
Heat oven to 300 degrees. Line a baking sheet with parchment paper.   Put the frozen cheese in a food processor/blender and pulse, until it's in tiny little pieces. In a large mixing bowl, beat egg whites and cream of tartar until very stiff peaks from. Gently fold in chopped cheese. Spoon mixture into a piping bag with ½-inch hole. Gently pipe "cheeto" shapes onto prepared pan. Sprinkle with parmesan cheese.   Bake 20-30 minutes. Turn off oven and leave the puffs inside another 30 minutes. Let cool completely and store in an airtight container.

Nutrition Info: Calories 102 Total Carbs 1g Protein 9g Fat 7g Sugar 0g Fiber 0g

126. Blt Stuffed Cucumbers

Servings: 4
Ingredients:
- 3 slices bacon, cooked crisp and crumbled
- 1 large cucumber
- ½ cup lettuce, diced fine
- ½ cup baby spinach, diced fine
- ¼ cup tomato, diced fine
- What you'll need from store cupboard:
- 1 tbsp. + ½ tsp fat-free mayonnaise
- ¼ tsp black pepper
- 1/8 tsp salt

Directions:

Peel the cucumber and slice in half lengthwise. Use a spoon to remove the seeds. In a medium bowl, combine remaining Ingredients and stir well. Spoon the bacon mixture into the cucumber halves. Cut into 2-inch pieces and serve.
Nutrition Info: Calories 95 Total Carbs 4g Net Carbs 3g Protein 6g Fat 6g Sugar 2g Fiber 1g

127. Espresso Chocolate Muffins

Servings: 8   Cooking Time: 15 Minutes
Ingredients:
- 120g all-purpose flour
- 60g cocoa powder
- 150g light brown sugar
- 2g baking powder
- 2g espresso coffee powder
- 3g of baking soda
- 1g of salt
- 1 large egg
- 170 ml of milk
- 5 ml vanilla extract
- 5 ml apple cider vinegar
- 80 ml of vegetable oil
- Nonstick Spray Oil

Directions:
Mix the flour, cocoa powder, sugar, baking powder, espresso coffee powder, baking soda and salt in a large bowl. Beat the egg, milk, vanilla, vinegar, and oil in a separate bowl. Mix the wet ingredients in the dry ones until they are well combined. Grease the muffin pans with oil spray and pour the mixture until they are filled to ¾. Preheat the air fryer for a few minutes and set the temperature to 150°C. Place the muffin molds carefully in the preheated air fryer. You may have to work in parts. Put the muffins in the air fryer previously preheated and set the time to 15 minutes at 150°C.
Nutrition Info: Calories: 374Fat: 0g Carbohydrates: 0g Protein: 0g Sugar: 0gCholesterol: 34mg

128. Coconutty Pudding Clouds

Servings: 4
Ingredients:
- 2 cup of heavy whipping cream
- ½ cup of reduced-fat cream cheese, soft
- ½ cup hazelnuts, ground
- 4 tbsp. unsweetened coconut flakes, toasted
- What you'll need from the store cupboard
- 2 tbsp. stevia, divided
- ½ tsp of vanilla
- ½ tsp of hazelnut extract
- ½ tsp of cacao powder, unsweetened

Directions:
In a medium bowl, beat cream, vanilla, and 1 tablespoon stevia until soft peaks form. In another mixing bowl, beat cream cheese, cocoa, remaining stevia, and hazelnut extract until smooth. In 4 glasses, place ground nuts on the bottom, add a layer of the cream cheese mixture, then the whip cream, and top with toasted coconut. Serve immediately.
Nutrition Info: Calories 396 Total Carbs 12g Net Carbs 11g Protein 6g Fat 35g Sugar 9g Fiber 1g

129. Freezer Fudge

Servings: 16   Cooking Time: 2 Hours
Ingredients:
- ¼ cup margarine
- ¼ cup creamed coconut
- What you'll need from store cupboard:
- 1 ¼ cup coconut oil
- 1 cup pecans, ground fine
- 6 tbsp. cocoa powder, unsweetened
- 2 tbsp. honey
- 1 tbsp. vanilla
- ¼ tsp sea salt

Directions:
Line an 8x8 inch glass baking dish with wax paper. Add the oil and margarine to a glass measuring cup. Fill a medium saucepan about half full of water and bring to a boil. Place the measuring cup in the pan and stir until they are melted and combined. Pour into a blender or food processor and add everything but the nuts. Process until smooth. And the nuts and pulse just to combine. Pour into the prepared pan and freeze until the fudge is set. Remove from the pan and cut into 32 pieces. Store in a plastic container in the freezer. Serving size is 2 pieces.
Nutrition Info: Calories 254 Total Carbs 7g Net Carbs 6g Protein 1g Fat 26g Sugar 5g Fiber 1g

130. Strawberry Sorbet

Servings: 4   Cooking Time: 4 Hours
Ingredients:
- 10 oz. strawberries, frozen
- What you'll need from store cupboard:
- 2cups water
- ¼ cup honey

Directions:
Place strawberries, water, and honey in a blender and process until smooth and creamy. Pour mixture into ice cream maker and process according to instructions. Transfer to a plastic container with an airtight lid and freeze 4 hours before serving.
Nutrition Info: Calories 38g Total Carbs 9g Net Carbs 7g Protein 0g Fat 0g Sugar 7g Fiber 2g

131. Italian Eggplant Rollups

Servings: 8   Cooking Time: 25 Minutes
Ingredients:
- 16 fresh spinach leaves
- 4 sun-dried tomatoes, rinsed, drained and diced fine
- 2 medium eggplants
- 1 green onion, diced fine
- 4 tbsp. fat-free cream cheese, soft
- 2 tbsp. fat-free sour cream
- What you'll need from store cupboard:
- 1 cup spaghetti sauce (chapter 16)
- 2 tbsp. lemon juice
- 1 tsp olive oil
- 1 clove garlic, diced fine
- ¼ tsp oregano
- 1/8 tsp black pepper

- Nonstick cooking spray

Directions:

Heat oven to 450 degrees. Spray 2 large cookie sheets with cooking spray. Trim the ends of the eggplant. Slice them lengthwise in ¼-inch slices. Discard the ones that are mostly skin, there should be about 16 slices. Arrange them in a single layer on prepared pans. In a small bowl, whisk together the lemon juice and oil and brush over both sides of the eggplant. Bake 20-25 minutes or until the eggplant starts to turn a golden brown color. Transfer to a plate to cool. In a mixing bowl, combine remaining Ingredients, except spinach, until thoroughly combined. To assemble, spread 1 teaspoon cream cheese mixture evenly over sliced eggplant, leaving ½-inch border around the edges .Top with a spinach leaf and roll up, starting at small end. Lay rolls, seam side down, on serving plate. Serve with warm spaghetti sauce (chapter 16).

Nutrition Info: Calories 78 Total Carbs 12g Net Carbs 6g Protein 3g Fat 3g Sugar 6g Fiber 6g

132. Chocolate Chip Muffins

Servings: 6-8   Cooking Time: 15 Minutes

Ingredients:
- 50g granulated sugar
- 125 ml of coconut milk or soymilk
- 60 ml coconut oil, liquid
- 5 ml vanilla extract
- 120g all-purpose flour
- 14g cocoa powder
- 4g baking powder
- 2g of baking soda
- A pinch of salt
- 85g chocolate chips
- 25g of pistachios, cracked (optional)
- Nonstick Spray Oil

Directions:

Put the sugar, coconut milk, coconut oil and vanilla extract in a small bowl, then set aside. Mix the flour, cocoa powder, baking powder, baking soda and salt in a separate bowl and set aside. Mix the dry ingredients with the wet ingredients gradually, until smooth. Then join with the chocolate and pistachio. Preheat the air fryer for a few minutes and set the temperature to 150°C. Grease the muffin pans with oil spray and pour the mixture until they are filled to ¾. Place the muffin molds carefully in the preheated air fryer. Set the time to 15 minutes at 150°C. Remove the muffins when finished cooking and let them cool for 10 minutes before serving.

Nutrition Info: Calories: 374 Fat: 17.31g Carbohydrates: 48.86g Protein: 9.41g Sugar: 7.73 Cholesterol: 45g

133. Banana Nut Cookies

Servings: 18   Cooking Time: 15 Minutes

Ingredients:
- 1 ½ cup banana, mashed
- What you'll need from store cupboard:
- 2 cup oats
- 1 cup raisins

- 1 cup walnuts
- 1/3 cup sunflower oil
- 1 tsp vanilla
- ½ tsp salt

Directions:

Heat oven to 350 degrees. In a large bowl, combine oats, raisins, walnuts, and salt. In a medium bowl, mix banana, oil, and vanilla. Stir into oat mixture until combined. Let rest 15 minutes. Drop by rounded tablespoonful onto 2 ungreased cookie sheets. Bake 15 minutes, or until a light golden brown. Cool and store in an airtight container. Serving size is 2 cookies.

Nutrition Info: Calories 148 Total Carbs 16g Net Carbs 14g Protein 3g Fat 9g Sugar 6g Fiber 2g

134. Tropical Fruit Tart

Servings: 8   Cooking Time: 10 Minutes

Ingredients:
- 1 mango, peeled, pitted and sliced thin
- 1 banana, sliced thin
- 2 egg whites
- What you'll need from store cupboard
- 15 ¼ oz. can pineapple chunks in juice, undrained
- 3 ½ oz. can sweetened flaked coconut
- 1 cup cornflakes, crushed
- 3 teaspoons Splenda
- 2 tsp cornstarch
- 1 tsp coconut extract
- Nonstick cooking spray

Directions:

Heat oven to 425 degrees. Spray a 9-inch springform pan with cooking spray. In a medium bowl, combine cornflakes, coconut, and egg whites. Toss until blended. Press firmly over the bottom and ½-inch up the sides of the prepared pan. Bake 8 minutes or until edges start to brown. Cool completely. Drain the juice from the pineapple into a small saucepan. Add cornstarch and stir until smooth. Bring to boil over high heat and let cook 1 minute, stirring constantly. Remove from heat and cool completely. Once cooled stir in Splenda and coconut extract. In a medium bowl, combine pineapple, mango, and banana. Spoon over crust and drizzle with pineapple juice mixture. Cover and chill at least 2 hours before serving.

Nutrition Info: Calories 120 Total Carbs 19g Net Carbs 17g Protein 2g Fat 4g Sugar 13g Fiber 2g

135. Chocolate And Nut Cake

Servings: 4   Cooking Time: 30 Minutes

Ingredients:
- 60g dark chocolate
- 2 butter spoons
- 1 egg
- 3 spoonful's of sugar
- 50g flour
- 1 envelope Royal yeast
- Chopped walnuts

Directions:

Melt the dark chocolate with the butter, over low heat. Once melted, put in a bowl. Incorporate the egg, sugar, flour, yeast (the latter passed through the sieve, to prevent lumps from forming) and finally the chopped nuts.   Beat well by hand until you get a uniform dough. Put the dough in a silicone mold or oven suitable for incorporation in the basket of the air fryer.   Preheat the air fryer a few minutes at 1800C.   Set the timer for 20 minutes at 1800C and when it has cooled down, unmold.

Nutrition Info: Calories: 108Fat: 12g Carbohydrates: 29g Protein: 4g Sugar: 100g Cholesterol: 3g

136. Pumpkin And Raspberry Muffins

Servings: 12 Muffins   Cooking Time: 25 Minutes

Ingredients:
- ¾ cup blanched almond flour
- ½ cup coconut flour
- 3 tablespoons tapioca
- 1 tablespoon cinnamon
- 1 tablespoon baking powder
- Pinch of nutmeg
- ½ cup stevia in raw
- ¼ teaspoon salt
- 1 cup puréed pumpkin
- 4 large eggs, whites and yolks separated
- 1½ teaspoons vanilla extract
- ½ cup coconut oil
- 10 drops liquid stevia
- 1½ cups frozen raspberries

Directions:
Preheat the oven to 350°F (180°C). Line a 12-cup muffin pan with paper muffin cups.   Combine the flours, tapioca, cinnamon, baking powder, nutmeg, stevia in raw, and salt in a large bowl. Stir to mix well.   Mix in the puréed pumpkin, egg yolks, vanilla extract, coconut oil, and liquid stevia until a batter forms. Divide the batter into the muffin cups.   Whip the egg whites in a separate large bowl until it forms the stiff peaks.   Top the batter with the beaten egg whites and raspberries. Place the muffin pan in the preheated oven and bake for 25 minutes or until a toothpick inserted in the center of the muffins comes out clean.   Remove the muffins from the oven and allow to cool for 5 minutes before serving.

Nutrition Info:(1 Muffin)calories: 223 fat: 15.6g protein: 4.4g carbs: 29.3g fiber: 2.9g sugar: 7.7g sodium: 76mg

137. Raspberry Lemon Cheesecake Squares

Servings: 12   Cooking Time: 40 Minutes

Ingredients:
- 2 cups raspberries
- 1 cup fat-free sour cream
- ¾ cup fat-free cream cheese, softened
- ½ cup egg substitute
- 2 tbsp. lemon juice
- 2 tsp lemon zest, divided
- What you'll need from store cupboard:
- ½ cup + 3 tbsp. Splenda
- 1 tsp vanilla
- Nonstick cooking spray

Directions:

Heat oven to 350°F. Spray 8-inch square baking pan with cooking spray.   In a large bowl, beat cream cheese, ½ cup Splenda, and vanilla on high speed until smooth. Add juice, 1 teaspoon zest, and egg substitute. Beat until thoroughly combined. Pour into prepared pan.   Bake 40 minutes or until firm to the touch. Remove from oven and cool completely.   In a small bowl, stir together the sour cream and 1 tablespoon Splenda until smooth. Spoon evenly over cooled cheesecake. Cover and refrigerate overnight.   minutes before serving, toss the berries and remaining 2 tablespoons Splenda in small bowl. Let sit. Just before serving, stir in the remaining zest and spoon the berry mixture over the top of the cheesecake. Cut into 12 bars and serve.

Nutrition Info: Calories 144 Total Carbs 18g Net Carbs 17g Protein 3g Fat 5g Sugar 14g Fiber 1g

138. Raspberry Almond Clafoutis

Servings: 8   Cooking Time: 1 Hour

Ingredients:
- 1 pint raspberries, rinse and pat dry
- 3 eggs
- ¾ cup almond milk, unsweetened
- ¼ cup half-n-half
- 4 tbsp. margarine
- What you'll need from store cupboard:
- ½ cup almond flour
- 1/3 cup Splenda
- ¼ cup almonds, sliced
- 1 tbsp. coconut flour
- 1 ½ tsp vanilla
- ½ tsp baking powder
- ¼ tsp allspice
- ¼ tsp almond extract
- Nonstick cooking spray

Directions:
Heat oven to 350 degrees. Spray a 9-inch pie dish with cooking spray and place on a baking sheet.   Place the berries, in a single layer, in the pie dish.   In a medium bowl, stir together the flours, baking powder, and allspice. Add the margarine to a small saucepan and melt over low heat. Once melted, remove from heat and whisk in Splenda until smooth.   Pour the margarine into a large bowl and whisk in eggs, one at a time. Add extracts and dry Ingredients. Stir in the almond milk and half-n-half, batter will be thin.   Pour over the raspberries and top with almonds. Bake 50-60 minutes, or center is set and top is lightly browned. Cool to room temperature before serving.

Nutrition Info:al Facts Per ServingCalories 273 Total Carbs 19g Net Carbs 13g Protein 7g Fat 19g Sugar 11g Fiber 6g

139. Fried Zucchini

Servings: 4   Cooking Time: 10 Minutes

Ingredients:
- 3 zucchini, slice ¼ - 1/8-inch thick
- 2 eggs
- What you'll need from store cupboard:
- ½ cup sunflower oil
- 1/3 cup coconut flour

- ¼ cup reduced fat Parmesan cheese
- 1 tbsp. water

Directions:
Heat oil in a large skillet over medium heat. In a shallow bowl whisk the egg and water together. In another shallow bowl, stir flour and parmesan together. Coat zucchini in the egg then flour mixture. Add, in a single layer, to the skillet. Cook 2 minutes per side until golden brown. Transfer to paper towel lined plate. Repeat. Serve immediately with your favorite dipping sauce.

Nutrition Info: Calories 138 Total Carbs 6g Net Carbs 4g Protein 6g Fat 11g Sugar 3g Fiber 2g

140. Fruity Coconut Energy Balls

Servings: 18   Cooking Time: None
Ingredients:
- 1 cup chopped almonds
- 1 cup dried figs
- ½ cup dried apricots, chopped
- ½ cup dried cranberries, unsweetened
- ½-teaspoon vanilla extract
- ¼-teaspoon ground cinnamon
- ½ cup shredded unsweetened coconut

Directions:
Place the almonds, figs, apricots, and cranberries in a food processor. Pulse the mixture until finely chopped. Add the vanilla extract and cinnamon then pulse to combine once more. Roll the mixture into 18 small balls by hand. Roll the balls in the shredded coconut and chill until firm.

Nutrition Info: Calories 100 Total Fat 0.7g, Saturated Fat 0.1g, Total Carbs 14.7g, Net Carbs 12.2g, Protein 2.1g, Sugar 2.2g, Fiber 2.5g, Sodium 1mg

141. Chewy Granola Bars

Servings: 36   Cooking Time: 35 Minutes
Ingredients:
- 1 egg, beaten
- 2/3 cup margarine, melted
- What you'll need from store cupboard:
- 3 ½ cup quick oats
- 1 cup almonds, chopped
- ½ cup honey
- ½ cup sunflower kernels
- ½ cup coconut, unsweetened
- ½ cup dried apples
- ½ cup dried cranberries
- ½ cup Splenda brown sugar
- 1 tsp vanilla
- ½ tsp cinnamon
- Nonstick cooking spray

Directions:
Heat oven to 350 degrees. Spray a large baking sheet with cooking spray. Spread oats and almonds on prepared pan. Bake 12-15 minutes until toasted, stirring every few minutes. In a large bowl, combine egg, margarine, honey, and vanilla. Stir in remaining Ingredients. Stir in oat mixture. Press into baking sheet and bake 13-18 minutes, or until edges are light

brown. Cool on a wire rack. Cut into bars and store in an airtight container.

Nutrition Info: Calories 119 Total Carbs 13g Net Carbs 12g Protein 2g Fat 6g Sugar 7g Fiber 1g

142. Blueberry No Bake Cheesecake

Servings: 8   Cooking Time: 3 Hours
Ingredients:
- 16 oz. fat free cream cheese, softened
- 1 cup sugar free frozen whipped topping, thawed
- ¾ cup blueberries
- 1 tbsp. margarine, melted
- What you'll need from store cupboard
- 8 zwieback toasts
- 1 cup boiling water
- 1/3 cup Splenda
- 1 envelope unflavored gelatin
- 1 tsp vanilla

Directions:
Place the toasts and margarine in a food processor. Pulse until mixture resembles coarse crumbs. Press on the bottom of a 9-inch springform pan. Place gelatin in a medium bowl and add boiling water. Stir until gelatin dissolved completely. In a large bowl, beat cream cheese, Splenda, and vanilla on medium speed until well blended. Beat in whipped topping. Add gelatin, in a steady stream, while beating on low speed. Increase speed to medium and beat 4 minutes or until smooth and creamy. Gently fold in berries and spread over crust. Cover and chill 3 hours or until set.

Nutrition Info: Calories 316 Total Carbs 20g Protein 6g Fat 23g Sugar 10g Fiber 0g

143. Honey Roasted Pumpkin Seeds

Servings: 8   Cooking Time: 30 Minutes
Ingredients:
- 2 cup raw fresh pumpkin seeds, wash and pat dry
- 1 tbsp. butter
- What you'll need from store cupboard:
- 3 tbsp. honey
- 1 tbsp. coconut oil
- 1 tsp cinnamon

Directions:
Heat oven to 275 degrees. Line a baking sheet with parchment paper, making sure it hangs over both ends. Place the pumpkin seeds in a medium bowl. In a small microwave safe bowl, add butter, coconut oil, and honey. Microwave until the butter melts and the honey is runny. Pour the honey mixture over the pumpkin seeds and stir. Add the cinnamon and stir again. Dump the pumpkin seeds into the middle of the paper and place it in the oven. Bake for 30-40 minutes until the seeds and honey are a deep golden brown, stirring every 10 minutes. When the seeds are roasted, remove from the oven and stir again. Stir a few times as they cool to keep them from sticking in one big lump. Enjoy the seeds once they are cool enough to eat. Store uncovered for up to one week. Serving size is ¼ cup.

Nutrition Info: Calories 267 Total Carbs 13g Net Carbs 12g Protein 8g Fat 22g Sugar 7g Fiber 1g

144. Fluffy Lemon Bars

Servings: 20   Cooking Time: 2 Hours
Ingredients:
- 8 oz. low fat cream cheese, soft
- 1/3 cup butter, melted
- 3 tbsp. fresh lemon juice
- What you'll need from store cupboard:
- 12 oz. evaporated milk
- 1 pkg. lemon gelatin, sugar free
- 1 ½ cup graham cracker crumbs
- 1 cup boiling water
- ¾ cup Splenda
- 1 tsp vanilla

Directions:
Pour milk into a large, metal bowl, place beaters in the bowl, cover and chill 2 hours.   In a small bowl, combine cracker crumbs and butter, reserve 1 tablespoon. Press the remaining mixture on the bottom of a 13x9-inch baking dish. Cover and chill until set.   In a small bowl, dissolve gelatin in boiling water. Stir in lemon juice and let cool.   In a large bowl, beat cream cheese, Splenda and vanilla until smooth. Add gelatin and mix well.   Beat the chilled milk until soft peaks form. Fold into cream cheese mixture. Pour over chilled crust and sprinkle with reserved crumbs. Cover and chill 2 hours before serving.
Nutrition Info: Calories 126 Total Carbs 15g Protein 3g Fat 5g Sugar 10g Fiber 0g

145. Gingerbread Cookies

Servings: 10   Cooking Time: 10 Minutes
Ingredients:
- 1 egg
- ¼ cup butter, soft
- What you'll need from store cupboard:
- 2 cup almond flour, sifted
- ¼ cup Splenda
- 1 tbsp. cinnamon
- 1 ½ tsp ginger
- 1 tsp vanilla
- ½ tsp baking powder
- ¼ tsp cloves
- ¼ tsp nutmeg

Directions:
In a medium bowl, stir together the almond flour, cinnamon, ginger, cloves, nutmeg, and baking powder. In a large bowl, beat the butter and Splenda for 1-2 minutes, until fluffy. Beat in the egg and vanilla. Beat in the almond flour mixture until a dough forms.   Form the dough into a ball, wrap with plastic wrap and refrigerate for at least 30 minutes.   Heat the oven to 350 degrees. Line a cookie sheet with parchment paper. Roll the dough out between two sheets of parchment paper to ¼-inch thick. Cut out desired shapes with cookie cutter and place on prepared pan. Or you can drop dough by teaspoonful onto pan.   Bake 10-15 minutes or until edges are golden brown. Remove to wire rack and cool. Store in airtight container. Serving size is 1 large, or 2 small cookies.

Nutrition Info: Calories 181 Total Carbs 9g Net Carbs 7g Protein 5g Fat 15g Sugar 6g Fiber 2g

146. Mini Eggplant Pizzas

Servings: 4   Cooking Time: 35 Minutes
Ingredients:
- 1 large eggplant, peeled and sliced into ¼ - inch circles
- 2 cup spaghetti sauce, (chapter 16)
- ½ cup reduced-fat mozzarella cheese, grated
- 2 eggs
- What you'll need from the store cupboard
- 1 ¼ cups Italian bread crumbs
- 1 tbsp. water
- ¼ tsp black pepper
- Nonstick cooking spray

Directions:
Heat oven to 350 degrees. Line 2 large cookie sheets with foil and spray well with cooking spray.   In a shallow dish, beat eggs, water and pepper. Place the bread crumbs in a separate shallow dish.   Dip eggplant pieces in egg mixture, then coat completely with bread crumbs. Place on prepared cookie sheets. Spray the tops with cooking spray and bake 15 minutes.   Turn the eggplant over and spray with cooking spray again. Bake another 15 minutes.   Remove from oven and top each piece with 1 tablespoon spaghetti sauce. Sprinkle cheese over sauce and bake another 4 – 5 minutes, or until sauce is bubbly and cheese is melted.
Nutrition Info: Calories 171 Total Carbs 24g Net Carbs 20g Protein 9g Fat 5g Sugar 6g Fiber 4g

147. Peanut Butter Pie

Servings: 8   Cooking Time: 4 Hours
Ingredients:
- 1 ½ cup skim milk
- 1 1/2 cup frozen fat-free whipped topping, thawed and divided
- 1 small pkg. sugar-free instant vanilla pudding mix
- 1 (1 ½ oz.) pkg. sugar-free peanut butter cups, chopped
- What you'll need from the store cupboard
- 1 (9-inch) reduced-fat graham cracker pie crust
- 1/3 cup reduced-fat peanut butter
- ½ tsp vanilla

Directions:
In a large bowl, whisk together milk and pudding mix until it thickens. Whisk in peanut butter, vanilla, and 1 cup whip cream. Fold in peanut butter cups.   Pour into pie crust and spread remaining whip cream over top. Cover and chill at least 4 hours before serving.
Nutrition Info: Calories 191 Total Carbs 27g Protein 4g Fat 6g Sugar 6g Fiber 0g

148. Dark Chocolate Almond Yogurt Cups

Servings: 6   Cooking Time: None
Ingredients:
- 3 cups plain nonfat Greek yogurt
- ½-teaspoon almond extract
- ¼-teaspoon liquid stevia extract (more to taste)

- 2 ounces 70% dark chocolate, chopped
- ½ cup slivered almonds

Directions:
Whisk together the yogurt, almond extract, and liquid stevia in a medium bowl. Spoon the yogurt into four dessert cups. Sprinkle with chopped chocolate and slivered almonds.
Nutrition Info: Calories 170Total Fat 0.7g, Saturated Fat 0.1g, Total Carbs 14.7g, Net Carbs 12.2g, Protein 2.1g, Sugar 2.2g, Fiber 2.5g, Sodium 41mg

149. Crispy Apple Chips

Servings: 4   Cooking Time: 2 Hours
Ingredients:
- 2 medium apples, sliced
- 1 teaspoon ground cinnamon

Directions:
Preheat the oven to 200°F (93°C). Line a baking sheet with parchment paper. Arrange the apple slices on the prepared baking sheet, then sprinkle with cinnamon. Bake in the preheated oven for 2 hours or until crispy. Flip the apple chips halfway through the cooking time. Allow to cool for 10 minutes and serve warm.
Nutrition Info:calories: 50   fat: 0g   protein: 0g carbs: 13.0g   fiber: 2.0g   sugar: 9.0g   sodium: 0mg

150. Zucchini Chips

Servings: 6   Cooking Time: 10 Minutes
Ingredients:
- 1 large zucchini, sliced into ¼-inch circle
- 1/4 cup reduced fat, Parmesan cheese, grated fine
- 3 tbsp. low-fat milk
- What you'll need from the store cupboard
- 1/3 cup whole wheat breadcrumbs
- ½ tsp garlic powder
- 1/8 tsp cayenne pepper
- Nonstick cooking spray

Directions:
After slicing zucchini pat dry with paper towels. Let sit for 60 minutes before using. Then pat dry again. Heat oven to 425 degrees. Spray a wire rack with cooking spray and place on cookie sheet. In a medium bowl combine all Ingredients except milk and zucchini. Pour milk into a shallow bowl. Dip zucchini into milk the coat with bread crumb mixture. Place on wire rack and bake 10 -15 minutes or until browned and crisp. Serve immediately.
Nutrition Info: Calories 25 Total Carbs 3g Protein 2g Fat 1g Sugar 1g Fiber 0g

151. Rum Spiced Nuts

Servings: 12   Cooking Time: 10 Minutes
Ingredients:
- 2 tbsp. Margarine
- What you'll need from store cupboard:
- 3 cups mixed nuts, unsalted
- 2 tbsp. dark rum
- 2 tbsp. Splenda
- 2 tsp curry powder
- 1 tsp salt
- 1 tsp ancho chili powder

- 1 tsp cinnamon
- 1 tsp cumin

Directions:
Place a medium, nonstick, skillet over medium heat. Add nuts and cook, stirring frequently, about 3-5 minutes, to lightly toast them. Add the margarine and rum and cook until most of the liquid evaporates. Combine the remaining Ingredients in a large bowl. Add the nuts and toss to coat. Dump out onto a large baking sheet to cool. Store in an airtight container. Serving size is ¼ cup.
Nutrition Info: Calories 254 Total Carbs 10g Net Carbs 8g Protein 6g Fat 22g Sugar 4g Fiber 2g

152. Tiramisu

Servings: 15   Cooking Time: 4 Hours
Ingredients:
- 2 (8 oz.) pkgs. reduced-fat cream cheese, soft
- 2 cup fat-free sour cream
- 2 (3 oz.) pkgs ladyfingers, split
- ¼ cup skim milk
- 2 tbsp. coffee liqueur
- What you'll need from store cupboard:
- ⅔ cup Splenda
- ½ cup strong brewed coffee
- 2 tbsp. unsweetened cocoa powder, sifted
- ½ tsp vanilla

Directions:
In a large bowl, combine sour cream, cream cheese, sugar substitute, milk, and vanilla. Beat on high until smooth. In a small bowl stir together coffee and liqueur. Place one package of lady fingers, cut side up, in a 2-quart baking dish. Brush with ½ the coffee mixture. Spread ½ the cheese mixture over top. Repeat layers. Sprinkle cocoa powder over top. Cover and chill 4 hours or overnight. Cut into squares to serve.
Nutrition Info: Calories 208 Total Carbs 24g Protein 6g Fat 8g Sugar 14g Fiber 0g

153. Raspberry Walnut Parfaits

Servings: 4   Cooking Time: 1 Hour
Ingredients:
- 1 can coconut milk, chilled (not low fat)
- ½ cup fresh raspberries, rinsed and dried
- What you'll need from store cupboard:
- ¼ cup walnuts, coarsely chopped
- 1 tbsp. Splenda
- 1 tsp vanilla

Directions:
In a medium bowl, combine the berries and walnuts. In a large bowl, beat coconut milk, Splenda and vanilla until combined. Let rest 5 minutes. In 4 small mason jars, spoon half the vanilla cream evenly. Top with berries. Repeat. Screw on the lids and chill at least one hour.
Nutrition Info: Calories 213 Total Carbs 8g Net Carbs 6g Protein 4g Fat 20g Sugar 4g Fiber 2g

154. Honey & Cinnamon Shortbread

Servings: 22   Cooking Time: 20 Minutes
Ingredients:
- ½ cup margarine, soft

- What you'll need from store cupboard:
- 1 2/3 cup flour
- 3 ½ tbsp. honey
- 1 tsp cinnamon
- 1/8 tsp baking powder

Directions:
Heat oven to 350 degrees. Line a baking sheet with parchment paper. In a large bowl, beat margarine and honey until smooth and creamy. Mix in the flour and baking powder to create a smooth dough. Shape dough into a rectangle, wrap with plastic wrap and chill 15 minutes. Roll dough out on a lightly floured surface to ¼-inch thick. Cut into rectangles and place on prepared baking sheet. If you like use a fork to make patterns on the dough. Chill 20 minutes. Bake 15-20 minutes, or until they start to turn golden brown. Transfer to wire rack to cool completely. Store in an airtight container.
Nutrition Info: Calories 82 Total Carbs 10g Protein 1g Fat 4g Sugar 3g Fiber 0g

155. Strawberry Cheesecake

Servings: 12   Cooking Time: 15 Minutes
Ingredients:
- 3 cups medium-size fresh strawberries, halved
- 2 1/2 packages fat-free cream cheese, soft
- 1 cup skim milk
- 1/3 cup margarine, melted
- What you'll need from store cupboard:
- 2 cups graham cracker crumbs
- ¾ cup + 2 tbsp. sugar substitute
- ¼ cup low-sugar strawberry spread
- 1 envelope unflavored gelatin
- 1 tbsp. lemon juice
- 2 tsp vanilla extract
- Nonstick cooking spray

Directions:
Heat oven to 350 degrees. Spray a 9-inch springform pan with cooking spray. In a medium bowl, combine cracker crumbs and margarine, stirring to combine. Press on bottom and up sides of prepared pan. Bake 8 minutes, let cool. Add milk to a small sauce pan and sprinkle gelatin over top, let stand 1 minutes. Cook over low heat, stirring constantly until gelatin dissolves, about 2 minutes. Let cool slightly. In a large bowl, beat cream cheese until smooth and creamy. Slowly add lemon juice and vanilla, beat well. Slowly beat in gelatin mixture, beating until smooth. Add ¾ cup sugar and beat just until blended. Pour into crust, cover and chill 3 hours. In a medium saucepan, combine berries, 2 tablespoons sugar, and strawberry spread. Cook over med-low heat, stirring constantly, until spread melts and berries are coated. Spoon over cheesecake. To serve, loosen cheese cake from side of pan and remove. Cut into wedges.
Nutrition Info: Calories 368 Total Carbs 30g Net Carbs 28g Protein 6g Fat 23g Sugar 20g Fiber 2g

156. Pistachio Cookies

Servings: 13-14   Cooking Time: 15 Minutes
Ingredients:
- 2 eggs, beaten

- What you'll need from store cupboard:
- 1 2/3 cup almond flour
- 1 cup + 2 tbsp. Splenda
- 3/4 cup + 50 pistachio nuts, shelled

Directions:
Add the ¾ cup nuts and 2 tablespoons Splenda to a food processor. Process until nuts are ground fine. Pour the ground nuts into a large bowl, and stir in flour and remaining Splenda until combined. Add eggs and mix Ingredients thoroughly. Wrap dough with plastic wrap and chill at least 8 hours or overnight. Heat oven 325 degrees. Line a cookie sheet with parchment paper. Roll teaspoonful of dough into small balls, about 1-inch in diameter. Place on prepared sheet. Smash cookie slightly then press a pistachio in the center. Bake 12-15 minutes or until the edges are lightly browned. Transfer to wire rack to cool completely. Store in airtight container. Serving size is 3 cookies.
Nutrition Info: Calories 108 Total Carbs 5g Net Carbs 3g Protein 4g Fat 8g Sugar 3g Fiber 2g

157. Peach Ice Cream

Servings: 32   Cooking Time: 4 Hours
Ingredients:
- 4 peaches, peel and chop
- 8 oz. fat free whipped topping
- 2 cup skim milk
- ¼ cup fresh lemon juice
- What you'll need from store cupboard:
- 2-12 oz. cans fat free evaporated milk
- 14 oz. can sweetened condensed milk
- 3.4 oz. pkg. sugar free instant vanilla pudding mix
- ½ cup Splenda
- 1 tsp vanilla
- ½ tsp almond extract
- 1/8 tsp salt

Directions:
In a large bowl, beat milk and pudding mix on low speed 2 minutes. Beat in remaining Ingredients, except whipped topping until thoroughly combined. Fold in whipped topping. Freeze in ice cream maker according to manufacturer's directions, this may take 2 batches. Transfer to freezer containers and freeze 4 hours before serving. Serving size is ½ cup.
Nutrition Info: Calories 106 Total Carbs 19g Protein 3g Fat 1g Sugar 15g Fiber 0g

158. Cheese Crisp Crackers

Servings: 4   Cooking Time: 10 Minutes
Ingredients:
- 4 slices pepper Jack cheese, quartered
- 4 slices Colby Jack cheese, quartered
- 4 slices cheddar cheese, quartered

Directions:
Heat oven to 400 degrees. Line a cooking sheet with parchment paper. Place cheese in a single layer on prepared pan and bake 10 minutes, or until cheese gets firm. Transfer to paper towel line surface to absorb excess oil. Let cool, cheese will crisp up more as it cools. Store in airtight container, or Ziploc bag. Serve with your favorite dip or salsa.

Nutrition Info: Calories 253 Total Carbs 1g Protein 15g Fat 20g Sugar 0g Fiber 0g

159. Chili Lime Tortilla Chips

Servings: 10   Cooking Time: 15 Minutes
Ingredients:
- 12 6-inch corn tortillas, cut into 8 triangles
- 3 tbsp. lime juice
- What you'll need from store cupboard:
- 1 tsp cumin
- 1 tsp chili powder

Directions:
Heat oven to 350 degrees.   Place tortilla triangles in a single layer on a large baking sheet.   In a small bowl stir together spices.   Sprinkle half the lime juice over tortillas, followed by ½ the spice mixture. Bake 7 minutes.   Remove from oven and turn tortillas over. Sprinkle with remaining lime juice and spices. Bake another 8 minutes or until crisp, but not brown. Serve with your favorite salsa, serving size is 10 chips.
Nutrition Info: Calories 65 Total Carbs 14g Net Carbs 12g Protein 2g Fat 1g Sugar 0g Fiber 2g

160. Sangria Jello Cups

Servings: 6   Cooking Time: 4 Hours
Ingredients:
- 1 cup raspberries
- 1 cup green grapes, halved
- What you'll need from store cupboard:
- 1 pkg. lemon gelatin, sugar free
- 1 pkg. raspberry gelatin, sugar free
- 11 oz. mandarin oranges, drain
- 1 ½ cup boiling water
- 1 cup cold water
- 1 cup white wine

Directions:
Place both gelatins in a large bowl and add boiling water. Stir to dissolve. Let rest 10 minutes.   Stir in cold water and wine, cover and refrigerate 45 minutes, or until partially set.   Fold in oranges, raspberries and grapes. Spoon evenly into 6 wine glasses. Cover and refrigerate 4 hours or until set.
Nutrition Info: Calories 88 Total Carbs 11g Net Carbs 9g Protein 3g Fat 0g Sugar 8g Fiber 2g

161. Mini Key Lime Tarts

Servings: 8   Cooking Time: 10 Minutes
Ingredients:
- 4 sheets phyllo dough*
- ¾ cup skim milk
- ¾ cup fat-free whipped topping, thawed
- ½ cup egg substitute
- ½ cup fat free sour cream
- 6 tbsp. fresh lime juice
- What you'll need from store cupboard
- 2 tbsp. cornstarch
- ½ cup Splenda
- Butter-flavored cooking spray

Directions:
In a medium saucepan, combine milk, juice, and cornstarch. Cook, stirring, over medium heat 2-3

minutes or until thickened. Remove from heat.   Add egg substitute and whisk 30 seconds to allow it to cook. Stir in sour cream and Splenda. Cover and chill until completely cool.   Heat oven to 350 degrees. Spray 8 muffin cups with cooking spray.   Lay 1 sheet of the phyllo on a cutting board and lightly spray it with cooking spray. Repeat this with the remaining sheets so they are stacked on top of each other.   Cut the phyllo into 8 squares and gently place them in the prepared muffin cups, pressing firmly on the bottom and sides. Bake 8-10 minutes or until golden brown. Remove them from the pan and let cool.   To serve: spoon the lime mixture evenly into the 8 cups and top with whipped topping. Garnish with fresh lime slices if desired.
Nutrition Info: Calories 82 Total Carbs 13g Net Carbs 12g Protein 3g Fat 1g Sugar 10g Fiber 1g

162. Pumpkin Spice Snack Balls

Servings: 10   Cooking Time: 10 Minutes
Ingredients:
- 1 ½ cups old-fashioned oats
- ½ cup chopped almonds
- ½ cup unsweetened shredded coconut
- ¾ cup canned pumpkin puree
- 2 tablespoons honey
- 2 teaspoons pumpkin pie spice
- ¼-teaspoon salt

Directions:
Preheat the oven to 300°F and line a baking sheet with parchment.   Combine the oats, almonds, and coconut on the baking sheet.   Bake for 8 to 10 minutes until browned, stirring halfway through.   Place the pumpkin, honey, pumpkin pie spice, and salt in a medium bowl.   Stir in the toasted oat mixture. Shape the mixture into 20 balls by hand and place on a tray.   Chill until the balls are firm then serve.
Nutrition Info: Calories 170 Total Fat 0.7g, Saturated Fat 0.1g, Total Carbs 14.7g, Net Carbs 12.2g, Protein 2.1g, Sugar 2.2g, Fiber 2.5g, Sodium 1mg

163. Chocolate Cherry Cake Roll

Servings: 10   Cooking Time: 15 Minutes
Ingredients:
- 10 maraschino cherries, drained and patted dry
- 4 eggs, room temperature
- 1 cup sugar-free Cool Whip, thawed
- ⅔ cup maraschino cherries, chop, drain and pat dry
- ½ cup cream cheese, soft
- What you'll need from the store cupboard
- ⅓ cup flour
- ½ cup Splenda for baking
- ¼ cup unsweetened cocoa powder
- 1 tablespoon sugar-free hot fudge ice cream topping
- ¼ tsp baking soda
- ¼ tsp salt
- Unsweetened cocoa powder
- Nonstick cooking spray

Directions:

Heat oven to 375 degrees. Spray a large sheet baking pan with cooking spray. Line bottom with parchment paper, spray and flour the paper.   In a small bowl, stir together flour, ¼ cup cocoa, baking soda, and salt.   In a large bowl, beat eggs on high speed for 5 minutes, Gradually add sweetener and continue beating until mixture is thick and lemon-colored.   Fold in dry Ingredients. Spread evenly into prepared pan. Bake 15 minutes or top springs back when touched lightly. Place a clean towel on a cutting board and sprinkle with cocoa powder. Turn cake onto towel and carefully remove parchment paper.   Starting at a short end, roll up towel. Cool on a wire rack for 1 hour.   Prepare the filling: in a small bowl, beat cream cheese until smooth. Add ½ cup whipped topping, beat on low until combined. Fold in another ½ cup whipped topping. Fold in the chopped cherries.   Unroll cake and remove the towel. Spread the filling to within 1 inch of the edges. Reroll cake and trim the ends. Cover and chill at least 2 hours or overnight.   To serve, warm up the fudge topping and drizzle over cake, garnish with whole cherries, then slice and serve.
Nutrition Info: Calories 163 Total Carbs 25g Protein 5g Fat 3g Sugar 12g Fiber 0g

164. Banana And Nut Bread

Servings: 1   Cooking Time: 40 Minutes
Ingredients:
- 28g unsalted butter, softened
- 100g of sugar
- 1 egg, beaten
- 2 ripe mashed bananas
- 2 ml of pure vanilla extract
- 20g all-purpose flour
- 3g baking soda
- 2g salt
- 40g chopped walnuts
- Nonstick Spray Oil

Directions:
Mix the butter with the sugar.   Mix the eggs, mashed bananas, and vanilla. Set aside   Preheat the air fryer for a few minutes and set the temperature to 150°C. Sift flour, baking soda and salt.   Join the dry ingredients in the moist ones until they combine. Then mix the chopped nuts.   Grease 1 mold for mini breads with oil spray and fill it with the mixture. Place in the preheated air fryer. Set to 40 minutes.
Nutrition Info:(Nutrition per Serving)Calories: 285 Fat: 11Carbohydrates: 38g Protein: 5g Sugar: 20g Cholesterol: 11mg

165. Soft Pretzel Bites

Servings: 8   Cooking Time: 15 Minutes
Ingredients:
- 3 cups mozzarella cheese, grated
- 3 large eggs
- ½ cup cream cheese
- What you'll need from the store cupboard
- 2 cups almond flour, super fine
- 1 tbsp. baking powder
- 1 tbsp. coarse salt

Directions:
Heat oven to 400 degrees. Line a large cookie sheet with parchment paper.   Stir almond flour and baking powder together in a small bowl.   Place the mozzarella and cream cheese in a large glass bowl. Be sure to surround the cream cheese with the mozzarella. Melt the cheese in 30 second intervals on high, stirring after each interval. Continue this step until they are completely melted, about 2 – 2 ½ minutes.   Place the cheese, 2 eggs, and flour mixture into a food processor with a dough blade. Pulse on high until the mixture forms a uniform dough.   Wrap a pastry board with plastic wrap making sure it is taut. Lightly coat your hands with vegetable oil and separate dough into 8 equal parts. Roll each into 1-inch thick ropes.   With a sharp knife, cut dough into ¾-inch pieces. Place on prepared cookie sheet.   In a small bowl, whisk the remaining egg. Brush the dough pieces with egg then sprinkle with salt. Bake 12 minutes, or until lightly browned. Set oven to broil and cook another 2 minutes to crisp up the outside of the pretzels. Serve warm by themselves or dip them in cheese sauce (chapter 16).
Nutrition Info: Calories 242 Total Carbs 6g Net Carbs 3g Protein 11g Fat 20g Sugar 1g Fiber 3g

166. Apple Crisp

Servings: 8   Cooking Time: 30 Minutes
Ingredients:
- 5 cups Granny Smith apples, peeled and sliced
- 3 tablespoons margarine
- What you'll need from the store cupboard
- ½ cup rolled oats
- ¼ cup + 2 tbsp. Splenda
- 3 tbsp. flour
- 1 tsp lemon juice
- ¾ teaspoon apple pie spice, divided

Directions:
Heat oven to 375.   In a large bowl, combine apples, 2 tablespoons Splenda, lemon juice, and ½ teaspoon apple pie spice. Mix to thoroughly coat apples.   Place apples in a 2-quart square baking pan.   In a medium bowl, combine oats, flour, ¼ Splenda, and remaining apple pie spice. With a pastry knife, cut in butter until mixture resembles coarse crumbs. Sprinkle evenly over apples.   Bake 30 – 35 minutes, or until apples are tender and topping is golden brown. Serve warm.
Nutrition Info: Calories 153 Total Carbs 27g Net Carbs 23g Protein 1g Fat 5g Sugar 18g Fiber 4g

167. Strawberry Lime Pudding

Servings: 4   Cooking Time: 10 Minutes
Ingredients:
- 2 cups plus 2 tablespoons fat-free milk
- 2 teaspoons flavorless gelatin
- 10 large strawberries, sliced
- 1-tablespoon fresh lime zest
- 2 teaspoons vanilla extract
- Liquid stevia extract, to taste

Directions:
Whisk together 2 tablespoons milk and gelatin in a medium bowl until the gelatin dissolves completely.

Place the strawberries in a food processor with the limejuice and vanilla extract. Blend until smooth then pour into a medium bowl. Warm the remaining milk in a small saucepan over medium heat. Stir in the lime zest and heat until steaming (do not boil). Gently whisk the gelatin mixture into the hot milk then stir in the strawberry mixture. Sweeten with liquid stevia to taste and chill until set. Servings cold.

Nutrition Info: Calories 70Total Fat 0.7g, Saturated Fat 0.1g, Total Carbs 14.7g, Net Carbs 12.2g, Protein 2.1g, Sugar 2.2g, Fiber 2.5g, Sodium 1mg

168. Pineapple Frozen Yogurt

Servings: 4   Cooking Time: 1 Hour
Ingredients:
- ½ cup half-and-half
- ½ cup plain reduced-fat yogurt
- ¼ cup egg substitute
- What you'll need from store cupboard:
- ¾ cup crushed pineapple, in juice
- ¼ cup Splenda

Directions:
In a medium bowl, beat egg substitute until thick and cream colored. Add remaining Ingredients and mix to thoroughly combine. Cover and chill completely, if using an ice cream maker. Once chilled add to ice cream maker and freeze according to manufacturer's directions. Or, you can pour the mixture into a shallow glass baking dish and freeze. Stir and scrape the mixture, every 10 minutes, with a rubber spatula until it reaches desired consistency, about 1 hour.

Nutrition Info: Calories 145 Total Carbs 20g Protein 5g Fat 4g Sugar 17g Fiber 0g

169. Cheesy Taco Chips

Servings: 6   Cooking Time: 40 Minutes
Ingredients:
- 1 cup Mexican blend cheese, grated
- 2 large egg whites
- What you'll need from store cupboard:
- 1 1/2 cup crushed pork rinds
- 1 tbsp. taco seasoning
- ¼ tsp salt

Directions:
Heat oven to 300 degrees. Line a large baking sheet with parchment paper. In a large bowl, whisk egg whites and salt until frothy. Stir in pork rinds, cheese, and seasoning and stir until thoroughly combined. Turn out onto prepared pan. Place another sheet of parchment paper on top and roll out very thin, about 12x12-inches. Remove top sheet of parchment paper, and using a pizza cutter, score dough in 2-inch squares, then score each square in half diagonally. Bake 20 minutes until they start to brown. Turn off oven and let them sit inside the oven until they are firm to the touch, about 10-20 minutes. Remove from oven and cool completely before breaking apart. Eat them as is or with your favorite dip.

Nutrition Info: Calories 260 Total Carbs 1g Protein 25g Fat 17g Sugar 0g Fiber 0g

170. Tex Mex Popcorn

Servings: 4   Cooking Time: 5 Minutes
Ingredients:
- ¼ cup cilantro, diced
- Refrigerated butter-flavor spray
- What you'll need from store cupboard:
- 4 cup popcorn
- 1 tsp chili powder
- ½ tsp salt
- ½ tsp cumin seeds
- ½ tsp garlic powder
- 1/8 tsp smoked paprika

Directions:
Place popcorn in a large bowl and spritz with butter spray. Add remaining Ingredients and toss to coat. Continue spritzing and tossing until popcorn is well coated. Store in an airtight container. Serving size is 1 cup.

Nutrition Info: Calories 32 Total Carbs 6g Net Carbs 5g Protein 1g Fat 0g Sugar 0g Fiber 1g

171. Pickled Cucumbers

Servings: 10   Cooking Time: 5 Minutes
Ingredients:
- 2 cucumbers, cut into 1/4-inch slices
- ½ onion, sliced thin
- What you'll need from the store cupboard
- 1 ½ cups vinegar
- 2 tbsp. stevia
- 1 tbsp. dill
- 2 cloves garlic, sliced thin
- 1 tsp peppercorns
- 1 tsp coriander seeds
- ½ tsp salt
- ¼ tsp red pepper flakes

Directions:
In a medium saucepan, combine vinegar and spices. Bring to a boil over high heat. Set aside. Place the cucumbers, onions, and garlic into a quart-sized jar, or plastic container, with an air tight lid. Pour hot liquid over the vegetables, making sure they are completely covered. Add the lid and chill at least a day before serving.

Nutrition Info: Calories 33 Total Carbs 6g Net Carbs 0g Protein 0g Fat 0g Sugar 4g Fiber 0g

172. Gingerbread Soufflés

Servings: 10   Cooking Time: 25 Minutes
Ingredients:
- 6 eggs, separated
- 1 cup skim milk
- 1 cup fat free whipped topping
- 2 tbsp. butter, soft
- What you'll need from store cupboard:
- ½ cup Splenda
- 1/3 cup molasses
- ¼ cup flour
- 2 tsp pumpkin pie spice
- 2 tsp vanilla
- 1 tsp ginger
- ¼ tsp salt

- 1/8 tsp cream of tartar
- Butter flavored cooking spray

Directions:

Heat oven to 350 degrees. Spray 10 ramekins with cooking spray and sprinkle with Splenda to coat, shaking out excess. Place on a large baking sheet.   In a large saucepan, over medium heat, whisk together milk, Splenda, flour and salt until smooth. Bring to a boil, whisking constantly. Pour into a large bowl and whisk in molasses, butter, vanilla, and spices. Let cool 15 minutes. Once spiced mixture has cooled, whisk in egg yolks.   In a large bowl, beat egg whites and cream of tartar on high speed until stiff peaks form. Fold into spiced mixture, a third at a time, until blended completely. Spoon into ramekins.   Bake 25 minutes until puffed and set. Serve immediately with a dollop of whipped topping.

Nutrition Info: Calories 170 Total Carbs 24g Protein 4g Fat 5g Sugar 18g Fiber 0g

173. Watermelon & Shrimp Ceviche

Servings: 14   Cooking Time: 1hour 30 Minutes

Ingredients:
- 1 lb. medium shrimp, peeled, deveined and tails removed
- 1 jalapeño pepper, diced fine
- 1 cup seedless watermelon, diced fine
- ½ cup + 2 tbsp. lime juice, divided
- ½ cup jicama, diced fine
- ½ cup red onion, diced fine
- ½ cup fresh cilantro, chopped
- What you'll need from store cupboard:
- Salt and pepper, to taste

Directions:

Chop shrimp into small pieces.   In a medium bowl, combine shrimp and ½ cup lime juice. Cover and chill 1 hour or until shrimp turn pink. Drain and discard juice. In a large mixing bowl, combine all Ingredients. Salt and pepper to taste. Cover and chill at least 30 minutes. Serve with, or on, your favorite crackers. Serving size is ¼ cup.

Nutrition Info: Calories 47 Total Carbs 3g Protein 8g Fat 1g Sugar 1g Fiber 0g

174. Chocolate Torte

Servings: 12   Cooking Time: 35 Minutes

Ingredients:
- 5 eggs, separated, room temperature
- ¾ cup margarine, sliced
- What you'll need from store cupboard:
- 1 pkg. semisweet chocolate chips
- ½ cup Splenda
- ¼ tsp cream of tartar
- Nonstick cooking spray

Directions:

Heat oven to 350 degrees. Spray a 6-7-inch springform pan with cooking spray.   In a microwave safe bowl, melt chocolate chips and margarine, in 30 second intervals.   In a large bowl, beat egg yolks till thick and lemon colored. Beat in chocolate.   In a separate large bowl, with clean beaters, beat egg whites and cream of tartar till foamy. Beat in Splenda, 1 tablespoon at a time,

till sugar is dissolved, continue beating till stiff glossy peaks form.   Fold ¼ of egg whites into chocolate mixture, then fold in the rest. Transfer to prepared pan. Bake 30-35 minutes, or center is set. Let cool completely before removing side of pan and serving.

Nutrition Info: Calories 181 Total Carbs 10g Protein 3g Fat 14g Sugar 10g Fiber 0g

175. Autumn Skillet Cake

Servings: 10   Cooking Time: 30 Minutes

Ingredients:
- 3 eggs, room temperature
- 1 cup of fresh cranberries
- 4 oz. cream cheese, soft
- 3 tbsp. fat free sour cream
- 2 tbsp. butter, melted
- What you'll need from store cupboard:
- 2 cup of almond flour, sifted
- ¾ cup Splenda
- ¾ cup pumpkin puree
- 1 ½ tbsp. baking powder
- 2 tsp cinnamon
- 1 tsp pumpkin spice
- 1 tsp ginger
- ¼ tsp nutmeg
- ¼ tsp salt
- Nonstick cooking spray

Directions:

Heat oven to 350 degrees. Spray a 9-inch cast iron skillet or cake pan with cooking spray.   In a large bowl, beat Splenda, butter and cream cheese until thoroughly combined. Add eggs, one at a time, beating after each. Add pumpkin and spices and combine. Add the dry Ingredients and mix well. Stir in the sour cream. Pour into prepared pan.   Sprinkle cranberries over batter and with the back of a spoon, push them half-way into the batter. Bake 30 minutes or the cake passes the toothpick test. Cool completely before serving.

Nutrition Info: Calories 280 Total Carbs 23g Net Carbs 20g Protein 7g Fat 17g Sugar 16g Fiber 3g

176. German Chocolate Cake Bars

Servings: 20   Cooking Time: 5 Minutes

Ingredients:
- 2 cup unsweetened coconut flakes
- 1 cup coconut milk, divided
- ¾ cup chopped pecans
- ¾ cup dark baking chocolate, chopped
- What you'll need from the store cupboard
- 1 ½ cup almond flour cracker crumbs (chapter 4)
- ½ cup + 2 tbsp. powdered sugar substitute
- ½ cup coconut oil
- Nonstick cooking spray

Directions:

Spray an 8x8-inch baking dish with cooking spray.   In a large bowl, combine the coconut, ½ cup sugar substitute, cracker crumbs and pecan, stir to combine. In a medium sauce pan, combine ½ cup milk and oil, cook over medium heat until oil is melted and mixture is heated through. Pour over coconut mixture and stir to combine. Press evenly in prepared baking dish and chill

1-2 hours. In a clean saucepan, place the chocolate and remaining milk over med-low heat. Cook, stirring constantly, until chocolate is melted and mixture is smooth. Add the 2 tablespoons sugar substitute and stir to combine. Pour chocolate over the coconut layer and chill 1 hour, or until set. Cut into squares to serve.

Nutrition Info: Calories 245 Total Carbs 12g Net Carbs 9g Protein 3g Fat 19g Sugar 7g Fiber 3g

177. Watermelon Ice

Servings: 8   Cooking Time: 8 Hours

Ingredients:
- 5 cup cubed watermelon, remove seeds
- ½ cup light cranberry juice cocktail
- What you'll need from store cupboard
- ½ cup Splenda
- 1 envelope unflavored gelatin

Directions:
Place watermelon in a food processor and pulse until almost smooth. In a small saucepan, over low heat, stir together Splenda and gelatin. Slowly add juice. Cook, stirring, until gelatin dissolves. Add to watermelon and process until combined. Pour into an 8-inch square dish, cover and freeze 5 hours, or until firm. Break watermelon mixture into chunks. Freeze another 3 hours. To serve; scrape and stir mixture with a fork to create an icy texture. Spoon into dessert dishes and serve.

Nutrition Info: Calories 94 Total Carbs 20g Protein 1g Fat 0g Sugar 18g Fiber 0g

178. Raspberry & Dark Chocolate Mini Soufflés

Servings: 6   Cooking Time: 10 Minutes

Ingredients:
- 1 cup fresh raspberries
- 4 egg whites
- What you'll need from store cupboard:
- ½ oz. dark chocolate, chopped
- 6 tsp Splenda
- 1 tsp margarine, soft

Directions:
Heat oven to 400 degrees. Use the margarine to grease 6 small ramekins. Puree the raspberries in a blender or food processor and press through a fine sieve to get all of the seeds out. Add 1 tablespoons Splenda and set aside. Beat egg whites until thickened and start adding the remaining Splenda, gradually, until the mixture forms stiff glossy peaks. Gently fold ⅓ of the egg whites into the raspberry puree. Once mixed, fold the raspberry puree mixture into the remaining egg whites and fold gently until there are no streaks of pink left. Spoon the raspberry mixture into the ramekins filling them half full. Divide the chocolate between the ramekins and then fill to the top with soufflé mixture. Place ramekins on a baking sheet. Bake for 9 minutes until golden brown and puffed up. Serve immediately.

Nutrition Info: Calories 60 Total Carbs 8g Net Carbs 7g Protein 3g Fat 1g Sugar 6g Fiber 1g

179. Chocolate Orange Bread Pudding

Servings: 8   Cooking Time: 35 Minutes

Ingredients:
- 4 cups French baguette cubes
- 1 ½ cups skim milk
- 3 eggs, lightly beaten
- 1-2 tsp orange zest, grated
- What you'll need from store cupboard
- ¼ cup Splenda
- ¼ cup sugar-free chocolate ice cream topping
- 3 tbsp. unsweetened cocoa powder
- 1 tsp vanilla
- ¾ tsp cinnamon

Directions:
Heat oven to 350°F. In medium bowl, stir together Splenda and cocoa. Stir in milk, eggs, zest, vanilla, and cinnamon until well blended. Place bread cubes in an 8-inch square baking dish. Pour milk mixture evenly over the top. Bake 35 minutes or until a knife inserted in the center comes out clean. Cool 5-10 minutes. Spoon into dessert dishes and drizzle lightly with ice cream topping. Serve.

Nutrition Info: Calories 139 Total Carbs 23g Net Carbs 22g Protein 6g Fat 2g Sugar 9g Fiber 1g

180. Fig Cookie Bars

Servings: 12   Cooking Time: 20 Minutes

Ingredients:
- ½ cup dried figs
- 1/8 cup reduced-fat cream cheese
- 3 tbsp. skim milk
- What you'll need from store cupboard:
- 2/3 cup flour
- ½ cup quick oats
- 1/3 cup powdered sugar substitute
- 6 tbsp. hot water
- 2 tbsp. sunflower oil
- 1 tbsp. Splenda
- ¾ tsp baking powder
- ½ tsp vanilla
- ¼ tsp salt
- Nonstick cooking spray

Directions:
Heat oven to 400 degrees. Spray a cookie sheet with cooking spray. Add the figs, water and Splenda to a blender and process until figs are finely chopped. In a large bowl, stir together flour, oats, baking powder, and salt. Add oil, and milk 1 tablespoon at a time, until mixture forms a ball. Roll dough out on a lightly floured surface to a 12x9-inch rectangle. Place on prepared pan. Spread fig mixture in a 2 ½-inch wide strip down the middle. At ½ inch intervals, use a sharp knife to cut the dough almost to the figs on both long sides. Fold strips over filling, overlapping and crossing in the middle. Bake 15-20 minutes or until light brown. Remove from oven and let cool. In a small bowl, beat cream cheese, powdered sugar substitute, and vanilla until smooth. Drizzle over bars and cut into 12 pieces.

Nutrition Info: Calories 105 Total Carbs 17g Net Carbs 16g Protein 2g Fat 3g Sugar 9g Fiber 1g

181. Cranberry & Almond Granola Bars

Servings: 12   Cooking Time: 20 Minutes

Ingredients:
- 1 egg
- 1 egg white
- What you'll need from store cupboard:
- 2 cup low-fat granola
- ¼ cup dried cranberries, sweetened
- ¼ cup almonds, chopped
- 2 tbsp. Splenda
- 1 teaspoon almond extract
- ½ tsp cinnamon

Directions:
Heat oven to 350 degrees. Line the bottom and sides of an 8-inch baking dish with parchment paper.   In a large bowl, combine dry Ingredients including the cranberries.   In a small bowl, whisk together egg, egg white and extract. Pour over dry Ingredients and mix until combined.   Press mixture into the prepared pan. Bake 20 minutes or until light brown.   Cool in the pan for 5 minutes. Then carefully lift the bars from the pan onto a cutting board. Use a sharp knife to cut into 12 bars. Cool completely and store in an airtight container.

Nutrition Info: Calories 85 Total Carbs 14g Net Carbs 13g Protein 3g Fat 3g Sugar 5g Fiber 1g

182. Onion Rings

Servings: 4   Cooking Time: 15 Minutes

Ingredients:
- 1 large onion, slice ½-inch thick
- 1 egg
- What you'll need from store cupboard:
- ¼ cup sunflower oil
- 2 tbsp. coconut flour
- 2 tbsp. reduced fat parmesan cheese
- ¼ tsp parsley flakes
- 1/8 tsp garlic powder
- 1/8 tsp cayenne pepper
- Salt to taste

Directions:
Heat oil in a large skillet over med-high heat.   In a shallow bowl, combine flour, parmesan, and seasonings. Beat the egg.   Separate onion slices into individual rings and place in large bowl, add beaten egg and toss to coat well. Let rest 1-2 minutes.   In small batches, coat onion in flour mixture and add to skillet. Cook 1-2 minutes per side, or until golden brown. Transfer to paper towel lined cookie sheet.   Serve with ketchup, (chapter 16), or your favorite dipping sauce.

Nutrition Info: Calories 184 Total Carbs 8g Net Carbs 5g Protein 3g Fat 16g Sugar 2g Fiber 3g

183. Coconut Milk Shakes

Servings: 2   Cooking Time: 5 Minutes

Ingredients:
- 1 ½ cup vanilla ice cream
- ½ cup coconut milk, unsweetened
- What you'll need from store cupboard:
- 2 ½ tbsp. coconut flakes
- 1 tsp unsweetened cocoa

Directions:
Heat oven to 350 degrees.   Place coconut on a baking sheet and bake, 2-3 minutes, stirring often, until coconut is toasted.   Place ice cream, milk, 2 tablespoons coconut, and cocoa in a blender and process until smooth.   Pour into glasses and garnish with remaining toasted coconut. Serve immediately.

Nutrition Info: Calories 323 Total Carbs 23g Net Carbs 19g Protein 3g Fat 24g Sugar 18g Fiber 4g

184. Coconut Macaroni

Servings: 5-6   Cooking Time: 15 Minutes

Ingredients:
- 100g of sweetened condensed milk
- 1 egg white
- 2 ml almond extract
- 2 ml vanilla extract
- A pinch of salt
- 175g unsweetened and shredded coconut

Directions:
Mix the condensed milk, egg white, almond extract, and salt in a bowl.   Add 160g of grated coconut and mix until well combined. The mixture must be able to maintain its shape.   Form 38 mm balls with your hands. In a separate dish, add 25 g of grated coconut. Roll the coconut macaroni in the grated coconut until they are covered.   Preheat the air fryer for a few minutes and set the temperature to 150°C.   Add the coconut macaroni to the preheated air fryer. Set the time to 15 minutes at 150°C.   Let the macaroni cool for 5-10 minutes and serve when they finish cooling.

Nutrition Info: Calories: 20 Fat: 0g Carbohydrates: 0g Protein: 0g Sugar: 0gCholesterol: 0mg

185. Crunchy Apple Fries

Servings: 8   Cooking Time: 10 Minutes

Ingredients:
- 3 apples, peeled, cored, and sliced into ½-inch pieces
- ¼ cup reduced fat margarine, melted
- 2 tbsp. walnuts, chopped
- What you'll need from the store cupboard
- ¼ cup quick oats
- 3 tbsp. light brown sugar
- 2 tbsp. whole wheat flour
- 1 tsp cinnamon
- 1/8 tsp salt

Directions:
Heat oven to 425 degrees. Put a wire rack on a large cookie sheet.   Add oats and walnuts to a food processor or blender and process until the mixture resembles flour.   Place the oat mixture in a shallow pan and add brown sugar, flour, cinnamon, and salt, mix well. Pour melted butter in a separate shallow pan. Dip apple slices in margarine, then roll in oat mixture to coat completely. Place on wire rack.   Bake 10 – 12 minutes or until golden brown. Let cool before serving.

Nutrition Info: Calories 146 Total Carbs 20g Net Carbs 17g Protein 1g Fat 7g Sugar 13g Fiber 3g

186. Whole-wheat Pumpkin Muffins

Servings: 36   Cooking Time: 15 Minutes

Ingredients:
- 1 ¾-cup whole-wheat flour
- 1-teaspoon baking powder
- 1-teaspoon baking soda
- 1-teaspoon ground cinnamon
- 1-teaspoon pumpkin pie spice
- ½-teaspoon salt
- 2 large eggs
- 1 cup canned pumpkin puree
- 1/3 cup unsweetened applesauce
- ¼-cup light brown sugar
- 1-teaspoon vanilla extract
- 1/3 cup fat-free milk
- Liquid stevia extract, to taste

Directions:
Preheat the oven to 350°F and grease two 24-cup mini muffin pans with cooking spray.   Whisk together the flour, baking powder, baking soda, cinnamon, pumpkin pie spice, and salt in a large mixing bowl.   In a separate bowl, whisk together the eggs, pumpkin, applesauce, brown sugar, vanilla extract, and milk.   Stir the wet ingredients into the dry until well combined.   Adjust sweetness to taste with liquid stevia extract, if desired. Spoon the batter into 36 cups and bake for 12 to 15 minutes until cooked through.

Nutrition Info: Calories 35,Total Fat 13.6gSaturated Fat 1.2g, Total Carbs 5.3g, Net Carbs 2.2g, Protein 5g, Sugar 1g,Fiber 3.1g, Sodium 53mg

187. Caramel Pecan Pie

Servings: 8   Cooking Time: 35 Minutes

Ingredients:
- 1 cup pecans, chopped
- ¾ cup almond milk, unsweetened
- 1/3 cup margarine, melted
- 1 tbsp. margarine, cold
- What you'll need from the store cupboard
- 2 cup almond flour
- ½ cup + 2 tablespoons Splenda for baking
- 1 tsp vanilla
- 1 tsp Arrowroot powder
- ¾ tsp sea salt
- ½ tsp vanilla
- ½ tsp maple syrup, sugar free
- Nonstick cooking spray

Directions:
Heat oven to 350 degrees. Spray a 9-inch pie pan with cooking spray.   In a medium bowl, combine flour, melted margarine, 2 tablespoons Splenda, and vanilla. Mix to thoroughly combine Ingredients. Press on bottom and sides of prepared pie pan. Bake 12 -15 minutes, or until edges start to brown. Set aside.   In a small sauce pan, combine milk, remaining Splenda, arrowroot, salt, ½ teaspoon vanilla, and syrup. Cook over medium heat until it starts to boil, stirring constantly. Keep cooking until it turns a gold color and starts to thicken, about 2-3 minutes. Remove from heat and let cool. Stir in ½ the pecans.   Pour the filling in the crust and top with remaining pecans. Bake about 15 minutes, or until filling starts to bubble. Cool completely before serving.

Nutrition Info: Calories 375 Total Carbs 20g Net Carbs 15g Protein 7g Fat 30g Sugar 14g Fiber 5g

188. Light Cheese Cake With Strawberry Syrup

Servings: 4   Cooking Time: 20 Minutes

Ingredients:
- 500g cottage cheese
- 3 whole eggs
- 2 tbsp. powdered sweetener
- 2 tbsp. oat bran
- ½ tbsp. baking yeast
- 2 tbsp. cinnamon
- 2 tbsp. vanilla aroma
- 1 lemon (the skin

Directions:
Mix in a bowl the cottage cheese, the sweetener, the cinnamon, the vanilla aroma, and the lemon zest. Mix very well until you get a homogeneous cream. Incorporate the eggs one by one.   Finally, add oats and yeast mixing well.   Put the whole mixture in a container to fit in the air fryer.   Preheat the air fryer a few minutes at 1800C.   Insert the mold into the basket of the air fryer and set the timer for about 20 minutes at 180°C.

Nutrition Info: Calories: 191 Fat: 12g Carbohydrates: 29g Protein: 4g Sugar: 100g Cholesterol: 7g

189. Peanut Butter Banana "ice Cream"

Servings: 6   Cooking Time: None

Ingredients:
- 4 medium bananas
- ½ cup whipped peanut butter
- 1-teaspoon vanilla extract

Directions:
Peel the bananas and slice them into coins.   Arrange the slices on a plate and freeze until solid.   Place the frozen bananas in a food processor.   Add the peanut butter and pulse until it is mostly smooth.   Scrape down the sides then add the vanilla extract.   Pulse until smooth then spoon into bowls to serve.

Nutrition Info: Calories 70Total Fat 0.7g, Saturated Fat 0.1g, Total Carbs 14.7g, Net Carbs 12.2g, Protein 2.1g, Sugar 2.2g, Fiber 2.5g, Sodium 1mg

190. Pumpkin Ice Cream With Candied Pecans

Servings: 8   Cooking Time: 1 Hour

Ingredients:
- 2 eggs
- 2 cup almond milk, unsweetened, divided
- 1 cup half-n-half
- What you'll need from store cupboard:
- 1 cup pumpkin
- 1 envelope unflavored gelatin
- ¾ cup Splenda
- ¾ cup Candied Pecans, (chapter 6)
- 2 tsp pumpkin pie spice

53

Directions:

Pour one cup almond milk into a small bowl. Sprinkle gelatin on top. Allow to sit for about 5 minutes. In a medium saucepan, whisk together Splenda and the eggs. Whisk in pumpkin and pumpkin spice. Whisk in gelatin. Bring the mixture just to a simmer, then remove from heat. Allow to cool about 5 minutes at room temperature, then refrigerate, uncovered for 45 minutes, stirring occasionally. Do not cool too long or the mixture will set. Remove pumpkin mixture from the refrigerator and whisk in half-n-half and remaining cup of almond milk. Pour into an ice-cream freezer and freeze according to manufactures instructions. When ice cream reaches the desired consistency, transfer to a freezer-safe container with a lid. Stir in candied pecans, cover, and place container in the freezer to further harden the ice cream.

Nutrition Info: Calories 254 Total Carbs 26g Net Carbs 24g Protein 5g Fat 13g Sugar 22g Fiber 2g

191. Chocolate Avocado Mousse

Servings: 3   Cooking Time: None

Ingredients:
- 1 large avocado, pitted and chopped
- ¼ cup fat-free milk
- ¼ cup unsweetened cocoa powder (dark)
- 2 teaspoons powdered stevia
- 1-teaspoon vanilla extract
- 2 tablespoons fat-free whipped topping

Directions:

Place the avocado in a food processor and blend smooth. In a small bowl, whisk together the milk and cocoa powder until well combined. Stir in the pureed avocado along with the stevia and vanilla extract. Spoon into bowls and serve with fat-free whipped topping

Nutrition Info: Calories 180Total Fat 0.7g, Saturated Fat 0.1g, Total Carbs 14.7g, Net Carbs 12.2g, Protein 2.1g, Sugar 2.2g, Fiber 2.5g, Sodium 23mg

192. Dark Chocolate Coffee Cupcakes

Servings: 24   Cooking Time: 20 Minutes

Ingredients:
- 2 eggs
- ½ cup fat free sour cream
- ½ cup butter, melted
- What you'll need from store cupboard:
- 2 cup Splenda
- 1 cup almond flour, sifted
- 1 cup strong coffee, room temperature
- 4 oz. unsweetened chocolate
- ½ cup coconut flour
- 3 tsp of baking powder
- ½ tsp-salt

Directions:

Heat oven to 350 degrees. Line two 12 cup muffin tins with cupcake liners. Melt the chocolate in a double broiler, set aside and allow to cool. Combine the Splenda, almond and coconut flours, baking powder and sea-salt. In a small bowl, combine the coffee, sour cream and butter. Add the butter mixture to the dry

Ingredients and beat on low speed until thoroughly combined. Add the eggs, one at a time, beating after each one. Fold in the chocolate until well blended. Spoon into prepared pans and bake 20-25 minutes or they pass the toothpick test. Cool completely before serving.

Nutrition Info: Calories 173 Total Carbs 20g Net Carbs 19g Protein 2g Fat 9g Sugar 16g Fiber 1g

193. Easy Banana Mug Cake

Servings: 1   Cooking Time: 1 Minutes

Ingredients:
- ½ ripe banana, mashed
- 3 tablespoons egg white
- 1 teaspoon oat flour
- ½ tablespoon vanilla protein powder
- 1 teaspoon rolled oats
- 1 teaspoon cocoa powder
- ½ teaspoon baking powder
- 2 tablespoons stevia
- 1 teaspoon olive oil
- 2 teaspoons chopped walnuts

Directions:

Whisk together the banana and egg whites in a bowl. Add the flour, vanilla protein powder, rolled oats, cocoa powder, baking powder, and stevia to the bowl. Stir to mix well. Grease a microwave-safe mug with olive oil. Pour the mixture in the bowl, then scatter with chopped walnuts. Microwave them for 1 minutes or until puffed. Serve immediately.

Nutrition Info:calories: 211 fat: 12.0g protein: 11.3g carbs: 46.7g fiber: 2.8g sugar: 6.6g sodium: 97mg

194. Cinnamon Toasted Almonds

Servings: 8   Cooking Time: 25 Minutes

Ingredients:
- 2 cups whole almonds
- 1-tablespoon olive oil
- 1-teaspoon ground cinnamon
- ½-teaspoon salt

Directions:

Preheat the oven to 325°F and line a baking sheet with parchment. Toss together the almonds, olive oil, cinnamon, and salt. Spread the almonds on the baking sheet in a single layer. Bake for 25 minutes, stirring several times, until toasted.

Nutrition Info: Calories 150,Total Fat 13.6gSaturated Fat 1.2g, Total Carbs 5.3g, Net Carbs 2.2g, Protein 5g, Sugar 1g,Fiber 3.1g, Sodium 148mg

195. Rosemary Potato Chips

Servings: 6   Cooking Time: 20 Minutes

Ingredients:
- 2 medium red potatoes, unpeeled cut in 1/16-inch slices
- 1 ¼ cup fat-free sour cream
- 2 tbsp. fresh rosemary, chopped fine
- What you'll need from store cupboard:
- 1 tbsp. olive oil
- ¼ tsp garlic salt

- 1/8 tsp black pepper
- Nonstick cooking spray

Directions:
Heat oven to 450 degrees. Spray 2 baking sheets with cooking spray. In a small bowl, combine rosemary, garlic salt, and pepper. Pat potatoes dry with paper towels. Arrange in single layer on prepared pans, spray with cooking spray. Bake 10 minutes. Flip over, brush with oil and sprinkle with herb mixture. Bake 5-10 minutes more until golden brown. Cool before serving. Serving size is about 10 chips with 3 tablespoons sour cream for dipping.
Nutrition Info: Calories 83 Total Carbs 14g Net Carbs 12g Protein 2g Fat 3g Sugar 1g Fiber 2g

196. Peanut Butter Oatmeal Cookies

Servings: 20   Cooking Time: 30 Minutes
Ingredients:
- 2 egg whites
- ½ cup margarine, soft
- What you'll need from store cupboard:
- 1 cup flour
- 1 cup quick oats
- ½ cup reduced-fat peanut butter
- 1/3 cup Splenda
- 1/3 Splenda brown sugar
- ½ tsp baking soda
- ½ tsp vanilla

Directions:
Heat oven to 350 degrees. In a large mixing bowl, combine dry Ingredients and stir to combine. In a separate bowl, beat together the egg whites and margarine. Add to dry Ingredients and mix well. Drop by teaspoonful onto nonstick cookie sheets. Bake 8-10 minutes or until edges start to brown. Remove to wire rack and cool completely. Store in an airtight container. Serving size is 2 cookies.
Nutrition Info: Calories 151 Total Carbs 17g Net Carbs 16g Protein 3g Fat 7g Sugar 7g Fiber 1g

197. Moist Butter Cake

Servings: 14   Cooking Time: 30 Minutes
Ingredients:
- 3 eggs
- ¾ cup margarine, divided
- ½ cup fat free sour cream
- What you'll need from store cupboard:
- 2 cup almond flour, packed
- 1 cup Splenda, divided
- 1 tsp baking powder
- 2 tbsp. water
- 1 tbsp. + 1 tsp vanilla, divided
- Butter flavored cooking spray

Directions:
Heat oven to 350 degrees. Spray a Bundt cake pan generously with cooking spray. In a large bowl, whisk together flour, sour cream, ½ cup margarine, 3 eggs, 2/3 cup Splenda, baking powder, and 1 teaspoon vanilla until thoroughly combined. Pour into prepared pan and bake 30-35 minutes, or it passes the toothpick test. Remove from oven. Melt ¼ cup margarine in a small saucepan over medium heat. Whisk in 1/3 cup Splenda, tablespoon vanilla, and water. Continue to stir until Splenda is completely dissolved. Use a skewer to poke several small holes in top of cake. Pour syrup mixture evenly over cake making sure all the holes are filled. Swirl the pan a couple of minutes until the syrup is absorbed into the cake. Let cool 1 hour. Invert onto serving plate, slice and serve.
Nutrition Info: Calories 259 Total Carbs 18g Net Carbs 16g Protein 4g Fat 17g Sugar 15g Fiber 2g

198. No Bake Lemon Tart

Servings: 8   Cooking Time: 2 Hours
Ingredients:
- ½ cup margarine, soft
- 1/3 cup + 3 tbsp. fresh lemon juice, divided
- 1/3 cup almond milk, unsweetened
- 4 ½ tbsp. margarine, melted
- 3-4 tbsp. lemon zest, grated fine
- What you'll need from store cupboard:
- 1 cup almond flour
- ¾ cup coconut, grated fine
- ¼ cup + 3 tbsp. Splenda
- 2 ½ tsp vanilla, divided
- 2 tsp lemon extract
- ¼ teaspoon salt

Directions:
Spray a 9-inch tart pan with cooking spray. In a medium bowl combine, flour, coconut, 3 tablespoons lemon juice, 2 tablespoons Splenda, melted margarine, 1 ½ teaspoons vanilla, and a pinch of salt until thoroughly combined. Dump into prepared pan and press evenly on bottom and halfway up sides. Cover and chill until ready to use. In a medium bowl, beat the soft margarine until fluffy. Add remaining Ingredients and beat until mixture is smooth. Taste and add more lemon juice or Splenda if desired. Pour the filling into the crust. Cover and chill until filling is set, about 2 hours.
Nutrition Info:al Facts Per ServingCalories 317 Total Carbs 17g Net Carbs 15g Protein 3g Fat 25g Sugar 13g Fiber 2g

199. Coconut Cream Pie

Servings: 8   Cooking Time: 10 Minutes
Ingredients:
- 2 cup raw coconut, grated and divided
- 2 cans coconut milk, full fat and refrigerated for 24 hours
- ½ cup raw coconut, grated and toasted
- 2 tbsp. margarine, melted
- What you'll need from store cupboard:
- 1 cup Splenda
- ½ cup macadamia nuts
- ¼ cup almond flour

Directions:
Heat oven to 350 degrees. Add the nuts to a food processor and pulse until finely ground. Add flour, ½ cup Splenda, and 1 cup grated coconut. Pulse until Ingredients are finely ground and resemble cracker crumbs. Add the margarine and pulse until mixture starts to stick together. Press on the bottom and sides of

55

a 9-inch pie pan. Bake 10 minutes or until golden brown. Cool   Turn the canned coconut upside down and open. Pour off the water and scoop the cream into a large bowl. Add remaining ½ cup Splenda and beat on high until stiff peaks form.   Fold in remaining 1 cup coconut and pour into crust. Cover and chill at least 2 hours. Sprinkle with toasted coconut, slice, and serve.

Nutrition Info:al Facts Per ServingCalories 329 Total Carbs 15g Net Carbs 4g Protein 4g Fat 23g Sugar 4g Fiber 11g

200. Grain-free Berry Cobbler

Servings: 10   Cooking Time: 25 Minutes

Ingredients:
- 4 cups fresh mixed berries
- ½-cup ground flaxseed
- ¼ cup almond meal
- ¼ cup unsweetened shredded coconut
- ½-tablespoon baking powder
- 1-teaspoon ground cinnamon
- ¼-teaspoon salt
- Powdered stevia, to taste
- 6 tablespoons coconut oil

Directions:
Preheat the oven to 375°F and lightly grease a 10-inch cast-iron skillet.   Spread the berries on the bottom of the skillet.   Whisk together the dry ingredients in a mixing bowl.   Cut in the coconut oil using a fork to create a crumbled mixture.   Spread the crumble over the berries and bake for 25 minutes until hot and bubbling.   Cool the cobbler for 5 to 10 minutes before serving.

Nutrition Info: Calories 215,Total Fat 13.6gSaturated Fat 1.2g, Total Carbs 5.3g, Net Carbs 2.2g, Protein 5g, Sugar 1g,Fiber 3.1g, Sodium 67mg

Beef, Pork & Lamb Recipes

201. Beef & Broccoli Skillet

Servings: 4   Cooking Time: 10 Minutes

Ingredients:
- 1 lb. lean ground beef
- 3 cups cauliflower rice, cooked
- 2 cups broccoli, chopped
- 4 green onions, sliced
- What you'll need from store cupboard:
- 1 cup teriyaki sauce (chapter 15)

Directions:
Cook beef in a large skillet over med-high heat until brown. Add the broccoli and white parts of the onion, cook, stirring for 1 minute.   Add the cauliflower and sauce and continue cooking until heated through and broccoli is tender-crisp, about 3-5 minutes. Serve garnished with green parts of the onion.

Nutrition Info: Calories 255 total carbs 9g Net carbs 6g Protein 37g Fat 7g Sugar 3g Fiber 3g

202. Balsamic Chicken & Vegetable Skillet

Servings: 4   Cooking Time: 20 Minutes

Ingredients:
- 1 lb. chicken breasts, cut in 1-inch cubes
- 1 cup cherry tomatoes, halved
- 1 cup broccoli florets
- 1 cup baby Bella mushrooms, sliced
- 1 tbsp. fresh basil, diced
- What you'll need from store cupboard:
- 1/2 recipe homemade pasta, cooked and drain well (chapter 14)
- ½ cup low sodium chicken broth
- 3 tbsp. balsamic vinegar
- 2 tbsp. olive oil, divided
- 1 tsp pepper
- ½ tsp garlic powder
- ½ tsp salt
- ½ tsp red pepper flakes

Directions:
Heat oil in a large, deep skillet over med-high heat. Add chicken and cook until browned on all sides, 8-10 minutes.   Add vegetables, basil, broth, and seasonings. Cover, reduce heat to medium and cook 5 minutes, or vegetables are tender.   Uncover and stir in cooked pasta and vinegar. Cook until heated through, 3-4 minutes. Serve.

Nutrition Info: Calories 386 Total Carbs 11g Net Carbs 8g Protein 43g Fat   18g Sugar 5g Fiber 3g

203. Russian Steaks With Nuts And Cheese

Servings: 4   Cooking Time: 20 Minutes

Ingredients:
- 800g of minced pork
- 200g of cream cheese
- 50g peeled walnuts
- 1 onion
- Salt
- Ground pepper
- 1 egg
- Breadcrumbs
- Extra virgin olive oil

Directions:
Put the onion cut into quarters in the Thermo mix glass and select 5 seconds speed 5.   Add the minced meat, cheese, egg, salt, and pepper.   Select 10 seconds, speed 5, turn left.   Add the chopped and peeled walnuts and select 4 seconds, turn left, speed 5.   Pass the dough to a bowl.   Make Russian steaks and go through breadcrumbs.   Paint the Russian fillets with extra virgin olive oil on both sides with a brush.   Put in the basket of the air fryer, without stacking the Russian fillets. Select 1800C, 15 minutes.

Nutrition Info: Calories: 1232Fat: 3.41g Carbohydrates: 0g Protein: 20.99g Sugar: 0gCholesterol: 63mg

204. Creamy Chicken Tenders

Servings: 4   Cooking Time: 15 Minutes

Ingredients:
- 1 lb. chicken breast tenders
- 1 cup half-n-half
- 4 tbsp. margarine
- What you'll need from store cupboard:
- 2 tsp garlic powder
- 2 tsp chili powder

Directions:
In a small bowl, stir together seasonings with a little salt if desired. Sprinkle over chicken to coat.   Heat 2 tablespoons margarine in a large skillet over medium heat. Cook chicken until no longer pink, 3-4 minutes per side. Transfer to a plate.   Add half-n-half and stir, scraping up the brown bits from the bottom of the skillet, and cook until it starts to boil. Reduce heat to med-low and simmer until sauce is reduced by half. Stir in remaining margarine and add chicken back to sauce to heat through. Serve.

Nutrition Info: Calories 281 Total Carbs 3g Protein 24g Fat 19g Sugar 0g Fiber 0g

205. Tangy Balsamic Beef

Servings: 8   Cooking Time: 6 – 8 Hours

Ingredients:
- 3-4 lb. beef roast, boneless
- ½ onion, diced fine
- What you'll need from store cupboard:
- 1 can low sodium beef broth
- ½ cup balsamic vinegar
- 5 cloves garlic, diced fine
- 3 tbsp. honey
- 1 tbsp. lite soy sauce
- 1 tbsp. Worcestershire sauce
- 1 tsp red chili flakes

Directions:
Place all Ingredients, except the roast, into the crock pot. Stir well. Add roast and turn to coat.   Cover and cook on low 6-8 hours. When the beef is done, remove to a plate and shred, using two forks. Add it back to the sauce and serve.

Nutrition Info: Calories 410 Total Carbs 9g Protein 45g Fat 20g Sugar 7g Fiber 0g

206. Sirloin Strips & "rice"

Servings: 6   Cooking Time: 30 Minutes
Ingredients:
- 1 ½ lbs. top sirloin steak, cut in thin strips
- 3 cup Cauliflower Rice, cook, (chapter 14)
- 2 onions, slice thin
- What you'll need from store cupboard:
- 14 ½ oz. tomatoes, diced, undrained
- ½ cup low sodium beef broth
- 1/3 cup dry red wine
- 1 clove garlic, diced
- 1 bay leaf
- 2 tsp olive oil, divided
- 1 tsp salt
- ½ tsp basil
- ½ tsp thyme
- ¼ tsp pepper

Directions:
Sprinkle beef strips with salt and pepper.   Heat oil in a large skillet over medium heat. Add steak and cook, stirring frequently, just until browned. Transfer to a plate and keep warm.   Add remaining oil to the skillet along with the onion and cook until tender. Add the garlic and cook 1 minute more.   Stir in remaining Ingredients, except the cauliflower, and bring to a boil. Reduce heat and simmer 10 minutes.   Return the steak back to the skillet and cook 2-4 minutes until heated through and tender. Discard bay leaf and serve over cauliflower rice.
Nutrition Info: Calories 278 Total Carbs 9g Net Carbs 6g Protein 37g Fat 9g Sugar 5g Fiber 3g

207. Spicy Bbq Beef Brisket

Servings: 14   Cooking Time: 5 Hours
Ingredients:
- 3 ½ lb. beef brisket
- ½ cup onion, diced fine
- 1 tsp lemon juice
- What you'll need from store cupboard:
- 2 cup barbecue sauce, (chapter 15)
- 1 pkt. Chili seasoning
- 1 tbsp. Worcestershire sauce
- 1 tsp garlic, diced fine

Directions:
Cut brisket in half and place in crock pot.   In a small bowl, combine remaining Ingredients, and pour over beef. Cover and cook on high heat 5-6 hours or until beef is fork tender.   Transfer brisket to a bowl. Use two forks and shred. Add the meat back to the crock pot and stir to heat through. Serve as is or on buns.
Nutrition Info: Calories 239 Total Carbs 7g Protein 34g Fat 7g Sugar 4g Fiber 0g

208. Slow Cooker Lemon Chicken With Gravy

Servings: 4   Cooking Time: 3 Hours
Ingredients:
- 1 lb. chicken tenderloins
- 3 tbsp. fresh lemon juice
- 3 tbsp. margarine, cubed
- 2 tbsp. fresh parsley, diced
- 2 tbsp. fresh thyme, diced
- 1 tbsp. lemon zest
- What you'll need from store cupboard:
- ¼ cup low sodium chicken broth
- 2 cloves garlic, sliced
- 2 tsp cornstarch
- 2 tsp water
- ½ tsp salt
- ½ tsp white pepper

Directions:
Add the broth, lemon juice, margarine, zest, garlic, salt and pepper to the crock pot, stir to combine. Add chicken, cover and cook on low heat 2 ½ hours.   Add the parsley and thyme and cook 30 minutes more, or chicken is cooked through.   Remove chicken to a plate and keep warm. Pour cooking liquid into a small saucepan and place over medium heat.   Stir water and cornstarch together until smooth. Add to sauce pan and bring to a boil. Cook, stirring, 2 minutes or until thickened. Serve with chicken.
Nutrition Info: Calories 303 Total Carbs 2g Protein 33g Fat 17g Sugar 0g Fiber 0g

209. Ritzy Beef Stew

Servings: 6   Cooking Time: 2 Hours
Ingredients:
- 2 tablespoons all-purpose flour
- 1 tablespoon Italian seasoning
- 2 pounds (907 g) top round, cut into ¾-inch cubes
- 2 tablespoons olive oil
- 4 cups low-sodium chicken broth, divided
- 1½ pounds (680 g) cremini mushrooms, rinsed, stems removed, and quartered
- 1 large onion, coarsely chopped
- 3 cloves garlic, minced
- 3 medium carrots, peeled and cut into ½-inch pieces
- 1 cup frozen peas
- 1 tablespoon fresh thyme, minced
- 1 tablespoon red wine vinegar
- ½ teaspoon freshly ground black pepper

Directions:
Combine the flour and Italian seasoning in a large bowl. Dredge the beef cubes in the bowl to coat well.   Heat the olive oil in a pot over medium heat until shimmering. Add the beef to the single layer in the pot and cook for 2 to 4 minutes or until golden brown on all sides. Flip the beef cubes frequently.   Remove the beef from the pot and set aside, then add ¼ cup of chicken broth to the pot. Add the mushrooms and sauté for 4 minutes or until soft. Remove the mushrooms from the pot and set aside. Pour ¼ cup of chicken broth in the pot. Add the onions and garlic to the pot and sauté for 4 minutes or until translucent.   Put the beef back to the pot and pour in the remaining broth. Bring to a boil.   Reduce the heat to low and cover. Simmer for 45 minutes. Stir periodically.   Add the carrots, mushroom, peas, and

thyme to the pot and simmer for 45 more minutes or until the vegetables are soft.   Open the lid, drizzle with red wine vinegar and season with black pepper. Stir and serve in a large bowl.

Nutrition Info:calories: 250   fat: 7.0g   protein: 25.0g   carbs: 24.0g   fiber: 3.0g   sugar: 5.0g sodium: 290mg

210. Pork Trinoza Wrapped In Ham

Servings: 6   Cooking Time: 20 Minutes

Ingredients:
- 6 pieces of Serrano ham, thinly sliced
- 454g pork, halved, with butter and crushed
- 6g of salt
- 1g black pepper
- 227g fresh spinach leaves, divided
- 4 slices of mozzarella cheese, divided
- 18g sun-dried tomatoes, divided
- 10 ml of olive oil, divided

Directions:
Place 3 pieces of ham on baking paper, slightly overlapping each other. Place 1 half of the pork in the ham. Repeat with the other half.   Season the inside of the pork rolls with salt and pepper.   Place half of the spinach, cheese, and sun-dried tomatoes on top of the pork loin, leaving a 13 mm border on all sides.   Roll the fillet around the filling well and tie with a kitchen cord to keep it closed.   Repeat the process for the other pork steak and place them in the fridge.   Select Preheat in the air fryer and press Start/Pause.   Brush 5 ml of olive oil on each wrapped steak and place them in the preheated air fryer.   Select Steak. Set the timer to 9 minutes and press Start/Pause.   Allow it to cool for 10 minutes before cutting.

Nutrition Info: Calories: 282 Fat: 23.41 Carbohydrates: 0g Protein: 16.59 Sugar: 0g Cholesterol: 73gm

211. Mississippi Style Pot Roast

Servings: 8   Cooking Time: 8 Hours

Ingredients:
- 3 lb. chuck roast
- What you'll need from store cupboard:
- 6-8 pepperoncini
- 1 envelope au jus gravy mix
- 1 envelope ranch dressing mix

Directions:
Place roast in crock pot. Sprinkle both envelopes of mixes over top. Place the peppers around the roast.   Cover and cook on low 8 hours, or high 4 hours.   Transfer roast to a large bowl and shred using 2 forks. Add it back to the crock pot and stir.   Remove the pepperoncini, chop and stir back into the roast. Serve.

Nutrition Info: Calories 379 Total Carbs 3g Protein 56g Fat 14g Sugar 1g Fiber 0g

212. Spicy Grilled Turkey Breast

Servings: 14   Cooking Time: 1 ½ Hours

Ingredients:
- 5 lb. turkey breast, bone in
- What you'll need from store cupboard:

- 1 cup low sodium chicken broth
- ¼ cup vinegar
- ¼ cup jalapeno pepper jelly
- 2 tbsp. Splenda brown sugar
- 2 tbsp. olive oil
- 1 tbsp. salt
- 2 tsp cinnamon
- 1 tsp cayenne pepper
- ½ tsp ground mustard
- Nonstick cooking spray

Directions:
Heat grill to medium heat. Spray rack with cooking spray. Place a drip pan on the grill for indirect heat.   In a small bowl, combine Splenda brown sugar with seasonings.   Carefully loosen the skin on the turkey from both sides with your fingers. Spread half the spice mix on the turkey. Secure the skin to the underneath with toothpicks and spread remaining spice mix on the outside.   Place the turkey over the drip pan and grill 30 minutes.   In a small saucepan, over medium heat, combine broth, vinegar, jelly, and oil. Cook and stir 2 minutes until jelly is completely melted. Reserve ½ cup of the mixture.   Baste turkey with some of the jelly mixture. Cook 1-1 ½ hours, basting every 15 minutes, until done, when thermometer reaches 170 degrees. Cover and let rest 10 minutes. Discard the skin. Brush with reserved jelly mixture and slice and serve.

Nutrition Info: Calories 314 Total Carbs 5g Protein 35g Fat 14g Sugar 5g Fiber 0g

213. Stuffed Cabbage And Pork Loin Rolls

Servings: 4   Cooking Time: 25 Minutes

Ingredients:
- 500g of white cabbage
- 1 onion
- 8 pork tenderloin steaks
- 2 carrots
- 4 tbsp. soy sauce
- 50g of olive oil
- Salt
- 8 sheets of rice

Directions:
Put the chopped cabbage in the Thermo mix glass together with the onion and the chopped carrot. Select 5 seconds, speed 5. Add the extra virgin olive oil. Select 5 minutes, varoma temperature, left turn, spoon speed.   Cut the tenderloin steaks into thin strips. Add the meat to the Thermomix glass. Select 5 minutes, varoma temperature, left turn, spoon speed. Without beaker   Add the soy sauce. Select 5 minutes, varoma temperature, left turn, spoon speed. Rectify salt. Let it cold down.   Hydrate the rice slices. Extend and distribute the filling between them.   Make the rolls, folding so that the edges are completely closed. Place the rolls in the air fryer and paint with the oil.   Select 10 minutes, 180oC.

Nutrition Info: Calories: 120 Fat: 3.41g Carbohydrates: 0g Protein: 20.99g Sugar: 0gCholesterol: 65mg

214. Cheesy Chicken & Spinach

Servings: 6   Cooking Time: 45 Minutes
Ingredients:
- 3 chicken breasts, boneless, skinless and halved lengthwise
- 6 oz. low fat cream cheese, soft
- 2 cup baby spinach
- 1 cup mozzarella cheese, grated
- What you'll need from store cupboard:
- 2 tbsp. olive oil, divided
- 3 cloves garlic, diced fine
- 1 tsp Italian seasoning
- Nonstick cooking spray

Directions:
Heat oven to 350 degrees. Spray a 9x13-inch glass baking dish with cooking spray.   Lay chicken breast cutlets in baking dish. Drizzle 1 tablespoon oil over chicken. Sprinkle evenly with garlic and Italian seasoning. Spread cream cheese over the top of chicken.   Heat remaining tablespoon of oil in a small skillet over medium heat. Add spinach and cook until spinach wilts, about 3 minutes. Place evenly over cream cheese layer. Sprinkle mozzarella over top.   Bake 35-40 minutes, or until chicken is cooked through. Serve.
Nutrition Info: Calories 363 Total Carbs 3g Protein 31g Fat 25g Sugar 0g Fiber 0g

215. Bbq Chicken & Noodles

Servings: 4   Cooking Time: 25 Minutes
Ingredients:
- 4 slices bacon, diced
- 1 chicken breast, boneless, skinless, cut into 1-inch pieces
- 1 onion, diced
- 1 cup low fat cheddar cheese, grated
- ½ cup skim milk
- What you'll need from store cupboard:
- 14 ½ oz. can tomatoes, diced
- 2 cup low sodium chicken broth
- ¼ cup barbecue sauce, (chapter 15)
- 2 cloves garlic, diced fine
- ¼ tsp red pepper flakes
- Homemade noodles, (chapter 14)
- Salt and pepper, to taste

Directions:
Place a large pot over med-high heat. Add bacon and cook until crispy. Drain fat, reserving 1 tablespoon. Stir in chicken and cook until browned on all sides, 3-5 minutes.   Add garlic and onion and cook, stirring often, until onions are translucent, 3-4 minutes.   Stir in broth, tomatoes, milk, and seasonings. Bring to boil, cover, reduce heat and simmer 10 minutes.   Stir in barbecue sauce, noodle, and cheese and cook until noodles are done and cheese has melted, 2-3 minutes. Serve.
Nutrition Info: Calories 331 Total Carbs 18g Net Carbs 15g Protein 34g Fat 13g Sugar 10g Fiber 3g

216. Homemade Flamingos

Servings: 4   Cooking Time: 20 Minutes
Ingredients:
- 400g of very thin sliced pork fillets c / n
- 2 boiled and chopped eggs
- 100g chopped Serrano ham
- 1 beaten egg
- Breadcrumbs

Directions:
Make a roll with the pork fillets. Introduce half-cooked egg and Serrano ham. So that the roll does not lose its shape, fasten with a string or chopsticks.   Pass the rolls through beaten egg and then through the breadcrumbs until it forms a good layer.   Preheat the air fryer a few minutes at 180° C.   Insert the rolls in the basket and set the timer for about 8 minutes at 1800 C.
Nutrition Info: Calories: 482 Fat: 23.41 Carbohydrates: 0g Protein: 16.59 Sugar: 0g Cholesterol: 173gm

217. Pesto Chicken

Servings: 6   Cooking Time: 20 Minutes
Ingredients:
- 1 ¾ lbs chicken breasts, skinless, boneless, and slice
- ½ cup mozzarella cheese, shredded
- ¼ cup pesto

Directions:
Add chicken and pesto in a mixing bowl and mix until well coated.   Place in refrigerator for 2-3 hours. Grill chicken over medium heat until completely cooked. Sprinkle cheese over chicken and serve.
Nutrition Info:303 Fat: 13g Carbohydrates: 1g Protein: 2Sugar: 1gCholesterol: 122mg

218. Breaded Chicken With Seed Chips

Servings: 4   Cooking Time: 40 Minutes
Ingredients:
- 12 chicken breast fillets
- Salt
- 2 eggs
- 1 small bag of seed chips
- Breadcrumbs
- Extra virgin olive oil

Directions:
Put salt to chicken fillets.   Crush the seed chips and when we have them fine, bind with the breadcrumbs. Beat the two eggs.   Pass the chicken breast fillets through the beaten egg and then through the seed chips that you have tied with the breadcrumbs.   When you have them all breaded, paint with a brush of extra virgin olive oil.   Place the fillets in the basket of the air fryer without being piled up.   Select 170 degrees, 20 minutes.   Take out and put another batch, repeat temperature and time. So, until you use up all the steaks.
Nutrition Info: Calories: 242 Fat: 13g Carbohydrates: 13.5g Protein: 18gSugar: 0g Cholesterol: 42mg

219. Turkey Meatballs With Spaghetti Squash

Servings: 4   Cooking Time: 35 Minutes
Ingredients:
- 1 lb. lean ground turkey

- 1 lb. spaghetti squash, halved and seeds removed
- 2 egg whites
- 1/3 cup green onions, diced fine
- ¼ cup onion, diced fine
- 2 ½ tbsp. flat leaf parsley, diced fine
- 1 tbsp. fresh basil, diced fine
- What you'll need from store cupboard:
- 14 oz. can no-salt-added tomatoes, crushed
- 1/3 cup soft whole wheat bread crumbs
- ¼ cup low sodium chicken broth
- 1 tsp garlic powder
- 1 tsp thyme
- 1 tsp oregano
- ½ tsp red pepper flakes
- ½ tsp whole fennel seeds

Directions:

In a small bowl, combine bread crumbs, onion, garlic, parsley, pepper flakes, thyme, and fennel. In a large bowl, combine turkey and egg whites. Add bread crumb mixture and mix well. Cover and chill 10 minutes. Heat the oven to broil. Place the squash, cut side down, in a glass baking dish. Add 3-4 tablespoons of water and microwave on high 10-12 minutes, or until fork tender. Make 20 meatballs from the turkey mixture and place on a baking sheet. Broil 4-5 minutes, turn and cook 4 more minutes. In a large skillet, combine tomatoes and broth and bring to a simmer over low heat. Add meatballs, oregano, basil, and green onions. Cook, stirring occasionally, 10 minutes or until heated through. Use a fork to scrape the squash into "strands" and arrange on a serving platter. Top with meatballs and sauce and serve.

Nutrition Info: Calories 253 Total Carbs 15g Net Carbs 13g Protein 27g Fat 9g Sugar 4g Fiber 2g

220. Spicy Lettuce Wraps

Servings: 6   Cooking Time: 5 Minutes

Ingredients:
- 12 Romaine lettuce leaves
- 1 lb. ground chicken
- 1/3 cup green onions, slice thin
- 2 tsp fresh ginger, grated
- What you'll need from store cupboard:
- 1/3 cup water chestnuts, diced fine
- 1/3 cup peanuts, chopped
- 2 cloves garlic, diced fine
- 3 tbsp. lite soy sauce
- 1 tbsp. cornstarch
- 1 tbsp. peanut oil
- ¼ tsp red pepper flakes

Directions:

In a large bowl, combine chicken, ginger, garlic, and pepper flakes. In a small bowl, stir together cornstarch and soy sauce until smooth. Heat oil in a large skillet over med-high heat, Add chicken and cook, stirring, 2-3 minutes, or chicken is cooked through. Stir in soy sauce and cook, stirring, until mixture starts to thicken, about 30 seconds. Add water chestnuts, green onions, and peanuts and heat through. Lay lettuce leaves out on a work surface. Divide filling evenly over them and roll up. Filling can also be made ahead of time

and reheated as needed. Serve warm with Chinese hot mustard for dipping, (chapter 15).

Nutrition Info: Calories 234 Total Carbs 13g Net Carbs 12g Protein 26g Fat 12g Sugar 6g Fiber 1g

221. Deconstructed Philly Cheesesteaks

Servings: 4   Cooking Time: 20 Minutes

Ingredients:
- 1 lb. lean ground beef
- 5-6 mushrooms, halved
- 4 slices provolone cheese
- 3 green bell peppers, quartered
- 2 medium onions, quartered
- What you'll need from store cupboard:
- ½ cup low sodium beef broth
- 1-2 tbsp. Worcestershire sauce
- 1 tsp olive oil
- Salt & pepper, to taste

Directions:

Heat oven to 400 degrees. Place vegetables in a large bowl and add oil. Toss to coat. Dump out onto a large baking sheet and bake 10-15 minutes, or until tender-crisp. Place beef in a large skillet and cook over med-high heat until no longer pink. Drain off fat. Add broth and Worcestershire. Cook, stirring occasionally, until liquid is absorbed, about 5 minutes. Salt and pepper beef if desired. Top with sliced cheese, remove from heat and cover until cheese melts. Divide vegetables evenly between 4 bowls. Top with beef and serve.

Nutrition Info: Calories 388 Total Carbs 15g Net Carbs 12g Protein 44g Fat 16g Sugar 9g Fiber 3g

222. Bbq Pork Tacos

Servings: 16   Cooking Time: 6 Hours

Ingredients:
- 2 lb. pork shoulder, trim off excess fat
- 2 onions, diced fine
- 2 cups cabbages, shredded
- What you'll need from store cupboard:
- 16 (6-inch) low carb whole wheat tortillas
- 4 chipotle peppers in adobo sauce, pureed
- 1 cup light barbecue sauce
- 2 cloves garlic, diced fine
- 1 ½ tsp paprika

Directions:

In a medium bowl, whisk together garlic, barbecue sauce and chipotles, cover and chill. Place pork in the crock pot. Cover and cook on low 8-10 hours, or on high 4-6 hours. Transfer pork to a cutting board. Use two forks and shred the pork, discarding the fat. Place pork back in the crock pot. Sprinkle with paprika then pour the barbecue sauce over mixture. Stir to combine, cover and cook 1 hour. Skim off excess fat. To assemble the tacos: place about ¼ cup of pork on warmed tortilla. Top with cabbage and onions and serve. Refrigerate any leftover pork up to 3 days.

Nutrition Info: Calories 265 Total Carbs 14g Net Carbs 5g Protein 17g Fat 14g Sugar 3g Fiber 9g

223. Beef Picadillo

Servings: 10   Cooking Time: 3-4 Hour

Ingredients:
- 1 ½ lbs. lean ground beef
- 1 onion, diced fine
- 1 red bell pepper, diced
- 1 small tomato, diced
- ¼ cup cilantro, diced fine
- What you'll need from store cupboard:
- 1 cup tomato sauce
- 3 cloves garlic, diced fine
- ¼ cup green olives, pitted
- 2 bay leaves
- 1 ½ tsp cumin
- ¼ tsp garlic powder
- Salt & pepper, to taste

Directions:
In a large skillet, over medium heat, brown ground beef. Season with salt and pepper. Drain fat. Add onion, bell pepper, and garlic and cook 3-4 minutes.   Transfer to crock pot and add remaining Ingredients. Cover and cook on high 3 hours.   Discard bay leaves. Taste and adjust seasonings as desired. Serve.

Nutrition Info: Calories 255 Total Carbs 6g Net Carbs 5g Protein 35g Fat 9g Sugar 3g Fiber 1g

224. Citrus Pork Tenderloin

Servings: 4   Cooking Time: 30 Minutes
Ingredients:
- ¼ cup freshly squeezed orange juice
- 2 teaspoons orange zest
- 1 teaspoon low-sodium soy sauce
- 1 teaspoon honey
- 1 teaspoon grated fresh ginger
- 2 teaspoons minced garlic
- 1½ pounds (680 g) pork tenderloin roast, fat trimmed
- 1 tablespoon extra-virgin olive oil

Directions:
Combine the orange juice and zest, soy sauce, honey, ginger, and garlic in a large bowl. Stir to mix well. Dunk the pork in the bowl and press to coat well. Wrap the bowl in plastic and refrigerate to marinate for at least 2 hours.   Preheat the oven to 400ºF (205ºC). Remove the bowl from the refrigerator and discard the marinade.   Heat the olive oil in an oven-safe skillet over medium-high heat until shimmering.   Add the pork and sear for 5 minutes. Flip the pork halfway through the cooking time.   Arrange the skillet in the preheated oven and roast the pork for 25 minutes or until well browned. Flip the pork halfway through the cooking time.   Transfer the pork on a plate. Allow to cool before serving.

Nutrition Info:calories: 228   fat: 9.0g   protein: 34.0g   carbs: 4.0g   fiber: 0g   sugar: 3.0g   sodium: 486mg

225. Beef Scallops

Servings: 4   Cooking Time: 20 Minutes
Ingredients:
- 16 veal scallops
- Salt
- Ground pepper
- Garlic powder
- 2 eggs
- Breadcrumbs
- Extra virgin olive oil

Directions:
Put the beef scallops well spread, salt, and pepper. Add some garlic powder.   In a bowl, beat the eggs.   In another bowl put the breadcrumbs.   Pass the Beef scallops for beaten egg and then for the breadcrumbs. Spray with extra virgin olive oil on both sides.   Put a batch in the basket of the air fryer. Do not pile the scallops too much.   Select 1800C, 15 minutes. From time to time, shake the basket so that the scallops move. When finishing that batch, put the next one and so on until you finish with everyone, usually 4 or 5 scallops enter per batch.

Nutrition Info: Calories: 330 Fat: 3.41g Carbohydrates: 0g Protein: 20.99g Sugar: 0gCholesterol:1 65mg

226. Chicken Pappardelle

Servings: 4   Cooking Time: 15 Minutes
Ingredients:
- ¾ lb. chicken breast, sliced lengthwise into ⅛-inch strips
- 1 small onion, sliced thin
- 8 cup spinach, chopped fine
- 4 cup low sodium chicken broth
- 1 cup fresh basil
- What you'll need from store cupboard:
- 2 quarts water
- ¼ cup reduced fat parmesan cheese, divided
- 6 cloves garlic, diced
- 1 tbsp. walnuts, chopped
- ¼ tsp cinnamon
- ¼ tsp paprika
- ¼ tsp red pepper flakes
- Salt
- Olive oil cooking spray

Directions:
Bring 2 quarts water to a simmer in a medium pot. Lightly spray a medium skillet with cooking spray and place over med-high heat. Add the garlic and cook until golden brown. Add the cinnamon, paprika, red pepper flakes, basil leaves, and onion. Cook until the onion has softened, about 2 minutes.   Add the spinach and cook until it has wilted and softened, another 2 minutes. Add the broth, bring to a simmer, cover, and cook until tender, about 5 minutes.   Add a pinch of salt to the now-simmering water. Turn off the heat and add the chicken and stir so that all the strips are separated. Cook just until the strips have turned white; they will be half-cooked. Using a slotted spoon, transfer the strips to a plate to cool. Check the spinach mixture; cook it until most of the broth has evaporated Stir in half the cheese and season with salt to taste. Add the chicken, toss to coat, and continue to cook until the chicken strips have cooked through, about 90 seconds. Spoon the mixture onto four plates, top with the remaining cheese and serve.

Nutrition Info: Calories 174 Total Carbs 7g Net Carbs 5g Protein 24g Fat 5g Sugar 2g Fiber 2g

227. One Pot Beef & Veggies

Servings: 10   Cooking Time: 8 Hours

Ingredients:
- 3 lb. beef roast
- 1 lb. red potatoes, cubed
- ¼ lb. mushrooms
- 1 green bell pepper, diced
- 1 parsnip, diced
- 1 red onion, diced
- What you'll need from store cupboard:
- 14 ½ oz. low sodium beef broth
- ¼ cup water
- 3 tbsp. cornstarch
- ¾ tsp salt
- ¾ tsp oregano
- ¼ tsp pepper

Directions:
Place the vegetables in a large crock pot. Cut roast in half and place on top of vegetables.   Combine broth, salt, oregano, and pepper, pour over meat.   Cover and cook on low heat 8 hours or until roast is tender.   Remove meat and vegetables to a serving platter, keep warm. Skim fat from cooking liquid and transfer to a small saucepan.   Place pan over medium heat and bring to a boil. Stir water and cornstarch together until smooth. Add to cooking liquid and stir 2 minutes until thickened. Serve with roast.

Nutrition Info: Calories 381 Total Carbs 28g Net Carbs 22g Protein 46g Fat 9g Sugar 12g Fiber 6g

228. Zesty Chicken & Asparagus Pasta

Servings: 4   Cooking Time: 15 Minutes

Ingredients:
- 2 chicken breasts, boneless, skinless, cut in 1-inch pieces
- 1 lb. asparagus, trim ends and cut in 2-inch pieces
- ½ cup half-n-half
- ½ cup mozzarella cheese, grated
- Juice and zest of one lemon
- 3 tbsp. margarine
- What you'll need from store cupboard:
- ½ recipe homemade pasta, (chapter 14) cook and drain
- 2/3 cup reduced fat parmesan cheese
- 1½ tbsp. olive oil
- 1½ tbsp. garlic, diced fine
- 1 tsp garlic powder
- ½ tsp oregano
- ½ tsp oregano
- ¼ tsp thyme
- Salt and black pepper, to taste

Directions:
Heat oil in a large skillet, over med-high heat. Add the chicken and salt and pepper to taste. Stir in oregano and cook 5 minutes, stirring occasionally until chicken is cooked through. Add 1 teaspoon diced garlic and cook 1 minute more. Transfer to plate.   Add margarine to the skillet and let melt. Add remaining garlic and asparagus and cook 1 minute, or until asparagus starts to turn bright green.   Whisk in the remaining Ingredients.

Cook, stirring frequently, until cheese melts and sauce thickens. Add the pasta and chicken, toss to coat and cook until heated through. Serve garnished with more parmesan cheese and chopped parsley if desired.

Nutrition Info: Calories 455 Total Carbs 15g Net Carbs 11g Protein 36g Fat 29g Sugar 6g Fiber 4g

229. Curried Chicken & Apples

Servings: 4   Cooking Time: 30 Minutes

Ingredients:
- 1 lb. chicken breasts, boneless, skinless, cut in 1-inch cubes
- 2 tart apples, peel and slice
- 1 sweet onion, cut in half and slice
- 1 jalapeno, seeded and diced
- 2 tbsp. cilantro, diced
- ½ tsp ginger, grated
- What you'll need from store cupboard:
- 14 ½ oz. tomatoes, diced and drained
- ½ cup water
- 3 cloves garlic, diced
- 2 tbsp. sunflower oil
- 1 tsp salt
- 1 tsp coriander
- ½ tsp turmeric
- ¼ tsp cayenne pepper

Directions:
Heat oil in a large skillet over med-high heat. Add chicken and onion, and cook until onion is tender. Add garlic and cook 1 more minute.   Add apples, water and seasonings and stir to combine. Bring to a boil. Reduce heat and simmer 12-15 minutes, or until chicken is cooked through, stirring occasionally.   Stir in tomatoes, jalapeno, and cilantro and serve.

Nutrition Info: Calories 371 Total Carbs 23g Net Carbs 18g Protein 34g Fat 16g Sugar 15g Fiber 5g

230. Arroz Con Pollo

Servings: 4   Cooking Time: 25 Minutes

Ingredients:
- 1 onion, diced
- 1 red pepper, diced
- 2 cup chicken breast, cooked and cubed
- 1 cup cauliflower, grated
- 1 cup peas, thaw
- 2 tbsp. cilantro, diced
- ½ tsp lemon zest
- What you'll need from store cupboard:
- 14 ½ oz. low sodium chicken broth
- ¼ cup black olives, sliced
- ¼ cup sherry
- 1 clove garlic, diced
- 2 tsp olive oil
- ¼ tsp salt
- ¼ tsp cayenne pepper

Directions:
Heat oil in a large skillet over med-high heat. Add pepper, onion and garlic and cook 1 minute. Add the cauliflower and cook, stirring frequently, until light brown, 4-5 minutes.   Stir in broth, sherry, zest and seasonings. Bring to a boil. Reduce heat, cover and simmer 15

minutes. Stir in the chicken, peas and olives. Cover and simmer another 3-6 minutes or until heated through. Serve garnished with cilantro.

Nutrition Info: Calories 161 Total Carbs 13g Net Carbs 9g Protein 14g Fat 5g Sugar 5g Fiber 4g

231. Tasty Harissa Chicken

Servings: 4   Cooking Time: 4 Hours 10 Minutes

Ingredients:
- 1 lb chicken breasts, skinless and boneless
- 1/2 tsp ground cumin
- 1 cup harissa sauce
- 1/4 tsp garlic powder
- 1/2 tsp kosher salt

Directions:
Season chicken with garlic powder, cumin, and salt. Place chicken to the slow cooker. Pour harissa sauce over the chicken. Cover slow cooker with lid and cook on low for 4 hours. Remove chicken from slow cooker and shred using a fork. Return shredded chicken to the slow cooker and stir well.

Nutrition Info: Calories: 235 Fat: 13g Carbohydrates: 1g Protein: 2Sugar: 1gCholesterol: 130mg

232. Pork Souvlakia With Tzatziki Sauce

Servings: 4   Cooking Time: 12 Minutes

Ingredients:
- ¼ cup lemon juice
- 1 tablespoon dried oregano
- ¼ teaspoon salt
- ¼ teaspoon ground black pepper
- 1 pound (454 g) pork tenderloin, cut into 1-inch cubes
- 1 tablespoon olive oil
- Tzatziki Sauce:
- ½ cup plain Greek yogurt
- 1 large cucumber, peeled, deseeded and grated
- 1 tablespoon fresh lemon juice
- 4 cloves garlic, minced or grated
- ¼ teaspoon ground black pepper
- Special Equipment:
- 8 bamboo skewers, soaked in water for at least 30 minutes

Directions:
Combine the lemon juice, oregano, salt, and ground black pepper in a large bowl. Stir to mix well. Dunk the pork cubes in the bowl of mixture, then toss to coat well. Wrap the bowl in plastic and refrigerate to marinate for 10 minutes or overnight. Preheat the oven to 450°F (235°C) or broil. Grease a baking sheet with the olive oil. Remove the bowl from the refrigerator. Run the bamboo skewers through the pork cubes. Set the skewers on the baking sheet, then brush with marinade. Broil the skewers in the preheated oven for 12 minutes or until well browned. Flip skewers at least 3 times during the broiling. Meanwhile, combine the ingredients for the tzatziki sauce in a small bowl. Remove the skewers from the oven and baste with the tzatziki sauce and serve immediately.

Nutrition Info:calories: 260 fat: 7.0g protein: 28.0g carbs: 21.0g fiber: 3.0g sugar: 3.0g sodium: 360mg

233. Salted Biscuit Pie Turkey Chops

Servings: 4   Cooking Time: 20 Minutes

Ingredients:
- 8 large turkey chops
- 300 gr of crackers
- 2 eggs
- Extra virgin olive oil
- Salt
- Ground pepper

Directions:
Put the turkey chops on the worktable, and salt and pepper. Beat the eggs in a bowl. Crush the cookies in the Thermo mix with a few turbo strokes until they are made grit, or you can crush them with the blender. Put the cookies in a bowl. Pass the chops through the beaten egg and then passed them through the crushed cookies. Press well so that the empanada is perfect. Paint the empanada with a silicone brush and extra virgin olive oil. Put the chops in the basket of the air fryer, not all will enter. They will be done in batches. Select 200 degrees, 15 minutes. When you have all the chops made, serve.

Nutrition Info: Calories: 126 Fat: 6g Carbohydrates 0gProtein: 18g Sugar: 0g

234. Cheesy Beef & Noodles

Servings: 4   Cooking Time: 15 Minutes

Ingredients:
- 1 lb. lean ground beef
- 1 onion, diced
- 2 cup mozzarella, grated
- ½ cup + 2 tbsp. fresh parsley diced
- What you'll need from store cupboard:
- Homemade Noodles, (chapter 15)
- 2 tbsp. tomato paste
- 1 tbsp. extra-virgin olive oil
- 1 tbsp. Worcestershire sauce
- 3 cloves garlic, diced fine
- 1 tsp red pepper flakes
- ½ tsp pepper
- Salt, to taste

Directions:
Heat oil in a large skillet over med-high heat. Add beef and cook, breaking up with a spatula, about 2 minutes. Reduce heat to medium and season with salt and pepper. Stir in garlic, onion, pepper flakes, Worcestershire, tomato paste, ½ cup parsley, and ½ cup water. Bring to a simmer and cook, stirring occasionally, 8 minutes. Stir in noodles and cook 2 minutes more. Stir in 1 cup of cheese, sprinkle the remaining cheese over the top and cover with lid, off the heat, until cheese melts. Serve garnished with remaining parsley.

Nutrition Info: Calories 372 Total Carbs 7g Net Carbs 6g Protein 44g Fat 18g Sugar 3g Fiber 1g

235. Chicken's Liver

Servings: 4   Cooking Time: 30 Minutes

Ingredients:
- 500g of chicken livers
- 2 or 3 carrots
- 1 green pepper
- 1 red pepper
- 1 onion
- 4 tomatoes
- Salt
- Ground pepper
- 1 glass of white wine
- ½ glass of water
- Extra virgin olive oil

Directions:
Peel the carrots, cut them into slices and add them to the bowl of the air fryer with a tablespoon of extra virgin olive oil 5 minutes.   After 5 minutes, add the peppers and onion in julienne. Select 5 minutes.   After that time, add the tomatoes in wedges and select 5 more minutes. Add now the chicken liver clean and chopped.   Season, add the wine and water.   Select 10 minutes.   Check that the liver is tender.

Nutrition Info:76 Fat: 13g Carbohydrates: 1g Protein: 2Sugar: 1gCholesterol: 130mg

236. Chutney Turkey Burgers

Servings: 4   Cooking Time: 15 Minutes
Ingredients:
- 1 lb. lean ground turkey
- 16 baby spinach leaves
- 4 slices red onion
- 2 green onions, diced
- ½ cup chutney, divided
- ¼ cup fresh parsley, diced
- 2 tsp lime juice
- What you'll need from store cupboard:
- 8 Flourless Burger Buns, (chapter 14)
- 1 tbsp. Dijon mustard
- ½ tsp salt
- ¼ tsp pepper
- Nonstick cooking spray.

Directions:
Heat grill to med-high heat. Spray rack with cooking spray.   In a small bowl, combine ¼ cup chutney, mustard, and lime juice.   In a large bowl, combine parsley, green onions, salt, pepper, and remaining chutney. Crumble turkey over mixture and mix well. Shape into 4 patties.   Place burgers on the grill and cook 5-7 minutes per side, or meat thermometer reaches 165 degrees.   Serve on buns with spinach leaves, sliced onions and reserved chutney mixture.

Nutrition Info: Calories 275 Total Carbs 15g Net Carbs 13g Protein 28g Fat 11g Sugar 2g Fiber 2g

237. Chicken Marsala

Servings: 4   Cooking Time: 25 Minutes
Ingredients:
- 4 boneless chicken breasts
- ½ lb. mushrooms, sliced
- 1 tbsp. margarine
- What you'll need from store cupboard:
- 1 cup Marsala wine
- ¼ cup flour
- 1 tbsp. oil
- Pinch of white pepper
- Pinch of oregano
- Pinch of basil

Directions:
On a shallow plate, combine flour and seasonings. Dredge the chicken in the flour mixture to coat both sides. In a large skillet, over medium heat, heat oil until hot. Add chicken and cook until brown on both sides, about 15 minutes. Transfer chicken to a plate.   Reduce heat to low and add mushrooms and ¼ cup of the wine. Cook about 5 minutes. Scrape bottom of pan to loosen any flour. Stir in reserved flour mixture and the remaining wine.   Simmer until mixture starts to thicken, stirring constantly. Add the chicken back to the pan and cook an additional 5 minutes. Serve.

Nutrition Info: Calories 327 Total Carbs 9g Net Carbs 8g Protein 21g Fat 14g Sugar 1g   Fiber 1g

238. Poblano & Cheese Burgers

Servings: 4   Cooking Time: 15 Minutes
Ingredients:
- 1 lb. lean ground beef
- 4 slices Monterey jack cheese
- 2 poblano peppers, seeded and chopped
- 1 egg
- 2 tbsp. margarine
- What you'll need from store cupboard
- 2 tbsp. dried minced onion
- 1 tbsp. liquid smoke
- 1 tbsp. Worcestershire sauce
- Salt & pepper to taste

Directions:
Heat up the grill.   In a large bowl, combine the beef, egg, onion, liquid smoke, Worcestershire, salt and pepper. Form into 6 patties and grill to desired doneness. Top with cheese.   Melt butter in a large skillet over med-high heat. Add pepper and cook until tender and it starts to char.   Place burgers on buns (chapter 14) top with peppers and your favorite burger toppings. Serve.

Nutrition Info: Calories 396 Total Carbs 4g Protein 43g Fat 22g Sugar 2g Fiber 0g

239. Ham And Cheese Stuffed Chicken

Burgers

Servings: 4   Cooking Time: 15 Minutes
Ingredients:
- ⅓ Cup soft bread crumbs
- 3 tablespoons milk
- 1 egg, beaten
- ½ teaspoon dried thyme
- Pinch salt
- Freshly ground black pepper
- 1¼ pounds ground chicken
- ¼ cup finely chopped ham
- ⅓ cup grated Havarti cheese
- Olive oil for misting

Directions:

In a medium bowl, combine the breadcrumbs, milk, egg, thyme, salt, and pepper. Add the chicken and mix gently but thoroughly with clean hands.   Form the chicken into eight thin patties and place on waxed paper.   Top four of the patties with the ham and cheese. Top with remaining four patties and gently press the edges together to seal, so the ham and cheese mixture is in the middle of the burger.   Place the burgers in the basket and mist with olive oil. Grill for 13 to 16 minutes or until the chicken is thoroughly cooked to 165°F as measured with a meat thermometer.   Beef, Pork, Lamb Recipes

Nutrition Info:324 Fat: 13g Carbohydrates: 1g Protein: 2Sugar: 1gCholesterol: 130mg

240. Turkey Stuffed Peppers

Servings: 8   Cooking Time: 55 Minutes
Ingredients:
- 1 lb. lean ground turkey
- 4 green bell peppers, halved and ribs and seeds removed
- 1 onion, diced
- 1 ½ cup mozzarella cheese
- 1 cup cauliflower, grated
- 1 cup mushrooms, diced
- What you'll need from store cupboard:
- 3 cups spaghetti sauce, (chapter 16)
- 3 cloves garlic, diced fine
- 2 tbsp. olive oil

Directions:
Heat the oil in a large skillet over med-high heat. Add the garlic, mushrooms, and onion. Add the turkey, cook, breaking up the turkey with a spatula, until turkey is cooked through, about 10 minutes.   Stir in the cauliflower, and cook, stirring frequently, 3-5 minutes. Add the spaghetti sauce and 1 cup mozzarella. Stir to combine and remove from heat.   Heat oven to 350 degrees. Place bell peppers in a large baking dish, skin side down. Fill the insides with the turkey mixture, place any extra filling around the peppers. Top each pepper with remaining mozzarella. Bake 40-45 minutes or the peppers are tender. Serve immediately.

Nutrition Info: Calories 214 Total Carbs 14g Net Carbs 10g Protein 20g Fat 11g Sugar 9g Fiber 4g

241. Sausage & Spinach Frittata

Servings: 6   Cooking Time: 40 Minutes
Ingredients:
- 8 eggs, beaten
- 1 1/3 cup sausage
- 1 ½ cup red bell pepper, diced
- ¾ cups baby spinach
- ¼ cup red onion, diced
- What you'll need from store cupboard:
- Salt and pepper, to taste
- Nonstick cooking spray

Directions:
Heat oven to 350 degrees. Spray a 9-inch pie pan with cooking spray.   Cook sausage in a medium skillet until no longer pink. Transfer to a large bowl with a slotted spoon.   Add remaining Ingredients and mix well. Pour into prepared pan and bake 30-35 minutes or until the center is completely set and top is starting to brown. Serve immediately.

Nutrition Info: Calories 156 Total Carbs 3g Net Carbs 2g Protein 12g Fat 10g Sugar 2g Fiber 1g

242. Crust Less Pizza

Servings: 4   Cooking Time: 25 Minutes
Ingredients:
- Pepperoni, ham, sausage, mushrooms, or toppings of your choice
- 8 oz. fat free cream cheese, soft
- 1 ½ cup mozzarella cheese, grated
- 2 eggs
- What you'll need from store cupboard:
- ½ cup lite pizza sauce
- ¼ cup reduced fat parmesan cheese
- 1 tsp garlic powder
- ¼ tsp pepper

Directions:
Heat oven to 350 degrees. Spray and 9x13-inch baking dish with cooking spray.   In a large bowl, beat cream cheese, eggs, pepper, garlic powder, and parmesan until combined. Spread in prepared dish and bake 12-15 minutes or until golden brown. Let cool 10 minutes. Spread pizza sauce over crust. Top with cheese and your favorite pizza toppings. Sprinkle lightly with garlic powder. Bake 8-10 minutes or until cheese melts. Cool 5 minutes before serving.

Nutrition Info: Calories 164 Total Carbs 4g Net Carbs 3g Protein 12g Fat 11g Sugar 1g Fiber 1g

243. Creamy Turkey & Peas With Noodles

Servings: 4   Cooking Time: 15 Minutes
Ingredients:
- 1 lb. lean ground turkey
- 1 lemon, juice and zest
- 1 ½ cup skim milk
- 1 cup low fat sharp cheddar cheese, grated
- 1 cup peas, frozen
- ¼ cup fresh parsley, diced
- 1 tbsp. margarine
- What you'll need from store cupboard:
- Homemade noodles, (chapter 14)
- ½ cup low sodium chicken broth
- 3 tbsp. flour
- 1 tbsp. olive oil
- 3 cloves garlic, diced fine
- ½ tsp ground mustard
- Pinch of nutmeg
- Salt and pepper, to taste

Directions:
Heat oil in a large skillet over med-high heat. Add turkey and season with salt and pepper. Cook, breaking up with a spatula, until no longer pink. Add garlic and cook 1 minute more.   Add the margarine and flour, and cook, stirring, 2 minutes until combined.   Stir in the broth and milk. Bring to a low boil, reduce heat to low and simmer until mixture starts to thicken.   Add the cheese and cook, stirring until it melts and combines into the sauce. Add the seasonings and peas, simmer 5 minutes, stirring occasionally.   Add the noodles and

lemon juice and cook another 2 minutes. Serve garnished with lemon zest and parsley.
Nutrition Info: Calories 427 Total Carbs 18g Net Carbs 16g Protein 40g Fat 22g Sugar 7g Fiber 2g

244. Classic Stroganoff

Servings: 5   Cooking Time: 20 Minutes
Ingredients:
- 5 ounces (142 g) cooked egg noodles
- 2 teaspoons olive oil
- 1 pound (454 g) beef tenderloin tips, boneless, sliced into 2-inch strips
- 1½ cups white button mushrooms, sliced
- ½ cup onion, minced
- 1 tablespoon all-purpose flour
- ½ cup dry white wine
- 1 (14.5-ounce / 411-g) can fat-free, low-sodium beef broth
- 1 teaspoon Dijon mustard
- ½ cup fat-free sour cream
- ¼ teaspoon salt
- ¼ teaspoon black pepper

Directions:
Put the cooked egg noodles on a large plate.   Heat the olive oil in a nonstick skillet over high heat until shimmering.   Add the beef and sauté for 3 minutes or until lightly browned. Remove the beef from the skillet and set on the plate with noodles.   Add the mushrooms and onion to the skillet and sauté for 5 minutes or until tender and the onion browns.   Add the flour and cook for a minute. Add the white wine and cook for 2 more minutes.   Add the beef broth and Dijon mustard. Bring to a boil. Keep stirring. Reduce the heat to low and simmer for another 5 minutes.   Add the beef back to the skillet and simmer for an additional 3 minutes. Add the remaining ingredients and simmer for 1 minute.   Pour them over the egg noodles and beef, and serve immediately.
Nutrition Info:calories: 275   fat: 7.0g   protein: 23.0g   carbs: 29.0g   fiber: 4.0g   sugar: 3.0g   sodium: 250mg

245. Ranch Chicken Casserole

Servings: 8   Cooking Time: 30 Minutes
Ingredients:
- 2 cup chicken, cooked & diced
- ½ lb. bacon, cooked & diced
- 4 eggs
- 1 cup reduced fat cheddar cheese, grated
- ½ cup half-n-half
- What you'll need from store cupboard:
- ½ cup fat free Ranch dressing
- Nonstick cooking spray

Directions:
Heat oven to 350 degrees. Lightly spray an 8x8-inch or 11x7-inch pan with cooking spray.   Spread chicken and bacon in the bottom of prepared pan. Top with cheese. Whisk together eggs, half-n-half, and ranch dressing. Pour on top of chicken mixture.   Bake, uncovered, for 30 to 35 minutes.

Nutrition Info: Calories 413 Total Carbs 2g Protein 38g Fat 27g Sugar 1g Fiber 0g

246. Healthy Turkey Chili

Servings: 4   Cooking Time: 45 Minutes
Ingredients:
- 1 lb. lean ground turkey
- 2 carrots, peeled and diced
- 2 stalks of celery, diced
- 1 onion, diced
- 1 zucchini, diced
- 1 red pepper, diced
- What you'll need from store cupboard:
- 14 oz. can tomato sauce
- 1 can black beans, drained and rinsed
- 1 can kidney beans, drained and rinsed
- 3 cups water
- 3 garlic cloves, diced fine
- 1 tbsp. chili powder
- 1 tbsp. olive oil
- 2 tsp salt
- 1 tsp pepper
- 1 tsp cumin
- 1 tsp coriander
- 1 bay leaf

Directions:
Heat oil in a heavy bottom soup pot over med-high heat. Add turkey and onion and cook until no longer pink, 5-10 minutes.   Add the vegetables and cook, stirring occasionally, 5 minutes. Add the garlic and spices and cook, stirring, 2 minutes.   Add the remaining Ingredients and bring to a boil. Reduce heat to low and simmer 30
Nutrition Info: Calories 218 Total Carbs 14g Net Carbs 10g Protein 25g Fat 9g Sugar 6g Fiber 4g

247. Roasted Vegetable And Chicken Tortillas

Servings: 4   Cooking Time: 20 Minutes
Ingredients:
- 1 red bell pepper, seeded and cut into 1-inch-wide strips
- ½ small eggplant, cut into ¼-inch-thick slices
- ½ small red onion, sliced
- 1 medium zucchini, cut lengthwise into strips
- 1 tablespoon extra-virgin olive oil
- Salt and freshly ground black pepper, to taste
- 4 whole-wheat tortilla wraps
- 2 (8-ounce / 227-g) cooked chicken breasts, sliced

Directions:
Preheat the oven to 400°F (205°C). Line a baking sheet with aluminum foil.   Combine the bell pepper, eggplant, red onion, zucchini, and olive oil in a large bowl. Toss to coat well.   Pour the vegetables into the baking sheet, then sprinkle with salt and pepper.   Roast in the preheated oven for 20 minutes or until tender and charred.   Unfold the tortillas on a clean work surface, then divide the vegetables and chicken slices on the tortillas.   Wrap and serve immediately.

Nutrition Info:calories: 483   fat: 25.0g   protein: 20.0g   carbs: 45.0g   fiber: 3.0g   sugar: 4.0g   sodium: 730mg

248. Beer Braised Brisket

Servings: 10   Cooking Time: 8 Hours
Ingredients:
- 5 lb. beef brisket
- 1 bottle of lite beer
- 1 onion, sliced thin
- What you'll need from store cupboard:
- 15 oz. can tomatoes, diced
- 3 cloves garlic, diced fine
- 1 tbsp. + 1 tsp oregano
- 1 tbsp. salt
- 1 tbsp. black pepper

Directions:
Place the onion on the bottom of the crock pot. Add brisket, fat side up. Add the tomatoes, undrained and beer. Sprinkle the garlic and seasonings on the top. Cover and cook on low heat 8 hours, or until beef is fork tender.
Nutrition Info: Calories 445 Total Carbs 4g Net Carbs 3g Protein 69g Fat 14g Sugar 2g Fiber 1g

249. Beef With Sesame And Ginger

Servings: 4-6   Cooking Time: 23 Minutes
Ingredients:
- ½ cup tamari or soy sauce
- 3 tbsp. olive oil
- 2 tbsp. toasted sesame oil
- 1 tbsp. brown sugar
- 1 tbsp. ground fresh ginger
- 3 cloves garlic, minced
- 1 to 1½ pounds skirt steak, boneless sirloin, or low loin

Directions:
Put together the tamari sauce, oils, brown sugar, ginger, and garlic in small bowl. Add beef to a quarter-size plastic bag and pour the marinade into the bag. Press on the bag as much air as possible and seal it.   Refrigerate for 1 to 1½ hours, turning half the time. Remove the meat from the marinade and discard the marinade. Dry the meat with paper towels. Cook at a temperature of 350°F for 20 to 23 minutes, turning halfway through cooking.
Nutrition Info: Calories: 381 Fat: 5g Carbohydrates: 9.6g Protein: 38g Sugar: 1.8gCholesterol: 0mg

250. Cheesy Beef Paseíllo

Servings: 15   Cooking Time: 20 Minutes
Ingredients:
- 1-2 tbsp. olive oil
- 2 pounds lean ground beef
- ½ chopped onion
- 2 cloves garlic, minced
- ½ tbsp. Adobo seasoning
- 2 tsp. dried oregano
- 1 packet of optional seasoning
- 2 tbsp. chopped cilantro
- ¼ cup grated cheese
- 15 dough disks

- 15 slices of yellow cheese

Directions:
In a large skillet over medium-high heat, heat the oil. Once the oil has warmed, add the meat, onions, and Adobo seasoning.   Brown veal, about 6-7 minutes. Drain the ground beef. Add the remaining seasonings and cilantro. Cook an additional minute. Add grated cheese, if desired. Melt the cheese.   On each dough disk, add a slice of cheese to the center and add 3-4 tablespoons of meat mixture over the slice of cheese. Fold over the dough disk and with a fork, fold the edges and set it aside.   Preheat the air fryer to 3700C for 3 minutes.   Once three minutes have passed, spray the air fryer pan with cooking spray and add 3-4 cupcakes to the basket. Close the basket, set to 3700C, and cook for 7 minutes. After 7 minutes, verify it. Cook up to 3 additional minutes, or the desired level of sharpness, if desired.   Repeat until finished.
Nutrition Info: Calories: 225 Fat: 3.41g Carbohydrates: 0g Protein: 20.99g Sugar: 0gCholesterol: 25mg

251. Pork Head Chops With Vegetables

Servings: 2-4   Cooking Time: 20 Minutes
Ingredients:
- 4 pork head chops
- 2 red tomatoes
- 1 large green pepper
- 4 mushrooms
- 1 onion
- 4 slices of cheese
- Salt
- Ground pepper
- Extra virgin olive oil

Directions:
Put the four chops on a plate and salt and pepper.   Put two of the chops in the air fryer basket.   Place tomato slices, cheese slices, pepper slices, onion slices and mushroom slices. Add some threads of oil.   Take the air fryer and select 1800C, 15 minutes.   Check that the meat is well made and take out.   Repeat the same operation with the other two pork chops.
Nutrition Info: Calories: 106 Fat: 3.41g Carbohydrates: 0g Protein: 20.99g Sugar: 0gCholesterol: 0mg

252. Easy Lime Lamb Cutlets

Servings: 4   Cooking Time: 8 Minutes
Ingredients:
- ¼ cup freshly squeezed lime juice
- 2 tablespoons lime zest
- 2 tablespoons chopped fresh parsley
- Sea salt and freshly ground black pepper, to taste
- 1 tablespoon extra-virgin olive oil
- 12 lamb cutlets (about 1½ pounds / 680 g in total)

Directions:
Combine the lime juice and zest, parsley, salt, black pepper, and olive oil in a large bowl. Stir to mix well. Dunk the lamb cutlets in the bowl of the lime mixture, then toss to coat well. Wrap the bowl in plastic and refrigerate to marinate for at least 4 hours.   Preheat

the oven to 450°F (235°C) or broil. Line a baking sheet with aluminum foil. Remove the bowl from the refrigerator and let sit for 10 minutes, then discard the marinade. Arrange the lamb cutlets on the baking sheet. Broil the lamb in the preheated oven for 8 minutes or until it reaches your desired doneness. Flip the cutlets with tongs to make sure they are cooked evenly. Serve immediately.

Nutrition Info:calories: 297 fat: 18.8g protein: 31.0g carbs: 1.0g fiber: 0g sugar: 0g sodium: 100mg

253. Hot Chicken Salad Casserole

Servings: 6   Cooking Time: 30 Minutes
Ingredients:
● 3 cup chicken breast, cooked and cut into cubes
● 6 oz. container plain low-fat yogurt
● 1 cup celery, diced
● 1 cup yellow or red sweet pepper, diced
● ¾ cup cheddar cheese, grated
● ¼ cup green onions, diced
● What you'll need from store cupboard:
● 1 can reduced-fat and reduced-sodium condensed cream of chicken soup
● ½ cup cornflakes, crushed
● ¼ cup almonds, sliced
● 1 tbsp. lemon juice
● ¼ teaspoon ground black pepper

Directions:
Heat oven to 400 degrees. In a large bowl, combine chicken, celery, red pepper, cheese, soup, yogurt, onions, lemon juice, and black pepper, stir to combine. Transfer to 2-quart baking dish. In a small bowl stir the cornflakes and almonds together. Sprinkle evenly over chicken mixture. Bake 30 minutes or until heated through. Let rest 10 minutes before serving.

Nutrition Info: Calories 238 Total Carbs 9g Net Carbs 8g Protein 27g Fat 10g Sugar 3g Fiber 1g

254. Horseradish Meatloaf

Servings: 8   Cooking Time: 45 Minutes
Ingredients:
● 1 ½ lbs. lean ground beef
● 1 egg, beaten
● ½ cup celery, diced fine
● ¼ cup onion, diced fine
● ¼ cup skim milk
● What you'll need from store cupboard:
● 4 slices whole wheat bread, crumbled
● ½ cup ketchup, (chapter 15)
● ¼ cup horseradish
● 2 tbsp. Dijon mustard
● 2 tbsp. chili sauce
● 1 ½ tsp Worcestershire sauce
● ½ tsp salt
● ¼ tsp pepper
● Nonstick cooking spray

Directions:
Heat oven to 350 degrees. Spray an 11x7-inch baking dish with cooking spray. In a large bowl, soak bread in milk for 5 minutes. Drain. Stir in celery, onion,

horseradish, mustard, chili sauce, Worcestershire, egg, salt, and pepper. Crumble beef over mixture and mix well. Shape into loaf in the prepared baking dish. Spread ketchup over the top. Bake 45-50 minutes or a meat thermometer reaches 160 degrees. Let rest 10 minutes before slicing and serving.

Nutrition Info: Calories 213 Total Carbs 8g Net Carbs 7g Protein 29g Fat 7g Sugar 2g Fiber 1g

255. Beef Tenderloin With Roasted Vegetables

Servings: 10   Cooking Time: 1 Hour
Ingredients:
● 3 lb. beef tenderloin
● 1 lb. Yukon gold potatoes, cut in 1-inch wedges
● 1 lb. Brussel sprouts, halved
● 1 lb. baby carrots
● 4 tsp fresh rosemary, diced
● What you'll need from store cupboard:
● ¾ cup dry white wine
● ¾ cup low sodium soy sauce
● 3 cloves garlic, sliced
● 4 tsp Dijon mustard
● 1 ½ tsp ground mustard
● Nonstick cooking spray

Directions:
Place beef in a large Ziploc bag. In a small bowl combine wine, soy sauce, rosemary, Dijon, ground mustard, and garlic. Pour half the mixture over the beef. Seal the bag and turn to coat. Refrigerate 4 ½ hours, turning occasionally. Cover and refrigerate remaining marinade. Heat oven to 425 degrees. Spray a 9x13-inch baking dish with cooking spray. Place the potatoes, Brussel sprouts and carrots in the prepared dish. Add reserved marinade and toss to coat. Cover and bake 30 minutes. Remove tenderloin and discard marinade. Place over vegetables and bake 30-45 minutes or until meat reaches desired doneness. Remove been and let stand 15 minutes. Check vegetables, if they are not tender bake another 10-15 minutes until done. Slice36 the beef and serve with vegetables.

Nutrition Info: Calories 356 Total Carbs 13g Net Carbs 10g Protein 43g Fat 13g Sugar 4g Fiber 3g

256. Ginger Chili Broccoli

Servings: 5   Cooking Time: 25 Minutes
Ingredients:
● 8 cups broccoli florets
● 1/2 cup olive oil
● 2 fresh lime juice
● 2 tbsp fresh ginger, grated
● 2 tsp chili pepper, chopped

Directions:
Add broccoli florets into the steamer and steam for 8 minutes. Meanwhile, for dressing in a small bowl, combine limejuice, oil, ginger, and chili pepper. Add steamed broccoli in a large bowl then pour dressing over broccoli. Toss well.

Nutrition Info: Calories 239 Fat 20.8 g, Carbohydrates 13.7 g, Sugar 3 g, Protein 4.5 g, Cholesterol 0 mg

257. Fried Pork Chops

Servings: 2   Cooking Time: 35 Minutes
Ingredients:
- 3 cloves of ground garlic
- 2 tbsp. olive oil
- 1 tbsp. of marinade
- 4 thawed pork chops

Directions:
Mix the cloves of ground garlic, marinade, and oil. Then apply this mixture on the chops.   Put the chops in the air fryer at 3600C for 35 minute
Nutrition Info: Calories: 118 Fat: 3.41g Carbohydrates: 0g Protein: 20.99g Sugar: 0gCholesterol: 39mg

258. Southwest Turkey Lasagna

Servings: 8   Cooking Time: 20 Minutes
Ingredients:
- 1 lb. lean ground turkey
- 1 onion, diced
- 1 green bell pepper, diced
- 1 red pepper, diced
- 8 oz. fat free cream cheese
- 1 cup Mexican cheese blend, grated
- ½ cup fat free sour cream
- What you'll need from store cupboard:
- 6 8-inch low carb whole wheat tortillas
- 10 oz. enchilada sauce
- ½ cup salsa, (chapter 16)
- 1 tsp chili powder
- Nonstick cooking spray

Directions:
Heat oven to 400 degrees. Spray a 13x9-inch baking dish with cooking spray.   In a large skillet, over medium heat, cook turkey, onion, and peppers until turkey is no longer pink. Drain fat.   Stir in cream cheese and chili powder.   Pour enchilada sauce into a shallow dish. Dip tortillas in sauce to coat. Place two tortillas in prepared dish. Spread with ½ the turkey mixture and sprinkle 1/3 of the cheese over turkey. Repeat layer. Top with remaining tortillas and cheese.   Cover with foil and bake 20-25 minutes, or until heated through. This can also be frozen up to 3 months.   Let rest 10 minutes before cutting. Serve topped with salsa and sour cream.
Nutrition Info: Calories 369 Total Carbs 36g Net Carbs 17g Protein 27g Fat 22g Sugar 4g Fiber 19g

259. Stuffed Grilled Pork Tenderloin

Servings: 6   Cooking Time: 25 Minutes
Ingredients:
- 2 ¾ lb. pork tenderloins
- ½ tsp fresh ginger, grated
- What you'll need from store cupboard:
- "Cornbread" Stuffing, (chapter 15)
- ¾ cup dry red wine
- 1/3 cup Splenda brown sugar
- ¼ cup ketchup, (chapter 16)

- 2 tbsp. low sodium soy sauce
- 2 cloves garlic, diced
- 1 tsp curry powder
- 1/5 tsp pepper
- Nonstick cooking spray

Directions:
Slice the tenderloins down the center lengthwise to within ½-inch of the bottom.   In a large Ziploc bag, combine wine, sugar, ketchup, soy sauce, garlic, curry powder, ginger and pepper. Add the pork, seal and turn to coat. Refrigerate 2-3 hours.   Heat the grill to med-high. Spray the grill rack with cooking spray.   Remove the pork from the bag and discard marinade. Open the tenderloins to lie flat, spread stuffing down the center of each. Tie closed with butcher string in 1 ½-inch intervals. Place tenderloins on the grill, cover and cook 25-40 minutes, or until a meat thermometer reaches 160 degrees. Let rest 5 minutes before slicing and serving.
Nutrition Info: Calories 452 Total Carbs 22g Net Carbs 19g Protein 36g Fat 18g Sugar 14g Fiber 3g

260. Pasta Bolognese

Servings: 8   Cooking Time: 2 Hours
Ingredients:
- 1 lb. lean ground beef
- 4 oz. pancetta, chopped
- 1 small onion, diced
- ½ cup celery, diced
- ½ cup carrots, diced
- ½ cup half-n-half
- ¼ cup fresh parsley, diced
- 1 tbsp. margarine
- What you'll need from store cupboard:
- 2 28 oz. cans tomatoes, crushed
- ¼ cup white wine
- 1 bay leaf
- Salt & fresh pepper, to taste
- Homemade pasta, cook and drain, (chapter 14)

Directions:
Place a heavy, deep saucepan over med-high heat. Add pancetta and cook, stirring occasionally, until fat melts. Add margarine, onions, celery and carrots, reduce heat to med-low and cook until soft, about 5 minutes. Increase heat to med-high, add meat, season with salt and pepper and sauté until browned.   Add wine and cook until it reduces down, about 3-4 minutes.   Add tomatoes and bay leaf. Reduce heat to low, cover and simmer, at least 1-1/2 to 2 hours, stirring occasionally. Stir in half & half and parsley, cook 2 minutes longer. Serve over pasta.
Nutrition Info: Calories 421 Total Carbs 23g Net Carbs 16g Protein 41g Fat 18g Sugar 13g Fiber 7g

261. Tasty Chicken Tenders

Servings: 4   Cooking Time: 25 Minutes
Ingredients:
- 1 ½ lbs chicken tenders
- 1 tbsp. extra virgin olive oil
- 1 tsp. rotisserie chicken seasoning
- 2 tbsp. BBQ sauce

Directions:

Add all ingredients except oil in a zip-lock bag. Seal bag and place in the refrigerator for 2-3 hours. Heat oil in a large pan over medium heat. Cook marinated chicken tenders in a pan until lightly brown and cooked.
Nutrition Info: Calories 365 Fat 16.1 g, Carbohydrates 2.8 g, Sugar 2 g, Protein 49.2 g, Cholesterol 151 mg

262. Creole Chicken

Servings: 2   Cooking Time: 25 Minutes
Ingredients:
- 2 chicken breast halves, boneless and skinless
- 1 cup cauliflower rice, cooked
- 1/3 cup green bell pepper, julienned
- ¼ cup celery, diced
- ¼ cup onion, diced
- What you'll need from store cupboard:
- 14 ½ oz. stewed tomatoes, diced
- 1 tsp sunflower oil
- 1 tsp chili powder
- ½ tsp thyme
- 1/8 tsp pepper

Directions:
Heat oil in a small skillet over medium heat. Add chicken and cook 5-6 minutes per side or cooked through. Transfer to plate and keep warm.   Add the pepper, celery, onion, tomatoes, and seasonings. Bring to a boil. Reduce heat, cover, and simmer 10 minutes or until vegetables start to soften.   Add chicken back to pan to heat through. Serve over cauliflower rice.
Nutrition Info: Calories 362 Total Carbs 14g Net Carbs 10g Protein 45g Fat 14g Sugar 8g Fiber 4g

263. Potatoes With Loin And Cheese(1)

Servings: 4   Cooking Time: 30 Minutes
Ingredients:
- 1kg of potatoes
- 1 large onion
- 1 piece of roasted loin
- Extra virgin olive oil
- Salt
- Ground pepper
- Grated cheese

Directions:
Peel the potatoes, cut the cane, wash, and dry.   Put salt and add some threads of oil, we bind well.   Pass the potatoes to the basket of the air fryer and select 180oC, 20 minutes.   Meanwhile, in a pan, put some extra virgin olive oil, add the peeled onion, and cut into julienne.   When the onion is transparent, add the chopped loin.   Sauté well and pepper.   Put the potatoes on a baking sheet.   Add the onion with the loin.   Cover with a layer of grated cheese.   Bake a little until the cheese takes heat and melts.
Nutrition Info: Calories: 332 Fat: 3.41g Carbohydrates: 0g Protein: 20.99g Sugar: 0gCholesterol: 0mg

264. Kielbasa & Lamb Cassoulet

Servings: 6   Cooking Time: 5 Hours 30 Minutes
Ingredients:
- 12 oz. lamb stew meat, cut into 1-inch cubes

- 8 oz. kielbasa, cut into 1/4-inch slices
- 1 eggplant, peeled and chopped
- 1 green pepper, coarsely chopped
- 1 tbsp. fresh thyme
- What you'll need from store cupboard:
- 2 cups low sodium beef broth
- 1 cup dried navy beans, rinsed well
- 6 oz. can tomato paste
- 3 cloves garlic, diced fine
- 1 tbsp. olive oil
- 1 bay leaf
- ¼ tsp whole black peppercorn
- Salt & pepper, to taste

Directions:
Place beans in a large saucepan. Add enough water to cover by 2 inches. Bring to a boil; reduce heat. Simmer, uncovered, for 10 minutes. Remove from heat. Cover and let stand for 1 hour. Drain and rinse beans.   Heat oil in a large skillet over med-high heat. Add lamb and cook until brown on all sides. Drain off fat. Transfer to a crock pot.   Add beans, broth, kielbasa, thyme, garlic, peppercorns, and bay leaf. Cover and cook on high 4 to 5 hours.   Add the eggplant, pepper and tomato paste, stir well. Cook another 30 minutes until vegetables are tender. Discard bay leaf and serve.
Nutrition Info: Calories 391 Total Carbs 35g Net Carbs 22g Protein 32g Fat 14g Sugar 8g Fiber 13g

265. Crock Pot Carnitas

Servings: 4   Cooking Time: 6 Hours
Ingredients:
- 4 lb. pork butt, boneless, trim the fat and cut into 2-inch cubes
- 1 onion, cut in half
- Juice from 1 orange, reserve orange halves
- 2 tbsp. fresh lime juice
- What you'll need from store cupboard:
- 2 cup water
- 1 ½ tsp salt
- 1 tsp cumin
- 1 tsp oregano
- 2 bay leaves
- ¾ tsp pepper

Directions:
Place pork and orange halves in the crock pot. In a medium bowl, combine remaining Ingredients and stir to combine. Pour over pork.   Cover and cook on high 5 hours. Pork should be tender enough to shred with a fork. If not, cook another 60 minutes.   Transfer pork to a bowl. Pour the sauce into a large saucepan and discard the bay leaves and orange halves.   Bring to a boil and cook until it thickens and resembles a syrup.   Use two forks to shred the pork. Add pork to the sauce and stir to coat. Serve.
Nutrition Info: Calories 464 Total Carbs 3g Protein 35g Fat 35g Sugar 1g Fiber 0g

266. Zucchini Lasagna

Servings: 4   Cooking Time: 1 Hour
Ingredients:
- 1 lb. lean ground beef

- 2 medium zucchini, julienned
- 3 tomatoes, blanch in hot water, remove skins and dice
- 1 onion, diced
- 1 serrano chili, remove seeds and dice
- 1 cup mushrooms, remove stems and dice
- ½ cup low-fat mozzarella, grated
- What you'll need from store cupboard:
- 2 cloves garlic, diced fine
- ½ cube chicken bouillon
- 1 tsp. paprika
- 1 tsp. dried thyme
- 1 tsp. dried basil
- Salt and pepper
- Nonstick cooking spray

Directions:
Lay zucchini on paper towel lined cutting board and sprinkle lightly with salt. Let sit for 10 minutes. Heat oven to broil. Blot zucchini with paper towels and place on baking sheet. Broil 3 minutes. Transfer to paper towels again to remove excess moisture. Lightly coat a deep skillet with cooking spray and place over med-high heat. Add garlic, onion, and chili and cook 1 minute. Add the tomatoes and mushrooms and cook, stirring frequently, about 4 minutes. Transfer vegetables to a bowl. Add the beef to the skillet with the paprika and cook until no longer pink. Add the vegetables and bouillon to the beef along with remaining spices and let simmer over low heat 25 minutes. Heat oven to 375 degrees. Line a small baking dish with parchment paper and place 1/3 of the zucchini in an even layer on the bottom. Top with 1/3 of the meat mixture. Repeat layers. Sprinkle cheese over top and bake 35 minutes. Let rest 10 minutes before serving.
Nutrition Info: Calories 272 Total Carbs 11g Net Carbs 8g Protein 38g Fat 8g Sugar 6g Fiber 3g

267. Stuffed Flank Steak

Servings: 6   Cooking Time: 30 Minutes
Ingredients:
- 1 ½ lb. flank steak
- ¼ cup fresh parsley, diced fine
- ¼ cup sun dried tomatoes
- What you'll need from store cupboard:
- ½ cup boiling water
- ½ cup reduced fat parmesan cheese
- 1 tbsp. horseradish, drain
- 2 tsp vegetable oil
- 1 tsp coarse black pepper
- Nonstick cooking spray

Directions:
Heat oven to 400 degrees. Line a shallow roasting pan with foil and spray it with cooking spray. Place tomatoes in a small bowl and pour boiling water over. Let stand 5 minutes. Drain the tomatoes and add cheese, parsley, horseradish, and pepper. Cut steak down the middle, horizontally, to within 1/2-inch of opposite side. Open up to lay flat and flatten to ¼-inch thick. Spread tomato mixture over steak leaving ½-inch edges. Roll up and tie with butcher string. Place in prepared pan and cook 30-40 minutes, or until meat reaches desired

doneness, 145 degrees on a meat thermometer is med-rare. Let rest 10-15 minutes then slice and serve.
Nutrition Info: Calories 267 Total Carbs 2g Protein 34g Fat 13g Sugar 0g Fiber 0g

268. Shepherd's Pie

Servings: 8   Cooking Time: 45 Minutes
Ingredients:
- 1 ½ lbs. ground lamb
- 3 carrots, grated
- 1 cauliflower, separated into small florets
- 1 red onion, diced
- 4 tbsp. margarine
- 2 tbsp. half-n-half
- ¼ cup low fat cheddar cheese, grated
- What you'll need from store cupboard:
- 1 2/3 cups canned tomatoes, diced
- 4 tbsp. low sodium beef broth
- 2 cloves garlic, diced fine
- 1 tbsp. olive oil
- Salt & pepper, to taste

Directions:
Heat oven to 350 degrees. Put a large saucepan of water on to boil. Heat the oil in a large saucepan over med-high heat. Add onion and cook until soft. Add the lamb and cook, stirring occasionally, until brown on all sides. Stir in the broth, tomatoes, and carrots. Reduce heat, and simmer 10 minutes, or until vegetables are tender and liquid evaporates. Add the cauliflower to the boiling water and cook until soft, about 8-10 minutes. Drain well. Add the margarine, half-n-half, salt, and pepper and use an immersion blender to puree until smooth. Pour the meat mixture into a large casserole dish. Top with cauliflower mash and sprinkle cheese over top. Bake 20 minutes, or until cheese is nicely browned. Serve.
Nutrition Info: Calories 262 Total Carbs 9g Net Carbs 6g Protein 27g Fat 13g Sugar 4g Fiber 3g

269. Lemon Chicken With Basil

Servings: 4   Cooking Time: 1h
Ingredients:
- 1kg chopped chicken
- 1 or 2 lemons
- Basil, salt, and ground pepper
- Extra virgin olive oil

Directions:
Put the chicken in a bowl with a jet of extra virgin olive oil. Put salt, pepper, and basil. Bind well and let stand for at least 30 minutes stirring occasionally. Put the pieces of chicken in the air fryer basket and take the air fryer Select 30 minutes. Occasionally remove. Take out and put another batch. Do the same operation.
Nutrition Info: Calories: 126 Fat: 6g Carbohydrates 0gProtein: 18g Sugar: 0g

270. Turkey & Pepper Skillet

Servings: 4   Cooking Time: 25 Minutes
Ingredients:
- 4 turkey cutlets, ¼-inch thick
- 1 red bell pepper, cut into strips

- 1 yellow bell pepper, cut into strips
- ½ large sweet onion, sliced
- What you'll need from store cupboard
- 14 oz. can crushed tomatoes, fire-roasted
- 2 tbsp. extra-virgin olive oil, divided
- 2 tsp red wine vinegar
- 1 tsp salt, divided
- ½ teaspoon Italian seasoning
- ¼ teaspoon black pepper

Directions:
Season turkey with ½ teaspoon salt. Heat 1 tablespoon oil in a large skillet over med-high heat. Add turkey, 2 cutlets at a time, and cook 1-3 minutes, then flip and cook until done, 1-2 more minutes. Transfer to a plate and keep warm while you cook the other 2 cutlets.   Add the onion, peppers, and remaining salt to the skillet. Cover and cook, stirring frequently, until vegetables are soft, about 5-7 minutes.   Add seasoning and pepper, and cook, stirring, 30 seconds. Add vinegar, and cook, stirring, until liquid has almost evaporated completely. Add tomatoes and bring to a simmer, stirring frequently. Add the turkey back to the skillet, reduce heat to med-low, and cook, turning cutlets to coat with sauce, 1-2 minutes. Serve garnished with fresh chopped basil if desired.
Nutrition Info: Calories 245 Total Carbs 14g Net Carbs 19g Protein 31g Fat 9g Sugar 9g Fiber 4g

271. Taco Casserole

Servings: 6   Cooking Time: 40 Minutes
Ingredients:
- 1 lb. lean ground beef
- 4 eggs
- 1 jalapeno, seeded and diced
- 2 oz. low fat cream cheese
- ½ cup cheddar cheese, grated
- ½ cup pepper jack cheese, grated
- ¼ cup onion, diced
- ¼ cup half-n-half
- What you'll need from store cupboard:
- 1 pkg. taco seasoning
- ¼ cup water
- ¼ cup salsa
- 1 tbsp. hot sauce
- Nonstick cooking spray

Directions:
Heat oven to 350 degrees. Spray an 8x8-inch baking dish with cooking spray.   Place a large skillet over medium heat and cook beef until no longer pink   Add onion and jalapeno and cook until onion is translucent. Drain off fat.   Stir in taco seasoning and water and cook 5 minutes. Add the cream cheese and salsa and stir to combine.   In a medium bowl, whisk the eggs, hot sauce and half-n-half together.   Pour the meat mixture into prepared pan and top with egg mixture. Sprinkle with both cheeses and bake 30 minutes, or until eggs are set.   Let cool 5 minutes before slicing and serving.
Nutrition Info: Calories 307 Total Carbs 6g Net Carbs 5g Protein 34g Fat 15g Sugar 1g Fiber 1g

272. Spicy Grilled Flank Steak

Servings: 6   Cooking Time: 15 Minutes
Ingredients:
- 1 ½ lb. flank steak
- What you'll need from store cupboard:
- 3 tbsp. lite soy sauce
- 3 tbsp. sherry
- 3 tbsp. red wine vinegar
- 3 tbsp. Splenda brown sugar
- 1 tbsp. vegetable oil
- 1 ½ tsp paprika
- 1 ½ tsp red pepper flakes
- 1 ½ tsp chili powder
- 1 ½ tsp Worcestershire sauce
- ¾ tsp parsley flakes
- ¾ tsp garlic powder
- ¾ tsp salt
- Nonstick cooking spray

Directions:
In a small bowl, combine all Ingredients except steak. Pour 1/3 cup marinade into a large Ziploc bag and add steak. Seal and turn to coat. Refrigerate 1-3 hours. Save remaining marinade for basting.   Heat grill to medium heat. Spray rack with cooking spray.   Place steak on the grill and cook 6-8 minutes per side, basting every few minutes. Let rest 10 minutes, then slice against the grain and serve.
Nutrition Info: Calories 271 Total Carbs 7g Protein 35g Fat 9g Sugar 7g Fiber 0g

273. Creamy And Aromatic Chicken

Servings: 4   Cooking Time: 30 Minutes
Ingredients:
- 4 (4-ounce / 113-g) boneless, skinless chicken breasts
- Salt and freshly ground black pepper, to taste
- 1 tablespoon extra-virgin olive oil
- ½ sweet onion, chopped
- 2 teaspoons chopped fresh thyme
- 1 cup low-sodium chicken broth
- ¼ cup heavy whipping cream
- 1 scallion, white and green parts, chopped

Directions:
Preheat the oven to 375°F (190°C).   On a clean work surface, rub the chicken with salt and pepper.   Heat the olive oil in an oven-safe skillet over medium-high heat until shimmering.   Put the chicken in the skillet and cook for 10 minutes or until well browned. Flip halfway through. Transfer onto a platter and set aside. Add the onion to the skillet and sauté for 3 minutes or until translucent.   Add the thyme and broth and simmer for 6 minutes or until the liquid reduces in half. Mix in the cream, then put the chicken back to the skillet. Arrange the skillet in the oven and bake for 10 minutes. Remove the skillet from the oven and serve them with scallion.
Nutrition Info:calories: 287   fat: 14.0g   protein: 34.0g   carbs: 4.0g   fiber: 1.0g   sugar: 1.0g   sodium: 184mg

274. Orange Chicken

Servings: 6   Cooking Time: 20 Minutes
Ingredients:
- 1 ½ lbs. chicken breast, cut into ½-inch pieces
- 1 medium orange, zest then cut in half
- ½ inch fresh ginger, peel and grate
- What you'll need from store cupboard:
- 1 cup pork rinds
- ½ cup coconut flour
- 2 cloves garlic, peeled
- 4 tbsp. coconut oil, divided
- 2 tbsp. Swerve confectioners
- 1 tsp black pepper
- 1 tsp salt

Directions:
Add the pork rinds, coconut flour and pepper to a food processor. Pulse until the mixture becomes a fine powder. Dump into a medium bowl.   Season the chicken with salt and pepper.   Heat 2 tablespoons oil in a large skillet over med-high heat. Add the chicken to the pork rind mixture and toss to coat. Add to skillet and cook, 2-3 minutes per side, or until browned. This will need to be done in batches. Transfer to paper towel lined plate. Add remaining oil to a small sauce pan and heat over med-high heat. Add swerve and stir to combine. Once the swerve has dissolved, lower the heat to medium and add zest, garlic, ginger, and the juice from half the orange. Stir and bring to a simmer, stirring occasionally. Remove from heat when it thickens and becomes glossy.   Place the chicken on serving plate. Pour the orange glaze over it, sprinkle with sesame seeds and serve.
Nutrition Info: Calories 377 Total Carbs 10g Net Carbs 9g Protein 37g Fat 23g Sugar 8g Fiber 1g

275. Cajun Chicken & Pasta

Servings: 4   Cooking Time: 20 Minutes
Ingredients:
- 3 chicken breasts, boneless, skinless, cut in 1-inch pieces
- 4 Roma tomatoes, diced
- 1 green bell pepper, sliced
- 1 red bell pepper, sliced
- ½ red onion, sliced
- 1 cup half-n-half
- 2 tbsp. margarine
- ¼ cup fresh parsley, diced
- What you'll need from store cupboard:
- ½ recipe homemade pasta, (chapter 14), cook and drain
- 2 cup low sodium chicken broth
- ½ cups white wine
- 2 tbsp. olive oil
- 3 tsp Cajun spice mix
- 3 cloves garlic, diced fine
- Cayenne pepper, to taste
- Freshly ground black pepper, to taste
- Salt, to taste

Directions:
Place chicken in a bowl and sprinkle with 1 ½ teaspoons Cajun spice, toss to coat.   Heat 1 tablespoon oil and 1 tablespoon margarine in a large cast iron skillet over high heat. add chicken, cooking in 2 batches, cook until brown on one side, about 1 minute, flip and brown the other side. Transfer to a plate with a slotted spoon.   Add remaining oil and margarine to the pan. Add peppers, onion, and garlic. Sprinkle remaining Cajun spice over vegetables and salt to taste. Cook, stirring occasionally, until vegetables start to turn black, 3-5 minutes. Add tomatoes and cook another 30 seconds. Transfer vegetables to a bowl with a slotted spoon.   Add wine and broth to the pan and cook, stirring to scrape up brown bits from the bottom, 3-5 minutes. Reduce heat to med-low and add half-n-half, stirring constantly. Cook until sauce starts to thicken. Taste and season with cayenne, pepper and salt, it should be spicy.   Add chicken and vegetables to the sauce and cook 1-2 minutes until hot. Stir in pasta and parsley and serve.
Nutrition Info: Calories 475 Total Carbs 21g Net Carbs 17g Protein 38g Fat 25g Sugar 10g Fiber 4g

276. Breaded Chicken Fillets

Servings: 4   Cooking Time: 25 Minutes
Ingredients:
- 3 small chicken breasts or 2 large chicken breasts
- Salt
- Ground pepper
- 3 garlic cloves
- 1 lemon
- Beaten eggs
- Breadcrumbs
- Extra virgin olive oil

Directions:
Cut the breasts into fillets.   Put in a bowl and add the lemon juice, chopped garlic cloves and pepper.   Flirt well and leave 10 minutes.   Beat the eggs and put breadcrumbs on another plate.   Pass the chicken breast fillets through the beaten egg and the breadcrumbs.   When you have them all breaded, start to fry.   Paint the breaded breasts with a silicone brush and extra virgin olive oil.   Place a batch of fillets in the basket of the air fryer and select 10 minutes 180 degrees. Turn around and leave another 5 minutes at 180 degrees.
Nutrition Info: Calories: 120 Fat: 6g Carbohydrates 0gProtein: 18g Sugar: 0g

277. Crunchy Grilled Chicken

Servings: 8   Cooking Time: 10 Minutes
Ingredients:
- 8 chicken breast halves, boneless and skinless
- 1 cup fat free sour cream
- ¼ cup lemon juice
- Butter flavored spray, refrigerated
- What you'll need from store cupboard:
- 2 cup stuffing mix, crushed
- 4 tsp Worcestershire sauce
- 2 tsp paprika
- 1 tsp celery salt
- 1/8 tsp garlic powder
- Nonstick cooking spray

Directions:

In a large Ziploc bag combine sour cream, lemon juice, Worcestershire, and seasonings. Add chicken, seal, and turn to coat. Refrigerate 1-4 hours.   Heat grill to medium heat. Spray rack with cooking spray.   Place stuffing crumbs in a shallow dish. Coat both sides of chicken with crumbs and spritz with butter spray. Place on grill and cook 4-7 minutes per side, or until chicken is cooked through. Serve.

Nutrition Info: Calories 230 Total Carbs 22g Net Carbs 21g Protein 25g Fat 3g Sugar 4g Fiber 1g

278. Hawaiian Chicken

Servings: 8   Cooking Time: 3 Hours
Ingredients:
- 8 chicken thighs, bone-in and skin-on
- 1 red bell pepper, diced
- 1 red onion, diced
- 2 tbsp. fresh parsley, chopped
- 2 tbsp. margarine
- What you'll need from store cupboard:
- 8 oz. can pineapple chunks
- 8 oz. can crushed pineapple
- 1 cup pineapple juice
- ½ cup low sodium chicken broth
- ¼ cup Splenda brown sugar
- ¼ cup water
- 3 tbsp. light soy sauce
- 2 tbsp. apple cider vinegar
- 2 tbsp. honey
- 2 tbsp. cornstarch
- 1 tsp garlic powder
- 1 tsp Sriracha
- ½ tsp ginger
- ½ tsp sesame seeds
- Salt & pepper to taste

Directions:
Season chicken with salt and pepper.   Melt butter in a large skillet over medium heat. Add chicken, skin side down, and sear both side until golden brown. Add chicken to the crock pot.   In a large bowl, combine pineapple juice, broth, Splenda, soy sauce, honey, vinegar, Sriracha, garlic powder, and ginger. Pour over chicken.   Top with kinds of pineapple. Cover and cook on high 2 hours. Baste the chicken occasionally.   Mix the cornstarch and water together until smooth. Stir into chicken and add the pepper and onion, cook another 60 minutes, or until sauce has thickened. Serve garnished with parsley and sesame seeds.

Nutrition Info: Calories 296 Total Carbs 24g Protein 17g Fat 13g Sugar 18g Fiber 1g

279. Lamb Ragu

Servings: 8   Cooking Time: 8 Hours
Ingredients:
- 2 lbs. lamb stew meat
- 2 onions, diced
- 1 carrot, peeled and sliced thin
- 4 sprigs fresh rosemary
- 3 tbsp. fresh sage
- What you'll need from store cupboard
- 28 oz. can whole plum tomatoes, peeled

- 2 cups red wine
- 8 cloves garlic, diced
- 2 tbsp. olive oil
- Salt & pepper, to taste

Directions:
Sprinkle lamb with salt and pepper.   Heat oil in a large skillet over med-high heat. Add lamb and cook until brown on all sides.   Add onion, reduce heat, and cook 10 minutes, until onion is golden brown. Transfer mixture to a crock pot.   Crush the tomatoes with a fork and add to the crock pot with remaining Ingredients. Cover and cook on low 8 hours.   Use two forks to shred any chunks of lamb and stir well. Serve.

Nutrition Info: Calories 331 Total Carbs 11g Net Carbs 9g Protein 34g Fat 12g Sugar 6g Fiber 2g

280. Turkey Roulade

Servings: 8   Cooking Time: 40 Minutes
Ingredients:
- 4 8 oz. turkey cutlets
- 5 oz. spinach, thaw and squeeze dry
- 1 egg, beaten
- 1 cup tart apple, peel and dice
- 1 cup mushrooms, diced
- ½ cup onion, diced fine
- 2 tbsp. lemon juice
- 2 tsp lemon zest
- What you'll need from store cupboard:
- ½ cup bread crumbs
- 2 tsp olive oil
- ¾ tsp salt, divided
- ¼ tsp pepper
- 1/8 tsp nutmeg
- Nonstick cooking spray

Directions:
Heat oven to 375 degrees. Spray 11x7-inch baking pan with cooking spray.   Heat oil in a large skillet over med-high heat. Add apple, mushrooms, and onion and cook until tender.   Remove from heat and stir in spinach, juice, zest, nutmeg, and ¼ teaspoon salt.   Cut the cutlets down the center to within ½ inch of the bottom. Open them so they lay flat and flatten to ¼-inch thickness. Sprinkle with salt and pepper.   Spread spinach mixture over cutlets leaving 1 inch around the edges. Roll up and tie closed with butcher string.   Place bread crumbs in a shallow dish. Dip each roulade in the egg then roll in bread crumbs. Place seam side down in prepared dish.   Bake 40-45 minutes or until turkey is cooked through. Let stand 5 minutes. Cut away the string and serve.

Nutrition Info: Calories 262 Total Carbs 10g Net Carbs 8g Protein 36g Fat 8g Sugar 4g Fiber 2g

281. Jalapeno Turkey Burgers

Servings: 4   Cooking Time: 10 Minutes
Ingredients:
- 1 lb. lean ground turkey
- 4 slices pepper Jack cheese
- 2 jalapeno peppers, seeded and diced
- 4 tbsp. lettuce, shredded
- 4 tbsp. fat free sour cream

- 2 tbsp. cilantro, diced
- 2 tbsp. light beer
- What you'll need from store cupboard:
- 4 low carb hamburger buns
- 2 cloves garlic, diced
- 4 tbsp. salsa
- ½ tsp pepper
- ¼ tsp hot pepper sauce
- ¼ tsp salt
- ¼ tsp cayenne pepper
- Nonstick cooking spray.

Directions:
Heat grill to medium heat. Spray the grill rack with cooking spray.   In a large bowl, combine jalapenos, cilantro, beer, pepper sauce, garlic, pepper, salt, and cayenne. Crumble turkey over mixture and combine thoroughly. Shape into 4 patties.   Place the burgers on the grill and cook 3-5 minutes per side, or until meat thermometer reaches 165 degrees. Top each with slice of cheese, cover, and cook until cheese melts.   Place patties on buns and top with salsa, sour cream and lettuce.
Nutrition Info: Calories 389 Total Carbs 20g Net Carbs 14g Protein 38g Fat 19g Sugar 4g Fiber 6g

282. Creamy Braised Oxtails

Servings: 6   Cooking Time: 4-6 Hours
Ingredients:
- 2 pounds oxtails
- 1 onion, diced
- ½ cup half-n-half
- 1 tsp margarine
- What you'll need from store cupboard:
- 1 cup low sodium beef broth
- ¼ cup sake
- 4 cloves garlic, diced
- 2 tbsp. chili sauce
- 1 tsp Chinese five spice
- Salt & pepper

Directions:
Melt the margarine in a large skillet over med-high heat. Sprinkle oxtails with salt and pepper and cook until brown on all sides, about 3-4 minutes per side.   Add onion and garlic and cook another 3-5 minutes. Add the sake to deglaze the skillet and cook until liquid is reduced, 1-2 minutes.   Transfer mixture to the crock pot. Add the broth, chili sauce, and five spice, stir to combine. Cover and cook on low 6 hours, or high 4 hours, or until meat is tender.   Stir in the half-n-half and continue cooking another 30-60 minutes or sauce has thickened. Serve.
Nutrition Info: Calories 447 Total Carbs 4g Protein 48g Fat 24g Sugar 1g Fiber 0g

283. North Carolina Style Pork Chops

Servings: 2   Cooking Time: 10 Minutes
Ingredients:
- 2 boneless pork chops
- 15 ml of vegetable oil
- 25g dark brown sugar, packaged
- 6g of Hungarian paprika

- 2g ground mustard
- 2g freshly ground black pepper
- 3g onion powder
- 3g garlic powder
- Salt and pepper to taste

Directions:
Preheat the air fryer a few minutes at 180oC.   Cover the pork chops with oil.   Put all the spices and season the pork chops abundantly, almost as if you were making them breaded.   Place the pork chops in the preheated air fryer.   Select Steak, set the time to 10 minutes. Remove the pork chops when it has finished cooking. Let it stand for 5 minutes and serve.
Nutrition Info: Calories: 118 Fat: 6.85g Carbohydrates: 0 Protein: 13.12g Sugar: 0gCholesterol: 39mg

284. Seared Duck Breast With Red Wine & Figs

Servings: 6   Cooking Time: 35 Minutes
Ingredients:
- 2 duck breasts, with skin still on
- ¼ onion, diced
- 1 sprig fresh rosemary
- What you'll need from store cupboard:
- ½ cup red wine
- 1 tbsp. sugar free fig preServings:
- ½ tbsp. red wine vinegar
- ½ clove garlic, diced
- 1/8 tsp Splenda
- Salt & pepper, to taste
- 1 pinch sugar

Directions:
Heat the oven to 450 degrees. Sprinkle the duck breasts with Splenda, salt and pepper.   Place a cast iron skillet over med-high heat. Place the duck breasts in the pan skin side down. Cook for 3 minutes, moving them around to make sure the skin doesn't burn.   Flip the breasts over and place the pan in the oven. Cook for 5 minutes. Then remove the breasts, and set aside. Return the skillet to the stove medium heat. Add the onions and cook for 10 minutes. Add the garlic and cook for 1 minute more.   Add the wine, vinegar, fig preserves, and herb sprig. Cook, stirring occasionally, for 15 minutes. Then strain the sauce into a small saucepan. With five minutes left in cooking the sauce, place the duck breasts back into the oven to warm.   Slice the duck into 1/2-inch thick pieces, and spoon on some of the sauce. Serve.
Nutrition Info: Calories 180 Total Carbs 4g Protein 18g Fat 7g Sugar 3g Fiber 0g

285. Alfredo Sausage & Vegetables

Servings: 6   Cooking Time: 15 Minutes
Ingredients:
- 1 pkg. smoked sausage, cut in ¼-inch slices
- 1 cup half-and-half
- ½ cup zucchini, cut in matchsticks
- ½ cup carrots, cut in matchsticks
- ½ cup red bell pepper, cut in matchsticks

- ½ cup peas, frozen
- ¼ cup margarine
- ¼ cup onion, diced
- 2 tbsp. fresh parsley, diced
- What you'll need from store cupboard:
- ½ recipe Homemade Pasta, cook & drain, (chapter 15)
- 1/3 cup reduced fat parmesan cheese
- 1 clove garlic, diced fine
- Salt & pepper, to taste

Directions:
Melt margarine in a large skillet over medium heat. Add onion and garlic and cook, stirring occasionally, 3-4 minutes or until onion is soft. Increase heat to med-high. Add sausage, zucchini, carrots, and red pepper. Cook, stirring frequently, 5-6 minutes, or until carrots are tender crisp. Stir in peas and half-n-half, cook 1-2 minutes until heated through. Stir in cheese, parsley, salt, and pepper. Add pasta nd toss to mix. Serve.
Nutrition Info: Calories 283 Total Carbs 18g Net Carbs 14g Protein 21g Fat 15g Sugar 8g Fiber 4g

286. Cheesesteak Stuffed Peppers

Servings: 4   Cooking Time: 35 Minutes
Ingredients:
- 4 slices low-salt deli roast beef, cut into 1/2-inch strips
- 4 slices mozzarella cheese, cut in half
- 2 large green bell peppers, slice in half, remove seeds, and blanch in boiling water 1 minute
- 1 ½ cup sliced mushrooms
- 1 cup thinly sliced onion
- 1 tbsp. margarine
- What you'll need from store cupboard:
- 1 tbsp. vegetable oil
- 2 tsp garlic, diced fine
- ¼ tsp salt
- ¼ tsp black pepper

Directions:
Heat oven to 400 degrees. Place peppers, skin side down, in baking dish. Heat oil and margarine in a large skillet over medium heat. Once hot, add onions, mushrooms, garlic, salt, and pepper, and cook, stirring occasionally, 10-12 minutes or mushrooms are tender. Remove from heat and stir in roast beef. Place a piece of cheese inside each pepper and fill with meat mixture. Cover with foil and bake 20 minutes. Remove the foil and top each pepper with remaining cheese. Bake another 5 minutes, or until cheese is melted.
Nutrition Info: Calories 191 Total Carbs 10g Net Carbs 8g Protein 12g Fat 12g Sugar 5g Fiber 2g

287. Chicken Soup

Servings: 6   Cooking Time: 1 Hour 20 Minutes
Ingredients:
- 4 lbs Chicken, cut into pieces
- 5 carrots, sliced thick
- 8 cups of water
- 2 celery stalks, sliced 1 inch thick
- 2 large onions, sliced

Directions:

In a large pot add chicken, water, and salt. Bring to boil. Add celery and onion in the pot and stir well. Turn heat to medium-low and simmer for 30 minutes. Add carrots and cover pot with a lid and simmer for 40 minutes. Remove Chicken from the pot and remove bones and cut Chicken into bite-size pieces. Return chicken into the pot and stir well.
Nutrition Info: Calories: 89 Fat: 6.33gCarbohydrates: 0g Protein: 7.56g Sugar: 0gCholesterol: 0mg

288. French Onion Chicken & Vegetables

Servings: 10   Cooking Time: 4 Hours
Ingredients:
- 1 lb. chicken breasts, boneless and skinless, cut in 1-inch pieces
- 1 lb. green beans, trim
- 1 lb. red potatoes, quartered
- ½ lb. mushrooms, halved
- ½ cup sweet onion, sliced
- 1 tsp lemon zest
- What you'll need from store cupboard:
- 2 14 ½ oz. cans low sodium chicken broth
- 2 tbsp. onion soup mix
- 1 tbsp. sunflower oil
- 2 tsp Worcestershire sauce
- ½ tsp lemon pepper
- ½ tsp salt
- ½ tsp pepper
- ¼ tsp garlic powder

Directions:
Sprinkle chicken with lemon pepper. Heat oil in a large skillet over medium heat. Cook chicken 4-5 minutes or until brown on all sides. Layer the green beans, potatoes, mushrooms, and onion in the crock pot. In a small bowl, combine remaining Ingredients and pour over vegetables. Top with chicken. Cover and cook on low heat 4-5 hours or until vegetables are tender. Serve.
Nutrition Info: Calories 256 Total Carbs 15g Net Carbs 12g Protein 30g Fat 8g Sugar 2g Fiber 3g

289. Pork On A Blanket

Servings: 4   Cooking Time: 10 Minutes
Ingredients:
- ½ puff pastry sheet, defrosted
- 16 thick smoked sausages
- 15 ml of milk

Directions:
Preheat la air fryer to 200°C and set the timer to 5 minutes. Cut the puff pastry into 64 x 38 mm strips. Place a cocktail sausage at the end of the puff pastry and roll around the sausage, sealing the dough with some water. Brush the top (with the seam facing down) of the sausages wrapped in milk and place them in the preheated air fryer. Cook at 200°C for 10 minutes or until golden brown.
Nutrition Info: Calories: 381 Fat: 5g Carbohydrates: 9.6g Protein: 38g Sugar: 1.8gCholesterol: 0mg

290. Chicken Thighs

Servings: 2   Cooking Time: 20 Minutes

Ingredients:
- 4 chicken thighs
- Salt to taste
- Pepper
- Mustard
- Paprika

Directions:
Before using the pot, it is convenient to turn on for 5 minutes to heat it. Marinate the thighs with salt, pepper, mustard and paprika. Put your thighs in the air fryer for 10 minutes at 3800F After the time, turn the thighs and fry for 10 more minutes. If necessary, you can use an additional 5 minutes depending on the size of the thighs so that they are well cooked

Nutrition Info:72 Fat: 13g Carbohydrates: 1g Protein: 2Sugar: 0gCholesterol: 39mg

291. Bacon & Cauliflower Casserole

Servings: 6   Cooking Time: 20 Minutes

Ingredients:
- 6 slices bacon, cooked and crumbled, divided
- 3 scallions, sliced thin, divided
- 5 cup cauliflower
- 2 cup cheddar cheese, grated and divided
- 1 cup fat free sour cream
- What you'll need from store cupboard:
- ½ tsp salt
- ¼ tsp fresh cracked pepper
- Nonstick cooking spray

Directions:
Heat oven to 350 degrees. Spray casserole dish with cooking spray.   Steam cauliflower until just tender. In a large bowl, combine cauliflower, sour cream, half the bacon, half the scallions and half the cheese. Stir in salt and pepper. Place in prepared baking dish and sprinkle remaining cheese over top.   Bake 18-20 minutes until heated through. Sprinkle remaining scallions and bacon over top and serve.

Nutrition Info: Calories 332 Total Carbs 15g Net Carbs 11g Protein 21g Fat 20g Sugar 6g Fiber 4g

292. Beef Tenderloin Steaks With Brandied Mushrooms

Servings: 4   Cooking Time: 20 Minutes

Ingredients:
- 4 beef tenderloin steaks, about ¾ inch thick
- 3 ½ cups Portobello mushrooms, sliced
- 1 tbsp. margarine
- What you'll need from store cupboard:
- ½ cup brandy, divided
- 1 tsp balsamic vinegar
- ½ tsp salt
- ½ tsp coarsely ground pepper
- ½ tsp instant coffee granules
- Nonstick cooking spray

Directions:
Heat oven to 200 degrees.   Salt and pepper both sides of the steaks and let sit 15 minutes.   In a small bowl, mix together coffee, vinegar, all but 1 tablespoon brandy, salt and pepper.   Spray a large skillet with cooking spray and place over med-high heat.   Spray the mushrooms with cooking spray and add to the hot pan. Cook 5 minutes or until most of the liquid is absorbed. Transfer the mushrooms to a bowl.   Add the steaks to the skillet and cook 3 minutes per side. Reduce heat to med-low and cook 2 more minutes or to desired doneness. Place on dinner plates, cover with foil and place in oven.   Add the brandy mixture to the skillet and bring to a boil. Boil 1 minute, or until reduced to about ¼ cup liquid. Stir in mushrooms and cook 1-2 minutes, or most of the liquid has evaporated. Remove from heat and stir in remaining 1 tablespoon brandy and the margarine.   Spoon evenly over steaks and serve immediately.

Nutrition Info: Calories 350 Total Carbs 1g Protein 44g Fat 12g Sugar 0g Fiber 0g

293. Turkey Stuffed Poblano Peppers

Servings: 2   Cooking Time: 40 Minutes

Ingredients:
- 2 Poblano peppers, halved lengthwise, cores and seeds removed
- 1 lb. ground turkey
- ½ cup low-fat cheddar cheese, grated
- 1 green onion, diced
- 1 tbsp. cilantro, chopped
- What you'll need from store cupboard:
- 8 oz. can tomato sauce
- 1 tbsp. olive oil
- 1 tsp oregano
- 1 tsp paprika
- 1 tsp ground cumin
- ½ tsp onion powder
- ½ tsp garlic paste or minced garlic
- Salt and pepper

Directions:
Heat oven to 350 degrees.   Use tongs to roast the skin of the peppers over an open flame until charred and blistered all over. Or place on a cookie sheet under the broiler until skin is charred.   Place peppers in a plastic bag to steam for 15 minutes.   In a small bowl, stir together tomato sauce, oregano, paprika, and cumin Heat oil in a large skillet over medium heat. Add turkey, onion powder, and garlic paste. Cook, stirring frequently, until meat has browned. Stir in 2 tablespoons of the sauce and season with salt and pepper.   Pour remaining sauce in the bottom of a baking dish.   With a butter knife, scrape the charred skin off the peppers, and place on sauce in dish.   Divide turkey mixture evenly over the peppers, sprinkle with cheese. Cover and bake 20 minutes.   Remove the foil, and bake until cheese starts to brown, about 5-7 minutes. Serve garnished with chopped green onion and cilantro.

Nutrition Info: Calories 665 Total Carbs 12g Net Carbs 9g Protein 71g Fat 36g Sugar 8g Fiber 3g

294. Hearty Beef Chili

Servings: 4   Cooking Time: 1 Hour

Ingredients:
- 1 lb. lean ground beef
- 1 large bell pepper, diced

- 1 cup onion, diced
- What you'll need from store cupboard:
- 4 oz. can green chilies, diced
- 1 cup tomato sauce
- 1 cup low sodium beef broth
- 1 tbsp. tomato paste
- 2 cloves garlic, diced fine
- 2 tsp chili powder
- 1 tsp salt
- 1 tsp Worcestershire
- 1 tsp cumin
- ½ tsp celery salt
- ¼ tsp pepper

Directions:
Heat a large pan over med-high heat. Add beef, onions, bell pepper and garlic and cook, stirring occasionally, until beef is no longer pink. Drain fat.   Add remaining Ingredients and bring to a simmer. Reduce heat to med-low and simmer 30 minutes to an hour. Taste and adjust seasonings if needed. Serve.

Nutrition Info: Calories 355 Total Carbs 30g Net Carbs 20g Protein 40g Fat 9g Sugar 18g Fiber 10g

295. Turkey Sloppy Joes

Servings: 8   Cooking Time: 4 Hours

Ingredients:
- 1 lb. lean ground turkey
- 1 onion, diced
- ½ cup celery, diced
- ¼ cup green bell pepper, diced
- What you'll need from store cupboard:
- 8 Flourless Burger Buns, (chapter 14)
- 1 can no salt added condensed tomato soup
- ½ cup ketchup, (chapter 14)
- 2 tbsp. yellow mustard
- 1 tbsp. Splenda brown sugar
- ¼ tsp pepper

Directions:
In a large saucepan, over medium heat, cook turkey, onion, celery, and green pepper until turkey is no longer pink. Transfer to crock pot.   Add remaining Ingredients and stir to combine. Cover, and cook on low heat 4 hours. Stir well and serve on buns.

Nutrition Info: Calories 197 Total Carbs 12g Net Carbs 11g Protein 17g Fat 8g Sugar 8g Fiber 1g

296. Chestnut Stuffed Pork Roast

Servings: 15   Cooking Time: 1 Hour 35 Minutes

Ingredients:
- 5 lb. pork loin roast, boneless, double tied
- ½ lb. ground pork
- ½ cup celery, diced fine
- ½ cup onion, diced fine
- 2 tbsp. fresh parsley, diced, divided
- 1 tbsp. margarine
- What you'll need from store cupboard:
- 15 oz. can chestnuts, drained
- 2 cup low sodium chicken broth
- 3 tbsp. flour
- 2 tbsp. brandy, divided
- ½ tsp salt

- ½ tsp pepper
- 1/8 tsp allspice
- Salt & black pepper, to taste

Directions:
Heat oven to 350 degrees.   Untie roast, open and pound lightly to even thickness.   Melt margarine in a skillet over med-high heat. Add celery and onion and cook until soft.   In a large bowl, combine ground pork, 1 tablespoon parsley, 1 tablespoon brandy and seasonings. Mix in celery and onion. Spread over roast. Lay a row of chestnuts down the center. Roll meat around filling and tie securely with butcher string. Roast in oven 1 ½ hours or until meat thermometer reaches 145 degrees. Remove and let rest 10 minutes. Measure out 2 tablespoons of drippings, discard the rest, into a saucepan. Place over medium heat and whisk in flour until smooth. Add broth and cook, stirring, until mixture thickens. Chop remaining chestnuts and add to gravy along with remaining brandy and parsley. Season with salt and pepper if desired. Slice the roast and serve topped with gravy.

Nutrition Info: Calories 416 Total Carbs 15g Protein 48g Fat 16g Sugar 0g Fiber 0g

297. Honey Bourbon Pork Chops

Servings: 4   Cooking Time: 4 Hours

Ingredients:
- 4 pork chops, cut thick
- What you'll need from store cupboard:
- 5 tbsp. honey
- 2 tbsp. lite soy sauce
- 2 tbsp. bourbon
- 2 cloves garlic, diced fine

Directions:
In a small bowl, whisk together honey, soy sauce and bourbon. Stir in garlic.   Place pork chops in crock pot and top with sauce. Turn to make sure the pork chops are coated.   Cover and cook on low heat for 4 hours, or until the chops reach desired doneness. Serve.

Nutrition Info: Calories 231 Total Carbs 24g Protein 23g Fat 3g Sugar 20g Fiber 0g

298. Pork Rind

Servings: 4   Cooking Time: 1h

Ingredients:
- 1kg of pork rinds
- Salt
- ½ tsp. black pepper coffee

Directions:
Preheat the air fryer. Set the time of 5 minutes and the temperature to 2000C.   Cut the bacon into cubes - 1 finger wide.   Season with salt and a pinch of pepper. Place in the basket of the air fryer. Set the time of 45 minutes and press the power button.   Shake the basket every 10 minutes so that the pork rinds stay golden brown equally.   Once they are ready, drain a little on the paper towel so they stay dry. Transfer to a plate and serve.

Nutrition Info:(Nutrition per Serving):Calories: 282 Fat: 23.41 Carbohydrates: 0g Protein: 16.59 Sugar: 0g Cholesterol: 73gm

299. Korean Chicken

Servings: 6   Cooking Time: 3-4 Hours
Ingredients:
- 2 lbs. chicken thighs, boneless and skinless
- 2 tbsp. fresh ginger, grated
- What you'll need from store cupboard:
- 4 cloves garlic, diced fine
- ¼ cup lite soy sauce
- ¼ cup honey
- 2 tbsp. Korean chili paste
- 2 tbsp. toasted sesame oil
- 2 tsp cornstarch
- Pinch of red pepper flakes

Directions:
Add the soy sauce, honey, chili paste, sesame oil, ginger, garlic and pepper flakes to the crock pot, stir to combine. Add the chicken and turn to coat in the sauce.   Cover and cook on low 3–4 hours or till chicken is cooked through.   When the chicken is cooked, transfer it to a plate.   Pour the sauce into a medium saucepan. Whisk the cornstarch and ¼ cup cold water until smooth. Add it to the sauce. Cook over medium heat, stirring constantly, about 5 minutes, or until sauce is thick and glossy.   Use 2 forks and shred the chicken. Add it to the sauce and stir to coat. Serve.

Nutrition Info: Calories 397 Total Carbs 18g Protein 44g Fat 16g Sugar 13g Fiber 0g

300. Dry Rub Chicken Wings

Servings: 4   Cooking Time: 30 Minutes
Ingredients:
- 9g garlic powder
- 1 cube of chicken broth, reduced sodium
- 5g of salt
- 3g black pepper
- 1g smoked paprika
- 1g cayenne pepper
- 3g Old Bay seasoning, sodium free
- 3g onion powder
- 1g dried oregano
- 453g chicken wings
- Nonstick Spray Oil
- Ranch sauce, to serve

Directions:
Preheat the air fryer. Set the temperature to 180 °C. Put ingredients in a bowl and mix well.   Season the chicken wings with half the seasoning mixture and sprinkle abundantly with oil spray.   Place the chicken wings in the preheated air fryer.   Select Chicken, set the timer to 30 minutes.   Shake the baskets halfway through cooking.   Transfer the chicken wings to a bowl and sprinkle them with the other half of the seasonings until they are well covered. Servings with ranch sauce

Nutrition Info: Calories: 120 Fat: 6g Carbohydrates 0gProtein: 18g Sugar: 0g

301. Tandoori Lamb

Servings: 6   Cooking Time: 30 Minutes
Ingredients:
- 1 leg of lamb, butterflied

- ½ cup plain Greek yogurt
- What you'll need from store cupboard:
- 1 tbsp. paprika
- 1 tsp cumin
- 1 tsp coriander
- 1 tsp onion powder
- 1 tsp garlic paste
- 1 tsp ginger paste
- Salt & pepper, to taste

Directions:
In a large Ziploc bag, combine yogurt and spices. Zip closed and squish to mix Ingredients. Add the lamb and massage the marinade into the meat. Chill 1 hour or overnight.   Heat oven to 325 degrees. Transfer lamb to a baking sheet. Season with salt and pepper and roast 30 minutes, or until lamb is medium rare.   Remove from oven and let rest 5 minutes. Slice and serve.

Nutrition Info: Calories 448 Total Carbs 2g Protein 68g Fat 17g Sugar 1g Fiber 0g

302. Turkey & Mushroom Casserole

Servings: 8   Cooking Time: 50 Minutes
Ingredients:
- 1 lb. cremini mushrooms, washed and sliced
- 1 onion, diced
- 6 cup cauliflower, grated
- 4 cup turkey, cooked and cut in bite size pieces
- 2 cup reduced fat Mozzarella, grated, divided
- 1 cup fat free sour cream
- What you'll need from store cupboard:
- ½ cup lite mayonnaise
- ¼ cup reduced fat parmesan cheese
- 2 tbsp. olive oil, divided
- 2 tbsp. Dijon mustard
- 1 ½ tsp thyme
- 1 ½ tsp poultry seasoning
- Salt and fresh-ground black pepper to taste
- Nonstick cooking spray

Directions:
Heat oven to 375 degrees. Spray a 9x13-inch baking dish with cooking spray.   In a medium bowl, stir together sour cream, mayonnaise, mustard, ½ teaspoon each thyme and poultry seasoning, 1 cup of the mozzarella, and parmesan cheese.   Heat 2 teaspoons oil in a large skillet over med-high heat. Add mushrooms and sauté until they start to brown and all liquid is evaporated. Transfer them to the prepared baking dish.   Add 2 more teaspoons oil to the skillet along with the onion and sauté until soft and they start to brown. Add the onions to the mushrooms.   Add another 2 teaspoons oil to the skillet with the cauliflower. Cook, stirring frequently, until it starts to get soft, about 3-4 minutes. Add the remaining thyme and poultry seasoning and cook 1 more minute.   Season with salt and pepper and add to baking dish. Place the turkey over the vegetables and stir everything together.   Spread the sauce mixture over the top and stir to combine. Sprinkle the remaining mozzarella over the top and bake 40 minutes, or until bubbly and cheese is golden brown. Let cool 5 minutes, then cut and serve.

Nutrition Info: Calories 351 Total Carbs 13g Net Carbs 10g Protein 37g Fat 16g Sugar 5g Fiber 3g

303. Meatloaf Reboot

Servings: 2   Cooking Time: 9 Minutes
Ingredients:
- 4 slices of leftover meatloaf, cut about 1-inch thick.

Directions:
Preheat your air fryer to 350 degrees.   Spray each side of the meatloaf slices with cooking spray. Add the slices to the air fryer and cook for about 9 to 10 minutes. Don't turn the slices halfway through the cooking cycle, because they may break apart. Instead, keep them on one side to cook to ensure they stay together

Nutrition Info: Calories: 201 Fat: 5g Carbohydrates: 9.6g Protein: 38g Sugar: 1.8gCholesterol: 10mg

304. Pork Loin With Onion Beer Sauce

Servings: 6   Cooking Time: 3 Hours
Ingredients:
- 1 ½ lb. pork loin
- 1 ½ cup dark beer
- 1 large onion, sliced
- What you'll need from store cupboard:
- 2 cloves garlic, diced fine
- 3 tbsp. water
- 2 tbsp. cornstarch
- 1 tbsp. olive oil
- 1 tbsp. Dijon mustard
- 2 bay leaves

Directions:
Heat oil in a large skillet over med-high heat. Add onions and cook until tender. Add the pork and brown on all sides. Transfer to the crock pot.   Add the beer, mustard, garlic, and bay leaves. Cover and cook on high 3 hours, or until pork is tender.   Transfer pork to a plate. Whisk together the corn starch and water and add to the crock pot, stir well. Let cook until sauce thickens, about 30 minutes.   Slice the pork and serve topped with sauce.

Nutrition Info: Calories 342 Total Carbs 7g Protein 31g Fat 18g Sugar 1g Fiber 0g

305. Mediterranean Stuffed Chicken

Servings: 6   Cooking Time: 45 Minutes
Ingredients:
- 6 chicken breast halves, boneless and skinless
- 10 oz. spinach, thaw and squeeze dry
- 4 green onions, slice thin
- 1 cup feta cheese, crumbled
- ½ cup sun dried tomatoes
- What you'll need from store cupboard:
- 1 cup boiling water
- 1 clove garlic, diced
- ¼ cup Greek olives, diced
- ¼ tsp salt
- ¼ tsp pepper
- Nonstick cooking spray

Directions:
Heat oven to 350 degrees. Spray 13x9-inch baking dish with cooking spray.   Place tomatoes in a bowl and add boiling water. Let set for 5 minutes.   In a medium bowl, combine spinach, cheese, onions, olive and garlic. Drain the tomatoes and chop, add to spinach mixture. Flatten chicken to ¼-inch thick and sprinkle with salt and pepper.   Spread spinach mixture over chicken and roll up, secure with toothpicks. Place in prepared dish and cover with foil.   Bake 30 minutes. Uncover, and bake 15-20 minutes, or until chicken is cooked through. Remove toothpicks before serving.

Nutrition Info: Calories 221 Total Carbs 6g Net Carbs 4g Protein 27g Fat 10g Sugar 1g Fiber 2g

306. Cajun Smothered Pork Chops

Servings: 4   Cooking Time: 25 Minutes
Ingredients:
- 4 pork chops, thick-cut
- 1 small onion, diced fine
- 1 cup mushrooms, sliced
- 1 cup fat free sour cream
- 2 tbsp. margarine
- What you'll need from store cupboard:
- 1 cup low sodium chicken broth
- 3 cloves garlic, diced fine
- 1 tbsp. Cajun seasoning
- 2 bay leaves
- 1 tsp smoked paprika
- Salt & pepper to taste

Directions:
Melt margarine in a large skillet over medium heat. Sprinkle chops with salt and pepper and cook until nicely browned, about 5 minutes per side. Transfer to a plate. Add onions and mushrooms and cook until soft, about 5 minutes. Add garlic and cook one minute more.   Add broth and stir to incorporate brown bits on bottom of the pan. Add a dash of salt and the bay leaves. Add pork chops back to sauce. Bring to a simmer, cover, and reduce heat. Cook 5-8 minutes, or until chops are cooked through.   Transfer chops to a plate and keep warm. Bring sauce to a boil and cook until it has reduced by half, stirring occasionally.   Reduce heat to low and whisk in sour cream, Cajun seasoning, and paprika. Cook, stirring frequently, 3 minutes. Add chops back to the sauce and heat through. Serve.

Nutrition Info: Calories   323 Total Carbs 13g Net Carbs 12g Protein 24g Fat 18g Sugar 5g Fiber 1g

307. Pork Liver

Servings: 4   Cooking Time: 15 Minutes
Ingredients:
- 500g of pork liver cut into steaks
- Breadcrumbs
- Salt
- Ground pepper
- 1 lemon
- Extra virgin olive oil

Directions:
Put the steaks on a plate or bowl.   Add the lemon juice, salt, and ground pepper.   Leave a few minutes to macerate the pork liver fillets.   Drain well and go through breadcrumbs, it is not necessary to pass the fillets through beaten egg because the liver is very moist,

the breadcrumbs are perfectly glued.   Spray with extra virgin olive oil. If you don't have a sprayer, paint with a silicone brush.   Put the pork liver fillets in the air fryer basket.   Program 1800C, 10 minutes.   Take out if you see them golden to your liking and put another batch. You should not pile the pork liver fillets, which are well extended so that the empanada is crispy on all sides.

Nutrition Info: Calories: 120 Fat: 3.41g Carbohydrates: 0g Protein: 20.99g Sugar: 0gCholesterol: 65mg

308. French Onion Casserole

Servings: 8   Cooking Time: 55 Minutes

Ingredients:
- 1 lb. lean ground beef
- 6 eggs
- 2 cup skim milk
- 1 cup Swiss cheese, grated
- ½ cup onion, diced
- What you'll need from store cupboard:
- 10 oz. can condensed French onion soup
- 6 oz. pkg. herb stuffing mix
- 1 tbsp. Worcestershire sauce
- 1 tbsp. olive oil
- 1 tbsp. chili sauce
- 2 tsp thyme
- Nonstick cooking spray

Directions:
Heat oven to 350 degrees. Spray a 13x9-inch baking dish with cooking spray.   Heat oil in a large skillet over medium heat. Add beef and cook, breaking up with spatula, until no longer pink.Add onion, Worcestershire, and chili sauce, and cook 3-5 minutes, until onions are soft.   In a large bowl, beat eggs, soup, milk, ½ cup cheese, and 1 teaspoon thyme. Add the dry stuffing mix and beef. Stir well, making sure to coat the stuffing mixture.   Transfer to prepared baking dish. Sprinkle with remaining cheese and thyme and let rest 15 minutes. Bake 45 minutes or until a knife inserted in center comes out clean. Serve.

Nutrition Info: Calories 327 Total Carbs 23g Net Carbs 22g Protein 30g Fat 12g Sugar 7g Fiber 1g

309. Cheesy Stuffed Chicken

Servings: 4   Cooking Time: 20 Minutes

Ingredients:
- 1 lb. chicken breasts, boneless and butterflied
- 2 cups fresh spinach, chopped
- 4 oz. low fat cream cheese, soft
- ¼ cup mozzarella cheese, grated
- What you'll need from store cupboard:
- ¼ cup reduced fat Parmesan cheese
- 1 tbsp. garlic, diced fine
- 1 tbsp. olive oil
- 1 tsp chili powder
- 1 tsp Italian seasoning
- ¾ tsp black pepper, divided
- ½ tsp salt

Directions:
In a medium bowl, combine spinach, cream cheese, parmesan, mozzarella, garlic, ½ teaspoon salt and ½

teaspoon pepper, stir to combine.   In a small bowl, stir together the chili powder, Italian seasoning, salt, and pepper, use it to season both sides of the chicken. Spoon ¼ of the cheese mixture into the middle of the chicken and fold over to seal it inside.   Heat oil in a large skillet over med-high heat. Add the chicken, cover and cook 9-10 minutes per side, or until cooked through. Serve.

Nutrition Info: Calories 256 Total Carbs 2g Net Carbs 1g Protein 29g Fat 14g Sugar 0g Fiber 1g

310. Middle East Chicken Skewers

Servings: 6   Cooking Time: 15 Minutes

Ingredients:
- 2 ½ lbs. chicken thighs, boneless, skinless, cut in large pieces
- 1 red onion, cut in wedges
- Zest & juice of 1 lemon
- 1 cup plain Greek yogurt
- What you'll need from store cupboard:
- 5 cloves garlic, diced
- 2 tbsp. olive oil
- 2 tsp paprika
- 1 ¾ tsp salt
- 1 tsp red pepper flakes
- ½ tsp pepper
- ½ tsp cumin
- 1/8 tsp cinnamon
- Nonstick cooking spray

Directions:
In a medium bowl, combine the yogurt, olive oil, paprika, cumin, cinnamon, red pepper flakes, lemon zest, lemon juice, salt, pepper and garlic.   Thread the chicken onto metal skewers, folding if the pieces are long and thin, alternating occasionally with the red onions. Place the kebabs on a baking sheet lined with aluminum foil. Spoon or brush the marinade all over the meat, coating well. Cover and refrigerate at least eight hours or overnight.   Heat the grill to medium-high heat. Spray the rack with cooking spray. Grill the kebabs until golden brown and cooked through, turning skewers occasionally, 10 to 15 minutes. Transfer the skewers to a platter and serve.

Nutrition Info: Calories 474 Total Carbs 14g Net Carbs 13g Protein 64g Fat 18g Sugar 12g Fiber 1g

311. Chicken Tuscany

Servings: 4   Cooking Time: 15 Minutes

Ingredients:
- 1½ lbs. chicken breasts, boneless, skinless and sliced thin
- 1 cup spinach, chopped
- 1 cup half-n-half
- What you'll need from store cupboard:
- ½ cup reduced fat parmesan cheese
- ½ cup low sodium chicken broth
- ½ cup sun dried tomatoes
- 2 tbsp. olive oil
- 1 tsp Italian seasoning
- 1 tsp garlic powder

Directions:

Heat oil in a large skillet over med-high heat. Add chicken and cook 3-5 minutes per side, or until browned and cooked through. Transfer to a plate.   Add half-n-half, broth, cheese and seasonings to the pan. Whisk constantly until sauce starts to thicken. Add spinach and tomatoes and cook, stirring frequently, until spinach starts to wilt, about 2-3 minutes.   Add chicken back to the pan and cook just long enough to heat through.
Nutrition Info: Calories 462 Total Carbs 6g Net Carbs 5g Protein 55g Fat 23g Sugar 0g Fiber 1g

312. Ritzy Jerked Chicken Breasts

Servings: 4   Cooking Time: 15 Minutes
Ingredients:
- 2 habanero chile peppers, halved lengthwise, seeded
- ½ sweet onion, cut into chunks
- 1 tablespoon minced garlic
- 1 tablespoon ground allspice
- 2 teaspoons chopped fresh thyme
- ¼ cup freshly squeezed lime juice
- ½ teaspoon ground nutmeg
- ¼ teaspoon ground cinnamon
- 1 teaspoon freshly ground black pepper
- 2 tablespoons extra-virgin olive oil
- 4 (5-ounce / 142-g) boneless, skinless chicken breasts
- 2 cups fresh arugula
- 1 cup halved cherry tomatoes

Directions:
Combine the habaneros, onion, garlic, allspice, thyme, lime juice, nutmeg, cinnamon, black pepper, and olive oil in a blender. Pulse to blender well.   Transfer the mixture into a large bowl or two medium bowls, then dunk the chicken in the bowl and press to coat well. Put the bowl in the refrigerator and marinate for at least 4 hours.   Preheat the oven to 400ºF (205ºC). Remove the bowl from the refrigerator, then discard the marinade.   Arrange the chicken on a baking sheet, then roast in the preheated oven for 15 minutes or until golden brown and lightly charred. Flip the chicken halfway through the cooking time.   Remove the baking sheet from the oven and let sit for 5 minutes. Transfer the chicken on a large plate and serve with arugula and cherry tomatoes.
Nutrition Info:calories: 226   fat: 9.0g   protein: 33.0g   carbs: 3.0g   fiber: 0g   sugar: 1.0g   sodium: 92mg

313. Lemon Chicken

Servings: 4   Cooking Time: 10 Minutes
Ingredients:
- 3 large boneless, skinless chicken breasts, cut into strips
- ¼ cup red bell pepper, cut into 2 inch strips
- ¼ cup green bell pepper, cut into 2 inch strips
- ¼ cup snow peas
- ¼ cup fresh lemon juice
- 1 tsp fresh ginger, peeled and diced fine
- What you'll need from store cupboard:
- ¼ cup + 1 tbsp. low sodium soy sauce, divided

- ¼ cup low-fat, low-sodium chicken broth
- 1 tbsp. Splenda
- 1 tbsp. vegetable oil
- 2 cloves garlic, diced fine
- 2 tsp cornstarch

Directions:
In a medium bowl, whisk together 1 teaspoon cornstarch and 1 tablespoon soy sauce. Add chicken, cover and chill about 10 minutes.   In a separate medium mixing bowl, stir together lemon juice, ¼ cup soy sauce, broth, ginger, garlic, Splenda, and remaining cornstarch until thoroughly combined.   Heat oil in a large skillet over med-high heat. Add chicken and cook, stirring frequently, 3-4 minutes or just until chicken is no longer pink.   Add sauce, peppers and peas. Cook 2 more minutes or until sauce thickens and vegetables are tender-crisp. Serve.
Nutrition Info: Calories 242 Total Carbs 9g Net Carbs 8g Protein 27g Fat 10g Sugar 5g Fiber 1g

314. Teriyaki Turkey Bowls

Servings: 4   Cooking Time: 15 Minutes
Ingredients:
- 1 lb. lean ground turkey
- 1 medium head cauliflower, separated into small florets
- What you'll need from store cupboard:
- 1 cup water, divided
- ¼ cup + 1 tbsp. soy sauce
- 2 tbsp. Hoisin sauce
- 2 tbsp. honey
- 1 ½ tbsp. cornstarch
- 1 tsp crushed red pepper flakes
- 1 tsp garlic powder
- Salt

Directions:
In a medium nonstick skillet, cook turkey over med-high heat until brown.   In a medium saucepan, combine ¾ cup water, ¼ cup soy sauce, hoisin, pepper flakes, honey, and garlic powder and cook over medium heat, stirring occasionally, until it starts to bubble.   In a small bowl whisk together ¼ cup water and cornstarch and add to the saucepan. Bring mixture to a full boil, stirring occasionally. Once it starts to boil, remove from heat and the turkey. Stir to combine.   Place the cauliflower florets in a food processor and pulse until it resembles rice.   Spray a nonstick skillet with cooking spray and add the cauliflower and 1 tablespoon soy sauce and cook until cauliflower starts to get soft, about 5-7 minutes. To serve, spoon cauliflower evenly into four bowls, top with turkey mixture and garnish with
Nutrition Info: Calories 267 Total Carbs 24g Net Carbs 20g Protein 26g Fat 9g Sugar 15g Fiber 4g

315. Garlic Honey Pork Chops

Servings: 6   Cooking Time: 10 Minutes
Ingredients:
- 6 boneless pork loin chops, trim excess fat
- What you'll need from store cupboard:
- ¼ cup lemon juice
- ¼ cup honey

- ¼ cup low sodium soy sauce
- ¼ cup dry white wine
- 2 tbsp. garlic, diced fine
- 1 tbsp. vegetable oil
- ¼ tsp black pepper

Directions:
Combine lemon juice, honey, soy sauce, wine, garlic, and pepper in a 9x13 baking dish. Mix well.   Add pork chops, turning to coat. Cover and refrigerate at least 4 hours, or overnight, turning chops occasionally.   Heat oil in a large skillet over med-high heat. Add chops and cook 2-3 minutes per side.   Pour marinade over chops and bring to a boil. Reduce heat to low and simmer 2-3 minutes, or chops are desired doneness. Serve topped with sauce.

Nutrition Info: Calories 436 Total Carbs 14g Protein 26g Fat 30g Sugar 12g Fiber 0g

316. Chicken Stuffed With Mushrooms

Servings: 4   Cooking Time: 3 Hours
Ingredients:
- 4 thin chicken breasts, boneless and skinless
- What you'll need from store cupboard:
- 1 small can mushrooms, drain and slice
- ½ cup + 2 tbsp. low sodium chicken broth
- ½ cup fine bread crumbs
- 1 tbsp. dry white wine
- 1 tbsp. cornstarch
- ½ tsp sage
- ½ tsp garlic powder
- ¼ tsp marjoram
- Salt & pepper to taste

Directions:
Place chicken between 2 sheets of plastic wrap and pound to 1/8-inch thick, working from the center to the edges.   In a small bowl, combine mushrooms, bread crumbs, 2 tablespoons broth and seasonings. Spoon one fourth stuffing mix onto short end of chicken breast. Fold long sides in and roll up. Secure with toothpick.   Place chicken in crock pot and add the ½ cup broth. Cover and cook on high 3 hours, or until chicken is cooked through. Transfer chicken to a plate and tent with foil to keep warm.   Strain cooking liquid through a sieve into a small saucepan. Place over medium heat. In a small bowl, whisk together the wine and cornstarch. Add to the saucepan and cook, stirring constantly, until sauce is bubbly and thick. Cook 2 minutes more. Spoon sauce over chicken and serve.

Nutrition Info: Calories   181 Total Carbs 13g Net Carbs 12g Protein 28g Fat 2g Sugar 1g Fiber 1g

317. Chicken Zucchini Patties With Salsa

Servings: 8   Cooking Time: 10 Minutes
Ingredients:
- 2 cup chicken breast, cooked, divided
- 1 zucchini, cut in ¾-inch pieces
- ¼ cup cilantro, diced
- What you'll need from store cupboard:
- 1/3 cup bread crumbs
- 1/3 cup lite mayonnaise
- 2 tsp olive oil

- ½ tsp salt
- ¼ tsp pepper
- Roasted Tomato Salsa, (chapter 15)

Directions:
Place 1 ½ cups chicken and zucchini into a food processor. Cover and process until coarsely chopped. Add bread crumbs, mayonnaise, pepper, cilantro, remaining chicken, and salt. Cover and pulse until chunky.   Heat oil in a large skillet over med-high heat. Shape chicken mixture into 8 patties and cook 4 minutes per side, or until golden brown. Serve topped with salsa.

Nutrition Info: Calories 146 Total Carbs 10g Net Carbs 8g Protein 12g Fat 7g Sugar 5g Fiber 2g

318. Roast Turkey & Rosemary Gravy

Servings: 18   Cooking Time: 1 ¾ Hours
Ingredients:
- 6 lb. turkey breast, bone in
- 2 apples, sliced
- 1 ½ cup leek, sliced, white parts only
- 3 tbsp. margarine
- 2 tsp fresh rosemary, diced, divided
- What you'll need from store cupboard:
- 2 ¼ cup low sodium chicken broth
- ¼ cup flour
- 1 tbsp. sunflower oil

Directions:
Heat oven to 325 degrees.   Place apples and leeks in the bottom of a large roasting pan, and pour in 1 cup of broth. Place turkey on top.   In a small bowl, combine oil and 1 ½ teaspoons rosemary. Loosen skin over turkey and rub rosemary mixture over the turkey. Secure skin to underside of turkey with toothpicks.   Bake 1 ¾-2 ¼ hours, basting every 30 minutes, until turkey is cooked through. If turkey starts to get too brown, cover with foil. Once turkey is done, cover and let rest 15 minutes before slicing. Discard apples and leeks. Save ¼ cup cooking liquid.   Melt margarine in a small saucepan over medium heat. Add flour and remaining rosemary and cook, stirring, until combined. Skim fat off the reserved cooking liquid and add to saucepan with remaining broth. Bring to a boil, cook, stirring, 1 minute until thickened. Serve with turkey.

Nutrition Info: Calories 306 Total Carbs 6g Net Carbs 5g Protein 33g Fat 14g Sugar 3g Fiber 1g

319. Beef Goulash

Servings: 6   Cooking Time: 1 Hour
Ingredients:
- 2 lb. chuck steak, trim fat and cut into bite-sized pieces
- 3 onions, quartered
- 1 green pepper, chopped
- 1 red pepper, chopped
- 1 orange pepper, chopped
- What you'll need from store cupboard:
- 3 cups water
- 1 can tomatoes, chopped
- 1 cup low sodium beef broth
- 3 cloves garlic, diced fine
- 2 tbsp. tomato paste

- 1 tbsp. olive oil
- 1 tbsp. paprika
- 2 tsp hot smoked paprika
- 2 bay leaves
- Salt & pepper, to taste

Directions:
Heat oil in a large soup pot over med-high. Add steak and cook until browned, stirring frequently. Add onions and cook 5 minutes, or until soft. Add garlic and cook another minute, stirring frequently. Add remaining Ingredients. Stir well and bring to a boil. Reduce heat to med-low and simmer 45-50 minutes, stirring occasionally. Goulash is done when steak is tender. Stir well before serving.

Nutrition Info: Calories 413 Total Carbs 14g Protein 53g Fat 15g Sugar 8g Fiber 3g

320. Herbed Chicken And Artichoke Hearts

Servings: 4   Cooking Time: 20 Minutes
Ingredients:
- 2 tablespoons olive oil, divided
- 4 (6-ounce / 170-g) boneless, skinless chicken breast halves
- ½ teaspoon dried thyme, divided
- 1 teaspoon crushed dried rosemary, divided
- ½ teaspoon ground black pepper, divided
- 2 (14-ounce / 397-g) cans water-packed, low-sodium artichoke hearts, drained and quartered
- ½ cup low-sodium chicken broth
- 2 garlic cloves, chopped
- 1 medium onion, coarsely chopped
- ¼ cup shredded Parmesan cheese
- 1 lemon, cut into 8 slices
- 2 green onions, thinly sliced

Directions:
Preheat the oven to 375°F (190°C). Grease a baking sheet with 1 teaspoon of olive oil.   Place the chicken breasts on the baking sheet and rub with ¼ teaspoon of thyme, ½ teaspoon of rosemary, ¼ teaspoon of black pepper, and 1 tablespoon of olive oil.   Combine the artichoke hearts, chicken broth, garlic, onion, and remaining thyme, rosemary, black pepper, and olive oil. Toss to coat well.   Spread the artichoke around the chicken breasts, then scatter with Parmesan and lemon slices.   Place the baking sheet in the preheated oven and roast for 20 minutes or until the internal temperature of the chicken breasts reaches at least 165°F (74°C).   Remove the sheet from the oven. Allow to cool for 10 minutes, then serve with green onions on top.

Nutrition Info:calories: 339   fat: 9.0g   protein: 42.0g   carbs: 18.0g   fiber: 1.0g   sugar: 2.0g   sodium: 667mg

321. Mediterranean Lamb Meatballs

Servings: 4   Cooking Time: 40 Minutes
Ingredients:
- 454g ground lamb
- 3 cloves garlic, minced
- 5g of salt
- 1g black pepper
- 2g of mint, freshly chopped

- 2g ground cumin
- 3 ml hot sauce
- 1g chili powder
- 1 scallion, chopped
- 8g parsley, finely chopped
- 15 ml of fresh lemon juice
- 2g lemon zest
- 10 ml of olive oil

Directions:
Mix the lamb, garlic, salt, pepper, mint, cumin, hot sauce, chili powder, chives, parsley, lemon juice and lemon zest until well combined.   Create balls with the lamb mixture and cool for 30 minutes.   Select Preheat in the air fryer and press Start/Pause.   Cover the meatballs with olive oil and place them in the preheated fryer. Select Steak, set the time to 10 minutes and press Start/Pause.

Nutrition Info:(Nutrition per Serving):Calories: 282 Fat: 23.41 Carbohydrates: 0g Protein: 16.59 Sugar: 0g Cholesterol: 73gm

322. Italian Pork Medallions

Servings: 2   Cooking Time: 15 Minutes
Ingredients:
- ½ lb. pork tenderloin
- ¼ cup onion, diced
- What you'll need from store cupboard:
- 1 clove garlic, diced
- 2 tbsp. Italian bread crumbs
- 1 tbsp. reduced fat parmesan cheese
- 2 tsp olive oil
- ¼ tsp salt
- 1/8 tsp pepper

Directions:
Slice the tenderloin into 4 equal pieces. Flatten each piece to ¼-inch thick.   In a large Ziploc bag, combine bread crumbs, cheese, salt, and pepper.   Heat oil in a large skillet over medium heat. Add pork to the Ziploc bag, one piece at a time, and turn to coat.   Add the pork to the skillet and cook 2-3 minutes per side, or until no longer pink. Transfer to a plate and keep warm.   Add onion to the skillet and cook, stirring, until tender. Add garlic and cook 1 minute more. Serve pork topped with onions.

Nutrition Info: Calories 244 Total Carbs 7g Net Carbs 6g Protein 31g Fat 10g Sugar 1g Fiber 1g

323. Pork Diane

Servings: 4   Cooking Time: 20 Minutes
Ingredients:
- 2 teaspoons Worcestershire sauce
- 1 tablespoon freshly squeezed lemon juice
- ¼ cup low-sodium chicken broth
- 2 teaspoons Dijon mustard
- 4 (5-ounce / 142-g) boneless pork top loin chops, about 1 inch thick
- Sea salt and freshly ground black pepper, to taste
- 1 teaspoon extra-virgin olive oil
- 2 teaspoons chopped fresh chives
- 1 teaspoon lemon zest

Directions:

Combine the Worcestershire sauce, lemon juice, broth, and Dijon mustard in a bowl. Stir to mix well.   On a clean work surface, rub the pork chops with salt and ground black pepper.   Heat the olive oil in a nonstick skillet over medium-high heat until shimmering.   Add the pork chops and sear for 16 minutes or until well browned. Flip the pork halfway through the cooking time. Transfer to a plate and set aside.   Pour the sauce mixture in the skillet and cook for 2 minutes or until warmed through and lightly thickened. Mix in the chives and lemon zest.   Baste the pork with the sauce mixture and serve immediately.
Nutrition Info:calories: 200 fat: 8.0g protein: 30.0g carbs: 1.0g fiber: 0g sugar: 1.0g sodium: 394mg

324. Turkey Noodle Casserole

Servings: 4   Cooking Time: 45 Minutes
Ingredients:
- 2 cup turkey breast, cooked and cubed
- 10 oz. spinach, thaw and squeeze dry
- 1 cup fat free cottage cheese
- ¾ cup mozzarella cheese, grated
- What you'll need from store cupboard:
- Homemade Noodles, (chapter 15)
- 1 can low fat condensed cream of chicken soup
- 1/8 tsp garlic salt
- 1/8 tsp rosemary
- 1/8 tsp paprika
- Nonstick cooking spray

Directions:
Heat oven to 350 degrees. Spray a 2-quart casserole dish with cooking spray.   In a large bowl combine turkey, soup, and seasonings.   In a separate bowl combine spinach, cottage cheese, and half the mozzarella cheese. Place ½ the noodles in the prepared dish. Add half the turkey mixture and half the spinach mixture. Repeat. Cover with foil and bake 35 minutes. Uncover and sprinkle remaining cheese over top. Bake 10-15 minutes longer until edges are lightly browned.   Let rest 5 minutes before sprinkling with paprika. Serve.
Nutrition Info: Calories 267 Total Carbs 12g Net Carbs 10g Protein 26g Fat 8g Sugar 4g Fiber 2g

325. Cheesy Chicken & "potato" Casserole

Servings: 6   Cooking Time: 40 Minutes
Ingredients:
- 4 slices bacon, cooked and crumbled
- 3 cups cauliflower
- 3 cups chicken, cooked and chopped
- 3 cups broccoli florets
- 2 cups reduced fat cheddar cheese, grated
- 1 cup fat free sour cream
- 4 tbsp. margarine, soft
- What you'll need from store cupboard
- 1 tsp salt
- ½ tsp black pepper
- ½ tsp garlic powder
- ½ tsp paprika
- Nonstick cooking spray

Directions:

In a large saucepan add 4-5 cups of water and bring to a boil. Add the cauliflower and cook about 4-5 minutes, or until it is tender drain well. Repeat with broccoli.   Heat oven to 350 degrees. Spray a baking dish with cooking spray.   In a medium bowl, mash the cauliflower with the margarine, sour cream and seasonings. Add remaining Ingredients, saving ½ the cheese, and mix well.   Spread mixture in prepared baking dish and sprinkle remaining cheese on top. Bake 20-25 minutes, or until heated through and cheese has melted. Serve.
Nutrition Info: Calories 346 Total Carbs 10g Net Carbs 8g Protein 28g Fat 15g Sugar 4g Fiber 2g

326. Beef & Veggie Quesadillas

Servings: 4   Cooking Time: 10 Minutes
Ingredients:
- ¾ lb. lean ground beef
- 2 tomatoes, seeded and diced
- 1 onion, diced
- 1 zucchini, grated
- 1 carrot, grated
- ¾ cup mushrooms, diced
- ½ cup mozzarella cheese, grated
- ¼ cup cilantro, diced
- What you'll need from store cupboard:
- 4 8-inch whole wheat tortillas, warmed
- 2 cloves garlic, diced
- 2 tsp chili powder
- ¼ tsp salt
- ¼ tsp hot pepper sauce
- Nonstick cooking spray

Directions:
Heat oven to 400 degrees. Spray a large baking sheet with cooking spray.   Cook beef and onions in a large nonstick skillet over medium heat, until beef is no longer pink, drain fat. Transfer to a bowl and keep warm. Add the mushrooms, zucchini, carrot, garlic, chili powder, salt and pepper sauce to the skillet and cook until vegetables are tender.   Stir in the tomatoes, cilantro and beef. Lay the tortillas on the prepared pan. Cover half of each with beef mixture, and top with cheese. Fold other half over filling. Bake 5 minutes. Flip over and bake 5-6 minute more or until cheese has melted. Cut into wedges and serve.
Nutrition Info: Calories 319 Total Carbs 31g Net Carbs 26g Protein 33g Fat 7g Sugar 5g Fiber 5g

327. Sumptuous Lamb And Pomegranate Salad

Servings: 8   Cooking Time: 30 Minutes
Ingredients:
- 1½ cups pomegranate juice
- 4 tablespoons olive oil, divided
- 1 tablespoon ground cinnamon
- 1 teaspoon cumin
- 1 tablespoon ground ginger
- 3 cloves garlic, chopped
- Salt and freshly ground black pepper, to taste
- 1 (4-pound / 1.8-kg) lamb leg, deboned, butterflied, and fat trimmed

- 2 tablespoons pomegranate balsamic vinegar
- 2 teaspoons Dijon mustard
- ½ cup pomegranate seeds
- 5 cups baby kale
- 4 cups fresh green beans, blanched
- ¼ cup toasted walnut halves
- 2 fennel bulbs, thinly sliced
- 2 tablespoons Gorgonzola cheese

Directions:
Mix the pomegranate juice, 1 tablespoon of olive oil, cinnamon, cumin, ginger, garlic, salt, and black pepper in a large bowl. Stir to mix well.   Dunk the lamb leg in the mixture, press to coat well. Wrap the bowl in plastic and refrigerate to marinate for at least 8 hours. Remove the bowl from the refrigerate and let sit for 20 minutes. Pat the lamb dry with paper towels.   Preheat the grill to high heat.   Brush the grill grates with 1 tablespoon of olive oil, then arrange the lamb on the grill grates.   Grill for 30 minutes or until the internal temperature of the lamb reaches at least 145ºF (63ºC). Flip the lamb halfway through the cooking time. Remove the lamb from the grill and wrap with aluminum foil. Let stand for 15 minutes.   Meanwhile, Combine the vinegar, mustard, salt, black pepper, and remaining olive oil in a separate large bowl. Stir to mix well.   Add the remaining ingredients and lamb leg to the bowl and toss to combine well. Serve immediately.
Nutrition Info:calories: 380   fat: 21.0g   protein: 32.0g   carbs: 16.0g   fiber: 5.0g   sugar: 6.0g   sodium: 240mg

328. Mediterranean Grilled Chicken

Servings: 4   Cooking Time: 10 Minutes
Ingredients:
- 4 chicken breasts, boneless, skinless
- What you'll need from store cupboard:
- 6 oz. pesto
- ¼ cup olive oil
- ¼ cup lemon juice
- 2 tbsp. red wine vinegar
- 2 tsp garlic, diced fine

Directions:
In a large freezer bag or a container mix together the olive oil, lemon juice, red wine vinegar, minced garlic and pesto. Add chicken and toss to coat. Place in refrigerator and marinate for 6 to 8 hours.   Heat grill to med-high. Cook chicken, 3-4 minutes per side, or until cooked through. Or, you can bake it in a 400 degree oven until no longer pink, about 30 minutes. Serve.
Nutrition Info: Calories 378 Total Carbs 2g Protein 36g Fat 25g Sugar 2g Fiber 0g

329. Air Fried Meatloaf

Servings: 2   Cooking Time: 20 Minutes
Ingredients:
- ½ lb. ground beef
- ½ lb. ground turkey
- 1 onion, chopped
- ¼ cup panko bread crumbs
- 3 Tbsp. ketchup
- ¼ cup brown sugar

- 1 egg, beaten
- Salt and pepper to taste

Directions:
Preheat air fryer to 400 degrees.   Let the ground beef and ground turkey sit on the counter for 10 to 15 minutes, as it will be easier to hand mix without being chilled from the refrigerator.   Combine all the ingredients.   Form into a loaf in a dish and place the dish in the frying basket. Spritz the top with a little olive oil.   Bake for 25 minutes, or until well browned. Let settle for about 10 minutes before serving.
Nutrition Info: Calories: 381 Fat: 5g Carbohydrates: 9.6g Protein: 38g Sugar: 1.8g   Cholesterol: 0mg

330. Honey Garlic Chicken

Servings: 6   Cooking Time: 6 Hours
Ingredients:
- 6 chicken thighs
- What you'll need from store cupboard:
- 2 tbsp. sugar free ketchup
- 2 tbsp. honey
- 2 tbsp. lite soy sauce
- 3 cloves garlic, diced fine

Directions:
Add everything, except chicken, to the crock pot. Stir to combine.   Lay chicken, skin side up, in a single layer. Cover and cook on low 6 hours, or high for 3 hours. Place chicken in a baking dish and broil 2-3 minutes to caramelize the outside. Serve.
Nutrition Info: Calories 57 Total Carbs 7g Protein 4g Fat 2g Sugar 6g Fiber 0g

331. Potatoes With Bacon, Onion And Cheese

Servings: 4   Cooking Time: 15 Minutes
Ingredients:
- 200g potatoes
- 150g bacon
- 1 onion
- Slices of cheese
- Extra virgin olive oil
- Salt

Directions:
Peel the potatoes, cut into thin slices, and wash them well. Drain and dry the potatoes, put salt and a few strands of extra virgin olive oil.   Stir well and place in the basket of the air fryer.   Cut the onion into julienne, put a little oil, and stir, place on the potatoes.   Finally, put the sliced bacon on the onion.   Take the basket to the air fryer and select 20 minutes, 1800C.   From time to time, remove the basket.   Take all the contents of the basket to a source and when it is still hot, place the slices of cheese on top.   You can let the heat of the potatoes melt the cheese or you can gratin a few minutes in the oven.
Nutrition Info: Calories: 120 Fat: 3.41g Carbohydrates: 0g Protein: 20.99g Sugar: 0gCholesterol: 65mg

332. Crock Pot Beef Roast With Gravy

Servings: 10   Cooking Time: 5 ½ Hours

Ingredients:
- 3 lb. beef sirloin tip roast
- What you'll need from store cupboard:
- ¼ cup lite soy sauce
- ¼ cup water
- 3 tbsp. balsamic vinegar
- 2 tbsp. cornstarch
- 2 tbsp. coarse ground pepper
- 1 tbsp. Worcestershire sauce
- 2 tsp ground mustard
- 1 ½ tsp garlic, diced fine

Directions:
Rub roast with garlic and pepper. Cut in half and place in crock pot.   Combine soy sauce, vinegar, Worcestershire, and mustard, pour over roast.   Cover and cook on low heat 5 ½-6 hours or until beef is tender. Remove roast and keep warm. Strain juices into a small sauce pan, skim off fat. Heat over medium heat.   Stir water and cornstarch together until smooth. Stir into beef juices. Bring to a boil, and cook, stirring, 2 minutes or until thickened. Serve with roast.

Nutrition Info: Calories 264 Total Carbs 3g Protein 37g Fat 12g Sugar 0g Fiber 0g

333. Pork Paprika

Servings: 6   Cooking Time: 40 Minutes

Ingredients:
- 1 lb. pork loin, trim fat and cut into 1-inch cubes
- 1 onion, diced fine
- 1 cup mushrooms, sliced thick
- 2/3 cup fat free sour cream
- What you'll need from store cupboard:
- 1 can petite tomatoes, diced
- ½ cup low sodium chicken broth
- 2 tbsp. olive oil
- 2 tbsp. sweet paprika, divided
- 1 tbsp. garlic, diced fine
- ½ tsp thyme
- ½ tsp caraway seeds, ground
- Salt & pepper to taste

Directions:
Place pork in large bowl and sprinkle 1 tablespoon paprika, salt and pepper over meat, toss to coat.   Heat 1 tablespoon oil in a large, deep skillet over med-high heat. Add pork and cook, stirring frequently until brown on all sides, about 5-6 minutes. Transfer to a plate. Add remaining tablespoon of oil to skillet and the mushrooms. Cook, stirring, till browned and no more liquid remains in the pan, about 5 minutes. Add the mushrooms to the pork.   Add more oil if needed and the onion. Cook about 3-5 minutes, or they just start to brown. Add garlic and spices and cook another 1-2 minutes. Add tomatoes with juice and broth, cook, stirring frequently, until mixture starts to thicken, about 5 minutes.   Stir the pork and mushrooms into the sauce. Reduce heat, cover, and simmer 15 minutes, or until pork is tender. Serve.

Nutrition Info: Calories 267 Total Carbs 8g Net Carbs 7g 23g Protein 15g Fat Sugar 3g Fiber 1g

334. Asian Roasted Duck Legs

Servings: 4   Cooking Time: 90 Minutes

Ingredients:
- 4 duck legs
- 3 plum tomatoes, diced
- 1 red chili, deseeded and sliced
- ½ small Savoy cabbage, quartered
- 2 tsp fresh ginger, grated
- What you'll need from store cupboard:
- 3 cloves garlic, sliced
- 2 tbsp. soy sauce
- 2 tbsp. honey
- 1 tsp five-spice powder

Directions:
Heat oven to 350 degrees.   Place the duck in a large skillet over low heat and cook until brown on all sides and most of the fat is rendered, about 10 minutes. Transfer duck to a deep baking dish.   Drain off all but 2 tablespoons of the fat.   Add ginger, garlic, and chili to the skillet and cook 2 minutes until soft. Add soy sauce, tomatoes and 2 tablespoons water and bring to a boil. Rub the duck with the five spice seasoning. Pour the sauce over the duck and drizzle with the honey. Cover with foil and bake 1 hour. Add the cabbage for the last 10 minutes.

Nutrition Info: Calories 211 Total Carbs 19g Net Carbs 16g Protein 25g Fat 5g Sugar 14g Fiber 3g

335. Chicken & Spinach Pasta Skillet

Servings: 4   Cooking Time: 15 Minutes

Ingredients:
- 1 lb. chicken, boneless, skinless, cut into 1-inch pieces
- 10 cup fresh spinach, chopped
- 1 lemon, juiced and zested
- What you'll need from store cupboard:
- ½ recipe homemade pasta, (chapter 14) cook and drain
- ½ cup dry white wine
- 4 cloves garlic, diced fine
- 4 tbsp. reduced fat parmesan cheese, divided
- 2 tbsp. extra-virgin olive oil
- ½ tsp salt
- ¼ tsp ground pepper

Directions:
Heat oil in a large, deep skillet over med-high heat. Add chicken, salt and pepper. Cook, stirring occasionally, until just cooked through, 5-7 minutes.   Add garlic and cook, stirring, until fragrant, about 1 minute.   Stir in wine, lemon juice and zest; bring to a simmer. Remove from heat. Stir in spinach and pasta. Cover and let stand until the spinach is just wilted. Divide among 4 plates and top each serving with 1 tablespoon Parmesan.

Nutrition Info: Calories 415 Total Carbs 12g Net Carbs 9g Protein 40g Fat 19g Sugar 4g Fiber 3g

336. Short Ribs

Servings: 6   Cooking Time: 6 Hours

Ingredients:
- 4 lbs. lean beef short ribs
- 1 tablespoon canola oil
- ¼ cup onion, chopped
- ½ cup celery, chopped
- 3 garlic cloves, minced
- 8 oz. can tomato sauce
- ¼ teaspoon paprika
- ½ teaspoon black pepper

Directions:
Heat oil in a skillet over high heat. Add ribs, cook and brown all sides. Add ribs to a slow cooker.   Mix the remaining ingredients in a bowl and add over the ribs. Cover and cook for 6 hours on high heat. Serve.
Nutrition Info: Calories: 769 Fat: 3.41g Carbohydrates: 0g Protein: 20.99g Sugar: 0g

337. Turkey Meatball And Vegetable Kabobs

Servings: 6   Cooking Time: 20 Minutes
Ingredients:
- 20 ounces (567 g) lean ground turkey (93% fat-free)
- 2 egg whites
- 2 tablespoons grated Parmesan cheese
- 2 cloves garlic, minced
- ½ teaspoon salt, or to taste
- ¼ teaspoon ground black pepper
- 1 tablespoon olive oil
- 8 ounces (227 g) fresh cremini mushrooms, cut in half to make 12 pieces
- 24 cherry tomatoes
- 1 medium onion, cut into 12 pieces
- ¼ cup balsamic vinegar
- Special Equipment:
- 12 bamboo skewers, soaked in water for at least 30 minutes

Directions:
Mix the ground turkey, egg whites, Parmesan, garlic, salt, and pepper in a large bowl. Stir to combine well. Shape the mixture into 12 meatballs and place on a baking sheet. Refrigerate for at least 30 minutes. Preheat the oven to 375°F (190°C). Grease another baking sheet with 1 tablespoon of olive oil.   Remove the meatballs from the refrigerator. Run the bamboo skewers through 2 meatballs, 1 mushroom, 2 cherry tomatoes, and 1 onion piece alternatively.   Arrange the kabobs on the greased baking sheet and brush with balsamic vinegar.   Grill in the preheated oven for 20 minutes or until an instant-read thermometer inserted in the middle of the meatballs reads at least 165°F (74°C). Flip the kabobs halfway through the cooking time. Allow the kabobs to cool for 10 minutes, then serve warm.
Nutrition Info:calories: 200   fat: 8.0g   protein: 22.0g   carbs: 7.0g   fiber: 1.0g   sugar: 4.0g   sodium: 120mg

338. Roasted Duck Legs With Balsamic Mushrooms

Servings: 4   Cooking Time: 1 Hour

Ingredients:
- 4 bone-in, skin-on duck legs
- 1/2 lb. cremini mushrooms, remove stems and cut caps into thick slices
- 1 green onion, sliced thin
- 1 small shallot, sliced thin
- 3-4 fresh thyme sprigs, crushed lightly
- What you'll need from store cupboard:
- 5 Tbs. extra-virgin olive oil
- 5 Tbs. balsamic vinegar
- 2 cloves garlic, sliced thin
- ½ tsp fresh thyme, chopped
- Kosher salt and freshly ground pepper

Directions:
Rinse duck and pat dry with paper towels.   In a shallow glass bowl, large enough to hold the duck, combine 3 tablespoons oil, 3 tablespoons vinegar, garlic, shallot, thyme sprigs, ½ teaspoon salt and some pepper. Add the duck, turning to coat. Cover and chill 3-4 hours turning legs once or twice.   Remove the duck from the marinade. Pour the marinade into a saucepan and bring to a boil over high heat. Remove from heat.   Place a footed rack on the bottom of a large pot, tall enough that the duck legs can stand 2 inches from the bottom. Add about 1 inch of water. Place the duck, skin side up on the rack. Cover and bring to a boil over med-high heat. Let steam until the skin is translucent, about 20 minutes. While duck is steaming, heat the oven to 450 degrees. Line a roasting pan large enough to hold the duck with foil. Place a flat rack in the pan.   When the duck is ready, transfer it skin side up to the prepared rack. Brush the skin with the glaze and roast, until skin is brown and crisp, about 20 minutes. Remove from oven and glaze the duck again. Let rest for 5 minutes.   In a large skillet, over med-high heat, heat the remaining oil. Add mushrooms and green onions and cook, stirring frequently about 2 minutes. Add the remaining vinegar, chopped thyme, salt and pepper to taste. Cook until mushrooms are soft and most of the liquid has evaporated.   To serve, place duck leg on a plate and spoon mushrooms over.
Nutrition Info: Calories 374 Total Carbs 4g Net Carbs 3g Protein 26g Fat 28g Sugar 1g Fiber 1g

339. South Of The Border Chicken Casserole

Servings: 10   Cooking Time: 30 Minutes
Ingredients:
- 1 lb. chicken breast, cooked and shredded
- 1 red bell pepper, diced
- 1 onion, diced
- 1 cup pepper Jack cheese, grated
- ½ cup fat free sour cream
- ¼ cup half-n-half
- 2 tbsp. cilantro, diced fine
- What you'll need from store cupboard:
- 1 cup salsa
- 2 tbsp. olive oil
- 1 tbsp. chili powder
- 1 tbsp. cumin
- 2 tsp oregano

- 2 tsp salt
- 1 tsp pepper

Directions:

Heat oven to 350 degrees.   Heat the oil in a large skillet over med-high heat. Add the pepper, onion, salt and pepper and cook until soft.   In a large bowl, stir together chili powder, cumin, and oregano. Add sour cream, salsa, veggies, and chicken and mix well.   Pour mixture into a 9x13-inch baking dish. Pour the half-n-half evenly over the top and sprinkle with the cheese. Bake 30 minutes, or until heated through and cheese is starting to brown. Serve garnished with cilantro.

Nutrition Info: Calories 240 Total Carbs 8g Net Carb 7g Protein 20g Fat 14g Sugar 3g Fiber 1g

340. Swedish Beef Noodles

Servings: 4   Cooking Time: 20 Minutes

Ingredients:
- 1 lb. lean ground beef
- 8 oz. cremini mushrooms, sliced
- 1 cup onion, sliced thin
- ½ cup sour cream
- What you'll need from store cupboard:
- 3 ½ cup low sodium beef broth
- 1 tsp garlic salt
- 1 tsp caraway seed
- Homemade noodles, (chapter 14)
- Nonstick cooking spray

Directions:

Spray a large pot with cooking spray and heat over med-high heat. Add beef and cook, breaking up with spatula, 2 minutes. Add onions and mushrooms and cook until beef is browned and onions are soft.   Add the garlic salt, caraway seeds, and broth. Bring to a boil. Cover, reduce heat and simmer 10 minutes. Add noodles and cook another 3-5 minutes or noodles are done.   Stir in sour cream until blended and serve.

Nutrition Info: Calories 368 Total Carbs 12g Net Carbs 11g Protein 46g Fat 13g Sugar 5g Fiber 1g

341. Grilled Cajun Beef Tenderloin

Servings: 12   Cooking Time: 1 Hour

Ingredients:
- 3 lb. beef tenderloin
- What you'll need from store cupboard:
- 1 tbsp. paprika
- 4 tsp salt
- 2 ¼ tsp onion powder
- 2 tsp cayenne pepper
- 1 ½ tsp garlic powder
- 1 ½ tsp white pepper
- 1 ½ tsp black pepper
- 1 tsp basil
- ½ tsp chili powder
- 1/8 tsp thyme
- 1/8 tsp ground mustard
- Dash of cloves
- Nonstick cooking spray.

Directions:

Heat grill to medium heat. Spray rack with cooking spray. In a small bowl combine spices.   Tie tenderloin with butcher string in 2-inch intervals. Rub outside of beef with spice mixture.   Place on the grill, cover and cook 50 minutes, or to desired doneness. Or roast in 425 degree oven 45-60 minutes.   Let rest 10 minutes before slicing and serving.

Nutrition Info: Calories 234 Total Carbs 2g Protein 33g Fat 10g Sugar 0g Fiber 0g

342. Cashew Chicken

Servings: 4   Cooking Time: 10 Minutes

Ingredients:
- 1 lb. skinless boneless chicken breast, cut in cubes
- 1/2 onion, sliced
- 2 tbsp. green onion, diced
- ½ tsp fresh ginger, peeled and grated
- What you'll need from store cupboard:
- 1 cup whole blanched cashews, toasted
- 1 clove garlic, diced fine
- 4 tbsp. oil
- 2 tbsp. dark soy sauce
- 2 tbsp. hoisin sauce
- 2 tbsp. water
- 2 tsp cornstarch
- 2 tsp dry sherry
- 1 tsp Splenda
- 1 tsp sesame seed oil

Directions:

Place chicken in a large bowl and add cornstarch, sherry, and ginger. Stir until well mixed.   In a small bowl, whisk together soy sauce, hoisin, Splenda, and water stirring until smooth.   Heat the oil in a wok or a large skillet over high heat. Add garlic and onion and cook, stirring until garlic sizzles, about 30 seconds.   Stir in chicken and cook, stirring frequently, until chicken is almost done, about 2 minutes.   Reduce heat to medium and stir in sauce mixture. Continue cooking and stirring until everything is blended together. Add cashews and cook 30 seconds.   Drizzle with sesame oil, and cook another 30 seconds, stirring constantly. Serve immediately garnished with green onions.

Nutrition Info: Calories 483 Total Carbs 19g Net Carbs 17g Protein 33g Fat 32g Sugar 6g Fiber 2g

343. Pork Chops With Creamy Marsala Sauce

Servings: 4   Cooking Time: 20 Minutes

Ingredients:
- 4 thin boneless pork loin chops, (about 1 pound), trimmed
- 4 thin slices prosciutto, (2 ounces), chopped
- 1 small onion, halve and slice thin
- 1 cup low-fat milk
- 3 tsp fresh oregano, chopped fine
- 3 tsp fresh chives, chopped fine
- What you'll need from store cupboard:
- ½ cup Marsala, (see Note), divided
- ¼ cup flour
- 2 tsp cornstarch
- 2 tsp extra-virgin olive oil
- ¼ tsp kosher salt

- ¼ tsp freshly ground pepper

Directions:
Mix 2 tablespoons of the wine with cornstarch, set aside. Place flour in a shallow dish. Sprinkle chops with salt and pepper then coat in flour.   Heat oil in nonstick skillet over med-high heat. Once it gets hot, reduce heat to medium and add pork. Cook until browned on both sides, 2 minutes per side. Transfer to a plate.   Add prosciutto to the pan and cook, stirring constantly, about 1 minute, until browned. Add onion and cook, stirring frequently, 2-3 minutes until it starts to get soft.   Add remaining wine, oregano, and 1 ½ teaspoons chives to the pan and bring to a boil. Add milk and cornstarch mix and adjust heat to make sure mixture stays at a simmer. Stir occasionally until sauce has thickened and reduced slightly, about 4-6 minutes.   Add pork chops to the sauce, turning to coat, and cook until heated through. Serve topped with sauce and garnished with remaining chives.

Nutrition Info: Calories 499 Total Carbs 14g Net Carbs 13g Protein 32g Fat 32g Sugar 5g Fiber 1g

344. Chicken Skewers With Yogurt

Servings: 2-4   Cooking Time: 10 Minutes
Ingredients:
- 123g of plain whole milk Greek yogurt
- 20 ml of olive oil
- 2g of paprika
- 1g cumin
- 1g crushed red pepper
- 1 lemon, juice and zest of the peel
- 5g of salt
- 1g freshly ground black pepper
- 4 cloves garlic, minced
- 454g chicken thighs, boneless, skinless, cut into 38 mm pieces
- 2 wooden skewers, cut in half
- Nonstick Spray Oil

Directions:
Mix the yogurt, olive oil, paprika, cumin, red paprika, lemon juice, lemon zest, salt, pepper, and garlic in a large bowl.   Add the chicken to the marinade and marinate in the fridge for at least 4 hours.   Select Preheat and press Start/Pause.   Cut the marinated chicken thighs into 38 mm pieces and spread them on skewers.   Place the skewers in the preheated air fryer.   Cook at 200°C for 10 minutes.

Nutrition Info: Calories: 113 Fat: 3.4Carbohydrates: 0g Protein: 20.6g

345. Provencal Ribs

Servings: 4   Cooking Time: 1h 20 Minutes
Ingredients:
- 500g of pork ribs
- Provencal herbs
- Salt
- Ground pepper
- Oil

Directions:
Put the ribs in a bowl and add some oil, Provencal herbs, salt, and ground pepper.   Stir well and leave in the

fridge for at least 1 hour.   Put the ribs in the basket of the air fryer and select 2000C, 20 minutes.   From time to time, shake the basket and remove the ribs.

Nutrition Info: Calories: 296 Fat: 3.41g Carbohydrates: 0g Protein: 20.99g Sugar: 0gCholesterol: 90mg

346. Garlic Butter Steak

Servings: 4   Cooking Time: 8 Minutes
Ingredients:
- 1 lb. skirt steak
- 1/4 cup fresh parsley, diced, divided
- 5 tbsp. margarine
- What you'll need from store cupboard:
- 6 tsp garlic, diced fine
- 1 tbsp. olive oil
- Salt and pepper for taste

Directions:
Cut the steak into 4 pieces. Pat dry then season both sides with salt and pepper   Heat oil in a large, heavy skillet over med-high heat. Add steak and sear both sides, 2-3 minutes for medium rare, until it reaches desired doneness. Transfer to plate and cover with foil to keep warm.   Melt the margarine in a separate skillet over low heat. Add garlic and cook, stirring, until garlic is a light golden brown.   Pour the garlic mixture into a bowl and season with salt to taste. Slice the steak against the grain and place on plates. Sprinkle parsley over steak then drizzle with garlic mixture. Serve immediately.

Nutrition Info: Calories 365 Total Carbs 2g Protein 31g Fat 25g Sugar 0g Fiber 0g

347. Blue Cheese Crusted Beef Tenderloin

Servings: 4   Cooking Time: 15 Minutes
Ingredients:
- 4 beef tenderloin steaks
- 2 tbsp. blue cheese, crumbled
- 4 ½ tsp fresh parsley, diced
- 4 ½ tsp chives, diced
- 1 ½ tsp butter
- What you'll need from store cupboard:
- ½ cup low sodium beef broth
- 4 ½ tsp bread crumbs
- 1 tbsp. flour
- 1 tbsp. Madeira wine
- ¼ tsp pepper
- Nonstick cooking spray

Directions:
Heat oven to 350 degrees. Spray a large baking sheet with cooking spray.   In a small bowl, combine blue cheese, bread crumbs, parsley, chives, and pepper. Press onto one side of the steaks.   Spray a large skillet with cooking spray and place over med-high heat.   Add steaks and sear 2 minutes per side. Transfer to prepared baking sheet and bake 6-8 minutes, or steaks reach desired doneness.   Melt butter in a small saucepan over medium heat. Whisk in flour until smooth. Slowly whisk in broth and wine. Bring to a boil, cook, stirring, 2 minutes or until thickened.   Plate the steaks and top with gravy. Serve.

Nutrition Info: Calories 263 Total Carbs 4g Protein 36g Fat 10g Sugar 0g Fiber 0g

348. Turkey Enchiladas

Servings: 8   Cooking Time: 35 Minutes
Ingredients:
- 3 cup turkey, cooked and cut in pieces
- 1 onion, diced
- 1 bell pepper, diced
- 1 cup fat free sour cream
- 1 cup reduced fat cheddar cheese, grated
- What you'll need from store cupboard:
- 8 6-inch flour tortillas
- 14 ½ oz. low sodium chicken broth
- ¾ cup salsa
- 3 tbsp. flour
- 2 tsp olive oil
- 1 ¼ tsp coriander
- ¼ tsp pepper
- Nonstick cooking spray

Directions:
Spray a large saucepan with cooking spray and heat oil over med-high heat. Add onion and bell pepper and cook until tender.   Sprinkle with flour, coriander and pepper and stir until blended. Slowly stir in broth. Bring to a boil and cook, stirring, 2 minutes or until thickened. Remove from heat and stir in sour cream and ¾ cup cheese.   Heat oven to 350 degrees. Spray a 13x9-inch pan with cooking spray.   In a large bowl, combine turkey, salsa, and 1 cup of cheese mixture. Spoon 1/3 cup mixture down middle of each tortilla and roll up. Place seam side down in prepared dish.   Pour remaining cheese mixture over top of enchiladas. Cover and bake 20 minutes. Uncover and sprinkle with remaining cheese. Bake another 5-10 minutes until cheese is melted and starts to brown.

Nutrition Info: Calories 304 Total Carbs 29g Net Carbs 27g Protein 23g Fat 10g Sugar 5g Fiber 2g

349. Easy Carbonara

Servings: 2   Cooking Time: 10 Minutes
Ingredients:
- 1 slice bacon, thick cut
- 1 egg
- ½ tbsp. fresh parsley, diced
- What you'll need from store cupboard:
- Homemade Noodles, chapter 15
- ¼ cup reduced fat parmesan cheese
- Black pepper, to taste

Directions:
Bring a large pot of salted water to a boil. Add the noodles and cook 1-2 minutes.   In a small bowl, beat the egg and parmesan cheese together.   Cook the bacon in a large pan until crispy. Remove the bacon (turn off the heat and leave the fat in the pan) and drain on a paper towel before cutting it into small pieces.   Once the noodles have boiled add them to the pan with the bacon fat. Pour the egg mixture over the hot pasta and toss together quickly (the heat from the pasta will cook the egg).   Add the chopped parsley, bacon and black pepper and continue tossing until combined. Serve.

Nutrition Info: Calories 237 Total Carbs 2g Protein 17g Fat 18g Sugar 0g Fiber 0g

350. Chicken Cordon Bleu

Servings: 8   Cooking Time: 25 Minutes
Ingredients:
- 8 chicken breast halves, boneless and skinless
- 8 slices ham
- 1 ½ cup mozzarella cheese, grated
- 2/3 cup skim milk
- ½ cup fat free sour cream
- What you'll need from store cupboard:
- 1 can low fat condensed cream of chicken soup
- 1 cup corn flakes, crushed
- 1 tsp lemon juice
- 1 tsp paprika
- ½ tsp pepper
- ½ tsp garlic powder
- ¼ tsp salt
- Nonstick cooking spray

Directions:
Heat oven to 350 degrees. Spray a 13x9-inch baking dish with cooking spray.   Flatten chicken to ¼-inch thick. Sprinkle with pepper and top with slice of ham and 3 tablespoons of cheese down the middle. Roll up, tuck ends under and secure with a toothpick.   Pour milk into a shallow bowl. In a separate shallow bowl, combine corn flakes and seasonings. Dip chicken in milk then roll in corn flake mixture and place in prepared dish.   Bake 25-30 minutes or until chicken is cooked through.   In a small saucepan, whisk together soup, sour cream, and lemon juice until combined. Cook over medium heat until hot.   Remove toothpicks from chicken and place on plates, top with sauce and serve.

Nutrition Info: Calories 382 Total Carbs 9g Net Carbs 8g Protein 50g Fat 14g Sugar 2g Fiber 1g

Meatless Recipes

351. Harvest Salad

Servings: 6   Cooking Time: 25 Minutes
Ingredients:
- 10 oz. kale, deboned and chopped
- 1 ½ cup blackberries
- ½ butternut squash, cubed
- ¼ cup goat cheese, crumbled
- What you'll need from store cupboard:
- Maple Mustard Salad Dressing (chapter 16)
- 1 cup raw pecans
- 1/3 cup raw pumpkin seeds
- ¼ cup dried cranberries
- 3 1/2 tbsp. olive oil
- 1 ½ tbsp. sugar free maple syrup
- 3/8 tsp salt, divided
- Pepper, to taste
- Nonstick cooking spray

Directions:
Heat oven to 400 degrees. Spray a baking sheet with cooking spray.   Spread squash on the prepared pan, add 1 ½ tablespoons oil, 1/8 teaspoon salt, and pepper to squash and stir to coat the squash evenly. Bake 20-25 minutes.   Place kale in a large bowl. Add 2 tablespoons oil and ½ teaspoon salt and massage it into the kale with your hands for 3-4 minutes.   Spray a clean baking sheet with cooking spray. In a medium bowl, stir together pecans, pumpkin seeds, and maple syrup until nuts are coated. Pour onto prepared pan and bake 8-10 minutes, these can be baked at the same time as the squash.   To assemble the salad: place all of the Ingredients in a large bowl. Pour dressing over and toss to coat. Serve.
Nutrition Info: Calories 436 Total Carbs 24g Net Carbs 17g Protein 9g Fat 37g Sugar 5g Fiber 7g

352. Spicy Potatoes

Servings: 4   Cooking Time: 30 Minutes
Ingredients:
- 400g potatoes
- 2 tbsp. spicy paprika
- 1 tbsp. olive oil
- cottage cheese
- Salt to taste

Directions:
Wash the potatoes with a brush. Unpeeled, cut vertically in a crescent shape, about 1 finger thick Place the potatoes in a bowl and cover with water. Let stand for about half an hour.   Preheat the air fryer. Set the timer of 5 minutes and the temperature to 2000C.   Drain the water from the potatoes and dry with paper towels or a clean cloth. Put them back in the bowl and pour the oil, salt and paprika over them. Mix well with your hands so that all of them are covered evenly with the spice mixture. Pour the spiced potatoes in the basket of the air fryer. Set the timer for 30 minutes and press the power button. Stir the potatoes in half the time.   Remove the potatoes from the air fryer, place on a plate.

Nutrition Info: Calories: 153 Cal Carbs: 2 g Fat: 11 g Protein: 4 g Fiber: 0 g

353. Buffalo Cauliflower Wings

Servings: 6   Cooking Time: 30 Minutes
Ingredients:
- 1-tablespoon almond flour
- 1 medium head of cauliflower
- 1 ½-teaspoon salt
- 4 tablespoons hot sauce
- 1-tablespoon olive oil

Directions:
Switch on the air fryer, insert fryer basket, grease it with olive oil, then shut with its lid, set the fryer at 400 degrees F and preheat for 5 minutes.   Meanwhile, cut cauliflower into bite-size florets and set aside.   Place flour in a large bowl, whisk in salt, oil and hot sauce until combined, add cauliflower florets and toss until combined.   Open the fryer, add cauliflower florets in it in a single layer, close with its lid and cook for 15 minutes until nicely golden and crispy, shaking halfway through the frying.   When air fryer beeps, open its lid, transfer cauliflower florets onto a serving plate and keep warm. Cook the remaining cauliflower florets in the same manner and serve.
Nutrition Info: Calories: 48 Cal Carbs: 2 g Fat: 11 g Protein: 4 g Fiber: 0.3 g

354. Asian Noodle Salad

Servings: 4
Ingredients:
- 2 carrots, sliced thin
- 2 radish, sliced thin
- 1 English cucumber, sliced thin
- 1 mango, julienned
- 1 bell pepper, julienned
- 1 small serrano pepper, seeded and sliced thin
- 1 bag tofu Shirataki Fettuccini noodles
- ¼ cup lime juice
- ¼ cup fresh basil, chopped
- ¼ cup fresh cilantro, chopped
- 2 tbsp. fresh mint, chopped
- What you'll need from the store cupboard
- 2 tbsp. rice vinegar
- 2 tbsp. sweet chili sauce
- 2 tbsp. roasted peanuts finely chopped
- 1 tbsp. Splenda
- ½ tsp sesame oil

Directions:
Pickle the vegetables: In a large bowl, place radish, cucumbers, and carrots. Add vinegar, coconut sugar, and lime juice and stir to coat the vegetables. Cover and chill 15 – 20 minutes.   Prep the noodles: remove the noodles from the package and rinse under cold water. Cut into smaller pieces. Pat dry with paper towels.   To assemble the salad. Remove the vegetables from the marinade, reserving marinade, and place in a large mixing bowl. Add noodles, mango, bell pepper, chili, and herbs.   In a small bowl, combine 2 tablespoons

marinade with the chili sauce and sesame oil. Pour over salad and toss to coat. Top with peanuts and serve.
Nutrition Info: Calories 158 Total Carbs 30g Net Carbs 24g Protein 4g Fat 4g Sugar 19g Fiber 6g

355. Cheesy Mushroom And Pesto Flatbreads

Servings: 2   Cooking Time: 13 To 17 Minutes
Ingredients:
- 1 teaspoon extra-virgin olive oil
- ½ red onion, sliced
- ½ cup sliced mushrooms
- Salt and freshly ground black pepper, to taste
- ¼ cup store-bought pesto sauce
- 2 whole-wheat flatbreads
- ¼ cup shredded Mozzarella cheese

Directions:
Preheat the oven to 350°F (180°C).   Heat the olive oil in a small skillet over medium heat. Add the onion slices and mushrooms to the skillet, and sauté for 3 to 5 minutes, stirring occasionally, or until they start to soften. Season with salt and pepper.   Meanwhile, spoon 2 tablespoons of pesto sauce onto each flatbread and spread it all over. Evenly divide the mushroom mixture between two flatbreads, then scatter each top with 2 tablespoons of shredded cheese.   Transfer the flatbreads to a baking sheet and bake until the cheese melts and bubbles, about 10 to 12 minutes.   Let the flatbreads cool for 5 minutes and serve warm.
Nutrition Info:calories: 346   fat: 22.8g   protein: 14.2g   carbs: 27.6g   fiber: 7.3g   sugar: 4.0g   sodium: 790mg

356. Honey Roasted Carrots

Servings: 2-4   Cooking Time: 12 Minutes
Ingredients:
- 454g of rainbow carrots, peeled and washed
- 15 ml of olive oil
- 30 ml honey
- 2 sprigs of fresh thyme
- Salt and pepper to taste

Directions:
Wash the carrots and dry them with a paper towel. Leave aside.   Preheat the air fryer for a few minutes an 1800C. Place the carrots in a bowl with olive oil, honey, thyme, salt, and pepper. Place the carrots in the air fryer at 1800C for 12 minutes. Be sure to shake the baskets in the middle of cooking.
Nutrition Info: Calories: 123Fat: 42g Carbohydrate: 9g Protein: 1g

357. Mushrooms Stuffed With Tomato

Servings: 4   Cooking Time: 50 Minutes
Ingredients:
- 8 large mushrooms
- 250g of minced meat
- 4 cloves of garlic
- Extra virgin olive oil
- Salt
- Ground pepper
- Flour, beaten egg and breadcrumbs
- Frying oil
- Fried Tomato Sauce

Directions:
Remove the stem from the mushrooms and chop it. Peel the garlic and chop. Put some extra virgin olive oil in a pan and add the garlic and mushroom stems.   Sauté and add the minced meat. Sauté well until the meat is well cooked and season.   Fill the mushrooms with the minced meat.   Press well and take the freezer for 30 minutes.   Pass the mushrooms with flour, beaten egg and breadcrumbs. Beaten egg and breadcrumbs. Place the mushrooms in the basket of the air fryer. Select 20 minutes, 1800C.   Distribute the mushrooms once cooked in the dishes.   Heat the tomato sauce and cover the stuffed mushrooms.
Nutrition Info: Calories: 160 Cal Carbs: 2 g Fat: 11 g Protein: 4 g Fiber: 0 g

358. Cheesy Summer Squash And Quinoa Casserole

Servings: 8   Cooking Time: 27 To 30 Minutes
Ingredients:
- 1 tablespoon extra-virgin olive oil
- 1 Vidalia onion, thinly sliced
- 1 large portobello mushroom, thinly sliced
- 6 yellow summer squash, thinly sliced
- 1 cup shredded Parmesan cheese, divided
- 1 cup shredded Cheddar cheese
- ½ cup tri-color quinoa
- ½ cup whole-wheat bread crumbs
- 1 tablespoon Creole seasoning

Directions:
Preheat the oven to 350°F (180°C).   Heat the olive oil in a large cast iron pan over medium heat.   Sauté the onion, mushroom, and squash in the oil for 7 to 10 minutes, stirring occasionally, or until the vegetables are softened.   Remove from the heat and add ½ cup of Parmesan cheese and the Cheddar cheese to the vegetables. Stir well.   Mix together the quinoa, bread crumbs, the remaining Parmesan cheese, Creole seasoning in a small bowl, then scatter the mixture over the vegetables.   Place the cast iron pan in the preheated oven and bake until browned and cooked through, about 20 minutes.   Cool for 10 minutes and serve on plates while warm.
Nutrition Info:calories: 184   fat: 8.9g   protein: 11.7g   carbs: 17.6g   fiber: 3.2g   sugar: 3.8g   sodium: 140mg

359. Eggplant Parmesan

Servings: 4   Cooking Time: 15 Minutes
Ingredients:
- 1/2 cup and 3 tablespoons almond flour, divided
- 1.25-pound eggplant, ½-inch sliced
- One tablespoon chopped parsley
- 1 teaspoon Italian seasoning
- 2 teaspoons salt
- 1-cup marinara sauce
- 1 egg, pastured

- 1-tablespoon water
- 3 tablespoons grated parmesan cheese, reduced-fat
- 1/4 cup grated mozzarella cheese, reduced-fat

Directions:
Slice the eggplant into ½-inch pieces, place them in a colander, sprinkle with 1 ½-teaspoon salt on both sides and let it rest for 15 minutes. Meanwhile, place ½-cup flour in a bowl, add egg and water and whisk until blended. Place remaining flour in a shallow dish, add remaining salt, Italian seasoning, and parmesan cheese and stir until mixed. Switch on the air fryer, insert fryer basket, grease it with olive oil, then shut with its lid, set the fryer at 360 degrees F and preheat for 5 minutes. Meanwhile, drain the eggplant pieces, pat them dry, and then dip each slice into the egg mixture and coat with flour mixture. Open the fryer; add coated eggplant slices in it in a single layer, close with its lid and cook for 8 minutes until nicely golden and cooked, flipping the eggplant slices halfway through the frying. Then top each eggplant slice with a tablespoon of marinara sauce and some of the mozzarella cheese and continue air frying for 1 to 2 minutes or until cheese has melted. When air fryer beeps, open its lid, transfer eggplants onto a serving plate and keep them warm. Cook remaining eggplant slices in the same manner and serve.
Nutrition Info: Calories: 123 Cal Carbs: 2 g Fat: 11 g Protein: 4 g Fiber: 6 g

360. Sweet Potato Salt And Pepper

Servings: 4   Cooking Time: 20 Minutes
Ingredients:
- 1 large sweet potato
- Extra virgin olive oil
- Salt
- Ground pepper

Directions:
Peel the sweet potato and cut into thin strips, if you have a mandolin it will be easier for you. Wash well and put salt. Add a little oil to impregnate the sweet potato in strips and place in the air fryer basket. Select 180oC, 30 minutes or so. From time to time, shake the basket so that the sweet potato moves. Pass to a tray or plate and sprinkle with fine salt and ground pepper.
Nutrition Info: Calories: 107 Fat: 0.6g Carbohydrates: 24.19g Protein: 1.61g Sugar: 5.95g Cholesterol: 0mg

361. Simple Sautéed Greens

Servings: 4   Cooking Time: 10 Minutes
Ingredients:
- 2 tablespoons extra-virgin olive oil
- 1 pound (454 g) Swiss chard, coarse stems removed and leaves chopped
- 1 pound (454 g) kale, coarse stems removed and leaves chopped
- ½ teaspoon ground cardamom
- 1 tablespoon freshly squeezed lemon juice
- Sea salt and freshly ground black pepper, to taste

Directions:
Heat the olive oil in a large skillet over medium-high heat. Add the Swiss chard, kale, cardamon, and lemon juice to the skillet, and stir to combine. Cook for about 10 minutes, stirring continuously, or until the greens are wilted. Sprinkle with the salt and pepper and stir well. Serve the greens on a plate while warm.
Nutrition Info:calories: 139   fat: 6.8g   protein: 5.9g carbs: 15.8g   fiber: 3.9g   sugar: 1.0g   sodium: 350mg

362. Sweet Potato Chips

Servings: 4   Cooking Time: 10 Minutes
Ingredients:
- 2 large sweet potatoes, cut into strips 25 mm thick
- 15 ml of oil
- 10g of salt
- 2g black pepper
- 2g of paprika
- 2g garlic powder
- 2g onion powder

Directions:
Cut the sweet potatoes into strips 25 mm thick. Preheat the air fryer for a few minutes. Add the cut sweet potatoes in a large bowl and mix with the oil until the potatoes are all evenly coated. Sprinkle salt, black pepper, paprika, garlic powder and onion powder. Mix well. Place the French fries in the preheated baskets and cook for 10 minutes at 205oC. Be sure to shake the baskets halfway through cooking.
Nutrition Info: Calories: 123 Cal Carbs: 2 g Fat: 11 g Protein: 4 g Fiber: 0 g

363. Chili Relleno Casserole

Servings: 8   Cooking Time: 35 Minutes
Ingredients:
- 3 eggs
- 1 cup Monterey jack pepper cheese, grated
- 3⁄4 cup half-n-half
- ½ cup cheddar cheese, grated
- What you'll need from store cupboard:
- 2 (7 oz.) cans whole green chilies, drain well
- ½ tsp salt
- Nonstick cooking spray

Directions:
Heat oven to 350 degrees. Spray an 8-inch baking pan with cooking spray. Slice each chili down one long side and lay flat. Arrange half the chilies in the prepared baking pan, skin side down, in single layer. Sprinkle with the pepper cheese and top with remaining chilies, skin side up. In a small bowl, beat eggs, salt, and half-n-half. Pour over chilies. Top with cheddar cheese. Bake 35 minutes, or until top is golden brown. Let rest 10 minutes before serving.
Nutrition Info: Calories 295 Total Carbs 36g Net Carbs 22g Protein 13g Fat 13g Sugar 21g Fiber 14g

364. Cauliflower Rice

Servings: 3   Cooking Time: 27 Minutes
Ingredients:
- 1 cup diced carrot
- 6 ounces tofu, extra-firm, drained
- 1/2 cup diced white onion
- 2 tablespoons soy sauce
- 1-teaspoon turmeric

- For the Cauliflower:
- 1/2 cup chopped broccoli
- 3 cups cauliflower rice
- 1 tablespoon minced garlic
- 1/2 cup frozen peas
- 1 tablespoon minced ginger
- 2 tablespoons soy sauce
- 1-tablespoon apple cider vinegar
- 1 1/2 teaspoons toasted sesame oil

Directions:
Switch on the air fryer, insert fryer pan, grease it with olive oil, then shut with its lid, set the fryer at 370 degrees F and preheat for 5 minutes.   Meanwhile, place tofu in a bowl, crumble it, then add remaining ingredients and stir until mixed.   Open the fryer, add tofu mixture in it, and spray with oil, close with its lid and cook for 10 minutes until nicely golden and crispy, stirring halfway through the frying.   Meanwhile, place all the ingredients for cauliflower in a bowl and toss until mixed. When air fryer beeps, open its lid, add cauliflower mixture, shake the pan gently to mix and continue cooking for 12 minutes, shaking halfway through the frying.

Nutrition Info: Calories: 258 Cal Carbs: 2 g Fat: 11 g Protein: 4 g Fiber: 7 g

365. Autumn Slaw

Servings: 8   Cooking Time: 2 Hours
Ingredients:
- 10 cup cabbage, shredded
- ½ red onion, diced fine
- ¾ cup fresh Italian parsley, chopped
- What you'll need from store cupboard:
- ¾ cup almonds, slice & toasted
- ¾ cup dried cranberries
- 1/3 cup vegetable oil
- ¼ cup apple cider vinegar
- 2 tbsp. sugar free maple syrup
- 4 tsp Dijon mustard
- ½ teaspoon salt
- Salt & pepper, to taste

Directions:
In a large bowl, whisk together vinegar, oil, syrup, Dijon, and ½ teaspoon salt. Add the onion and stir to combine. Let rest 10 minutes, or cover and refrigerate until ready to use.   After 10 minutes, add remaining Ingredients to the dressing mixture and toss to coat. Taste and season with salt and pepper if needed. Cover and chill 2 hours before serving.

Nutrition Info: Calories 133   Total Carbs 12g net Carbs 8g Protein 2g Fat 9g Sugar 5g Fiber 4g

366. Pizza Stuffed Portobello's

Servings: 4   Cooking Time: 10 Minutes
Ingredients:
- 8 Portobello mushrooms, stems removed
- 1 cup mozzarella cheese, grated
- 1 cup cherry tomatoes, sliced
- ½ cup crushed tomatoes
- ½ cup fresh basil, chopped
- What you'll need from store cupboard:

- 2 tbsp. balsamic vinegar
- 1 tbsp. olive oil
- 1 tbsp. oregano
- 1 tbsp. red pepper flakes
- ½ tbsp. garlic powder
- ¼ tsp pepper
- Pinch salt

Directions:
Heat oven to broil. Line a baking sheet with foil.   Place mushrooms, stem side down, on foil and drizzle with oil. Sprinkle with garlic powder, salt and pepper. Broil for 5 minutes.   Flip mushrooms over and top with crushed tomatoes, oregano, parsley, pepper flakes, cheese and sliced tomatoes. Broil another 5 minutes.   Top with basil and drizzle with balsamic. Serve.

Nutrition Info: Calories 113 Total Carbs 11g Net Carbs 7g Protein 9g Fat 5g Sugar 3g Fiber 4g

367. Cajun Style French Fries

Servings: 4   Cooking Time: 28 Minutes
Ingredients:
- 2 reddish potatoes, peeled and cut into strips of 76 x 25 mm
- 1 liter of cold water
- 15 ml of oil
- 7g of Cajun seasoning
- 1g cayenne pepper
- Tomato sauce or ranch sauce, to serve

Directions:
Cut the potatoes into 76 x 25 mm strips and soak them in water for 15 minutes.   Drain the potatoes, rinse with cold, dry water with paper towels.   Preheat the air fryer, set it to 195°C.   Add oil and spices to the potatoes, until they are completely covered.   Add the potatoes to the preheated air fryer and set the timer to 28 minutes.   Be sure to shake the baskets in the middle of cooking Remove the baskets from the air fryer when you have finished cooking and season the fries with salt and pepper.

Nutrition Info: Calories: 158 Cal Carbs: 2 g Fat: 11 g Protein: 4 g Fiber: 0 g

368. Avocado & Citrus Shrimp Salad

Servings: 4   Cooking Time: 5 Minutes
Ingredients:
- 1 lb. medium shrimp, peeled and deveined, remove tails
- 8 cup salad greens
- 1 lemon
- 1 avocado, diced
- 1 shallot, diced fine
- What you'll need from store cupboard:
- ½ cup almonds, sliced and toasted
- 1 tbsp. olive oil
- Salt and freshly ground black pepper

Directions:
Cut the lemon in half and squeeze the juice, from both halves, into a small bowl, set aside. Slice the lemon into thin wedges.   Heat the oil in a skillet over medium heat. Add lemon wedges and let cook, about 1 minute, to infuse the oil with the lemons.   Add the shrimp and

cook, stirring frequently, until shrimp turn pink. Discard the lemon wedges and let cool.   Place the salad greens in a large bowl. Add the shrimp, with the juices from the pan, and toss to coat. Add remaining Ingredients and toss to combine. Serve.
Nutrition Info: Calories 425 Total Carbs 17 Net Carbs 8g Protein 35 Fat 26 Sugar 2 Fiber 9

369. Florentine Pizza

Servings: 2   Cooking Time: 20 Minutes
Ingredients:
- 1 3/4 cup grated mozzarella cheese
- ½ cup frozen spinach, thaw
- 1 egg
- 2 tbsp. reduced fat parmesan cheese, grated
- 2 tbsp. cream cheese, soft
- What you'll need from the store cupboard
- ¾ cup almond flour
- ¼ cup light Alfredo sauce
- ½ tsp Italian seasoning
- ¼ tsp red pepper flakes
- Pinch of salt

Directions:
Heat oven to 400 degrees.   Squeeze all the excess water out of the spinach.   In a glass bowl, combine mozzarella and almond flour. Stir in cream cheese. Microwave 1 minute on high, then stir. If the mixture is not melted, microwave another 30 seconds.   Stir in the egg, seasoning, and salt. Mix well. Place dough on a piece of parchment paper and press into a 10-inch circle. Place directly on the oven rack and bake 8-10 minutes or until lightly browned.   Remove the crust and spread with the Alfredo sauce, then add spinach, parmesan and red pepper flakes evenly over top. Bake another 8-10 minutes. Slice and serve.
Nutrition Info: Calories 441 Total Carbs 14g Net Carbs 9g Protein 24g Fat 35g Sugar 4g Fiber 5g

370. Vegetables In Air Fryer

Servings: 2   Cooking Time: 30 Minutes
Ingredients:
- 2 potatoes
- 1 zucchini
- 1 onion
- 1 red pepper
- 1 green pepper

Directions:
Cut the potatoes into slices.   Cut the onion into rings. Cut the zucchini slices   Cut the peppers into strips. Put all the ingredients in the bowl and add a little salt, ground pepper and some extra virgin olive oil.   Mix well.   Pass to the basket of the air fryer.   Select 1600C, 30 minutes.   Check that the vegetables are to your liking.
Nutrition Info: Calories: 135Cal Carbs: 2 g Fat: 11 g Protein: 4 g Fiber: 05g

371. Tofu Bento

Servings: 4   Cooking Time: 10 Minutes
Ingredients:
- 1 pkg. extra firm tofu

- 1 red bell pepper, sliced
- 1 orange bell pepper, sliced
- 2 cup cauliflower rice, cooked
- 2 cups broccoli, chopped
- ¼ cup green onion, sliced
- What you'll need from store cupboard:
- 2 tbsp. low-sodium soy sauce
- 1 tbsp. olive oil
- 1 tsp ginger,
- 1 tsp garlic powder
- 1 tsp onion powder
- 1 tsp chili paste

Directions:
Remove tofu from package and press with paper towels to absorb all excess moisture, let set for 15 minutes. Chop tofu into cubes. Add tofu and seasonings to a large Ziploc bag and shake to coat.   Heat oil in a large skillet over medium heat. Add tofu and vegetables and cook, stirring frequently, 5-8 minutes, until tofu is browned on all sides and vegetables are tender.   To serve, place ½ cup cauliflower rice on 4 plates and top evenly with tofu mixture.
Nutrition Info: Calories 93 Total Carbs 12g Net Carbs 8g Protein 7g Fat 3g Sugar 5g Fiber 4g

372. Tofu In Peanut Sauce

Servings: 4   Cooking Time: 1 Hour 25 Minutes
Ingredients:
- 1 pkg. extra firm tofu, pressed 15 minutes and cut into cubes
- 1 pkg. fresh baby spinach
- 2 limes
- 1 tbsp. margarine
- What you'll need from store cupboard:
- ½ cup raw peanut butter
- 2 tbsp. lite soy sauce
- 3 cloves garlic, chopped fine
- ½ tsp ginger
- ¼ tsp red pepper flakes

Directions:
Melt margarine in a large saucepan. Add tofu and garlic and cook, stirring occasionally, 5-10 minutes, or until tofu starts to brown.   Add remaining Ingredients, except spinach and bring to simmer. Reduce heat, cover and cook, stirring occasionally 30-35 minutes.   Stir in the spinach and cook 15 minutes more. Serve.
Nutrition Info: Calories 325 Total Carbs 15g Net Carbs 10g Protein 18g Fat 24g Sugar 5g Fiber 5g

373. Mexican Scrambled Eggs & Greens

Servings: 4   Cooking Time: 5 Minutes
Ingredients:
- 8 egg whites
- 4 egg yolks
- 3 tomatoes, cut in ½-inch pieces
- 1 jalapeno pepper, slice thin
- ½ avocado, cut in ½-inch pieces
- ½ red onion, diced fine
- ½ head Romaine lettuce, torn
- ½ cup cilantro, chopped
- 2 tbsp. fresh lime juice

97

- What you'll need from store cupboard:
- 12 tortilla chips, (chapter 5), broken into small pieces
- 2 tbsp. water
- 1 tbsp. olive oil
- ¾ tsp pepper, divided
- ½ tsp salt, divided

Directions:
In a medium bowl, combine tomatoes, avocado, onion, jalapeno, cilantro, lime juice, ¼ teaspoon salt, and ¼ teaspoon pepper.   In a large bowl, whisk egg whites, egg yolks, water, and remaining salt and pepper. Stir in tortilla chips.   Heat oil in a large skillet over medium heat. Add egg mixture and cook, stirring frequently, 3-5 minutes, or desired doneness.   To serve, divide lettuce leaves among 4 plates. Add scrambled egg mixture and top with salsa.

Nutrition Info: Calories 280 Total Carbs 10g Net Carbs 6g Protein 15g Fat 21g Sugar 4g Fiber 4g

374. Sweet Potato Cauliflower Patties

Servings: 7   Cooking Time: 40 Minutes
Ingredients:
- 1 green onion, chopped
- 1 large sweet potato, peeled
- 1 teaspoon minced garlic
- 1-cup cilantro leaves
- 2-cup cauliflower florets
- ¼-teaspoon ground black pepper
- 1/4 teaspoon salt
- 1/4 cup sunflower seeds
- 1/4 teaspoon cumin
- 1/4 cup ground flaxseed
- 1/2 teaspoon red chili powder
- 2 tablespoons ranch seasoning mix
- 2 tablespoons arrowroot starch

Directions:
Cut peeled sweet potato into small pieces, and then place them in a food processor and pulse until pieces are broken up.   Then add onion, cauliflower florets, and garlic, pulse until combined, add remaining ingredients and pulse more until incorporated.   Tip the mixture in a bowl, shape the mixture into seven 1 ½ inch thick patties, each about ¼ cup, then place them on a baking sheet and freeze for 10 minutes.   Switch on the air fryer, insert fryer basket, grease it with olive oil, then shut with its lid, set the fryer at 400 degrees F and preheat for 10 minutes.   Open the fryer, add patties in it in a single layer, close with its lid and cook for 20 minutes until nicely golden and cooked, flipping the patties halfway through the frying.   When air fryer beeps, open its lid, transfer patties onto a serving plate and keep them warm. Cook the remaining patties in the same manner and serve.

Nutrition Info: Calories: 85Cal Carbs: 2 g Fat: 11 g Protein: 4 g Fiber: 5 g

375. Healthy Taco Salad

Servings: 4   Cooking Time: 10 Minutes
Ingredients:
- 2 whole Romaine hearts, chopped

- 1 lb. lean ground beef
- 1 whole avocado, cubed
- 3 oz. grape tomatoes, halved
- ½ cup cheddar cheese, cubed
- 2 tbsp. sliced red onion
- What you'll need from the store cupboard
- 1/2 batch Tangy Mexican Salad Dressing (chapter 16)
- 1 tsp ground cumin
- Salt and pepper to taste

Directions:
Cook ground beef in a skillet over medium heat. Break the beef up into little pieces as it cooks. Add seasonings and stir to combine. Drain grease and let cool for about 5 minutes.   To assemble the salad, place all Ingredients into a large bowl. Toss to mix then add dressing and toss. Top with reduced-fat sour cream and/or salsa if desired.

Nutrition Info: Calories 449 Total Carbs 9g Net Carbs 4g Protein 40g Fat 22g Sugar 3g Fiber 5g

376. Wilted Dandelion Greens With Sweet Onion

Servings: 4   Cooking Time: 12 Minutes
Ingredients:
- 1 tablespoon extra-virgin olive oil
- 1 Vidalia onion, thinly sliced
- 2 garlic cloves, minced
- 2 bunches dandelion greens, roughly chopped
- ½ cup low-sodium vegetable broth
- Freshly ground black pepper, to taste

Directions:
Heat the olive oil in a large skillet over low heat.   Cook the onion and garlic for 2 to 3 minutes until tender, stirring occasionally.   Add the dandelion greens and broth and cook for 5 to 7 minutes, stirring frequently, or until the greens are wilted.   Transfer to a plate and season with black pepper. Serve warm.

Nutrition Info:calories: 81   fat: 3.8g   protein: 3.1g   carbs: 10.7g   fiber: 3.8g   sugar: 2.0g   sodium: 72mg

377. Asian Fried Eggplant

Servings: 4   Cooking Time: 40 Minutes
Ingredients:
- 1 large eggplant, sliced into fourths
- 3 green onions, diced, green tips only
- 1 tsp fresh ginger, peeled & diced fine
- What you'll need from store cupboard:
- ¼ cup + 1 tsp cornstarch
- 1 ½ tbsp. soy sauce
- 1 ½ tbsp. sesame oil
- 1 tbsp. vegetable oil
- 1 tbsp. fish sauce
- 2 tsp Splenda
- ¼ tsp salt

Directions:
Place eggplant on paper towels and sprinkle both sides with salt. Let for 1 hour to remove excess moisture. Pat dry with more paper towels.   In a small bowl, whisk together soy sauce, sesame oil, fish sauce, Splenda, and 1 teaspoon cornstarch.   Coat both sides of the eggplant

with the ¼ cup cornstarch, use more if needed. Heat oil in a large skillet, over med-high heat. Add ½ the ginger and 1 green onion, then lay 2 slices of eggplant on top. Use ½ the sauce mixture to lightly coat both sides of the eggplant. Cook 8-10 minutes per side. Repeat. Serve garnished with remaining green onions.

Nutrition Info: Calories 155 Total Carbs 18g Net Carbs 13g Protein 2g Fat 9g Sugar 6g Fiber 5g

378. Chicken Guacamole Salad

Servings: 6   Cooking Time: 20 Minutes
Ingredients:
- 1 lb. chicken breast, boneless & skinless
- 2 avocados
- 1-2 jalapeno peppers, seeded & diced
- 1/3 cup onion, diced
- 3 tbsp. cilantro, diced
- 2 tbsp. fresh lime juice
- What you'll need from store cupboard:
- 2 cloves garlic, diced
- 1 tbsp. olive oil
- Salt & pepper, to taste

Directions:
Heat oven to 400 degrees. Line a baking sheet with foil. Season chicken with salt and pepper and place on prepared pan. Bake 20 minutes, or until chicken is cooked through. Let cool completely.   Once chicken has cooled, shred or dice and add to a large bowl. Add remaining Ingredients and mix well, mashing the avocado as you mix it in. Taste and season with salt and pepper as desired. Serve immediately.

Nutrition Info: Calories 324 Total Carbs 12g Net Carbs 5g Protein 23g Fat 22g Sugar 1g Fiber 7g

379. Warm Portobello Salad

Servings: 4   Cooking Time: 10 Minutes
Ingredients:
- 6 cup mixed salad greens
- 1 cup Portobello mushrooms, sliced
- 1 green onion, sliced
- What you'll need from store cupboard:
- Walnut or Warm Bacon Vinaigrette (chapter 16)
- 1 tbsp. olive oil
- 1/8 tsp ground black pepper

Directions:
Heat oil in a nonstick skillet over med-high heat. Add mushrooms and cook, stirring occasionally, 10 minutes, or until they are tender. Stir in onions and reduce heat to low.   Place salad greens on serving plates, top with mushrooms and sprinkle with pepper. Drizzle lightly with your choice of vinaigrette.

Nutrition Info: Calories 81 Total Carbs 9g Protein 4g Fat 4g Sugar 0g Fiber 0g

380. Layered Salad

Servings: 10   Cooking Time:
Ingredients:
- 6 slices bacon, chopped and cooked crisp
- 2 tomatoes, diced
- 2 stalks celery, sliced
- 1 head romaine lettuce, diced

- 1 red bell pepper, diced
- 1 cup frozen peas, thawed
- 1 cup sharp cheddar cheese, grated
- 1/4 cup red onion, diced fine
- What you'll need from the store cupboard
- 1 cup fat-free ranch dressing

Directions:
Use a 9x13- inch glass baking dish and layer half the lettuce, pepper, celery, tomatoes, peas, onion, cheese, bacon, and dressing. Repeat. Serve or cover and chill until ready to serve.

Nutrition Info: Calories 130 Total Carbs 14g Net Carbs 12g Protein 6g Fat 6g Sugar 5g Fiber 2g

381. Hassel Back Potatoes

Servings: 2   Cooking Time: 40 Minutes
Ingredients:
- 4 medium reddish potatoes washed and drained
- 30 ml of olive oil
- 12g of salt
- 1g black pepper
- 1g garlic powder
- 28g melted butter
- 8g parsley, freshly chopped, to decorate

Directions:
Wash and scrub potatoes. Let them dry with a paper towel.   Cut the slits, 6 mm away, on the potatoes, stopping before you cut them completely, so that all the slices are connected approximately 13 mm at the bottom of the potato.   Preheat the air fryer for 6 minutes, set it to 175°C.   Cover the potatoes with olive oil and season evenly with salt, black pepper, and garlic powder.   Add the potatoes in the air fryer and cook for 30 minutes at 175°C.   Brush the melted butter over the potatoes and cook for another 10 minutes at 175 ° C.   Garnish with freshly chopped parsley.

Nutrition Info: Calories: 415 Fat: 42g Carbohydrate: 9g Protein: 1g

382. Baked "potato" Salad

Servings: 8   Cooking Time: 15 Minutes
Ingredients:
- 2 lb. cauliflower, separated into small florets
- 6-8 slices bacon, chopped and fried crisp
- 6 boiled eggs, cooled, peeled, and chopped
- 1 cup sharp cheddar cheese, grated
- ½ cup green onion, sliced
- What you'll need from the store cupboard
- 1 cup reduced-fat mayonnaise
- 2 tsp yellow mustard
- 1 ½ tsp onion powder, divided
- Salt and fresh-ground black pepper to taste

Directions:
Place cauliflower in a vegetable steamer, or a pot with a steamer insert, and steam 5-6 minutes.   Drain the cauliflower and set aside.   In a small bowl, whisk together mayonnaise, mustard, 1 teaspoon onion powder, salt, and pepper.   Pat cauliflower dry with paper towels and place in a large mixing bowl. Add eggs, salt, pepper, remaining ½ teaspoon onion powder, then dressing. Mix gently to combine Ingredients together.

Fold in the bacon, cheese, and green onion. Serve warm or cover and chill before serving.

Nutrition Info: Calories 247 Total Carbs 8g Net Carbs 5g Protein 17g Fat 17g Sugar 3g Fiber 3g

383. Butternut Noodles With Mushroom Sauce

Servings: 4   Cooking Time: 15 Minutes

Ingredients:
- ¼ cup extra-virgin olive oil
- ½ red onion, finely chopped
- 1 pound (454 g) cremini mushrooms, sliced
- 1 teaspoon dried thyme
- ½ teaspoon sea salt
- 3 garlic cloves, minced
- ½ cup dry white wine
- Pinch red pepper flakes
- 4 cups butternut noodles
- 4 ounces (113 g) Parmesan cheese, grated (optional)

Directions:
Heat the olive oil in a large skillet over medium-high heat until shimmering.   Add the onion, mushrooms, thyme, and salt to the skillet. Sauté for 6 minutes, stirring occasionally, or until the mushrooms begin to brown. Stir in the garlic and cook for 30 seconds until fragrant. Fold in the wine and red pepper flakes and whisk to combine.   Add the butternut noodles to the skillet and continue cooking for 5 minutes, stirring occasionally, or until the noodles are softened.   Divide the mixture among four bowls. Sprinkle the grated Parmesan cheese on top, if desired.

Nutrition Info:calories: 243   fat: 14.2g   protein: 3.7g   carbs: 21.9g   fiber: 4.1g   sugar: 2.1g   sodium: 157mg

384. Caprese Salad

Servings: 4   Cooking Time: 10 Minutes

Ingredients:
- 3 medium tomatoes, cut into 8 slices
- 2 (1-oz.) slices mozzarella cheese, cut into strips
- ¼ cup fresh basil, sliced thin
- What you'll need from store cupboard:
- 2 tsp extra-virgin olive oil
- 1/8 tsp salt
- Pinch black pepper

Directions:
Place tomatoes and cheese on serving plates. Sprinkle with salt and pepper. Drizzle oil over and top with basil. Serve.

Nutrition Info: Calories 77 Total Carbs 4g Protein 5g Fat 5g Sugar 2g Fiber 1g

385. Asparagus Avocado Soup

Servings: 4   Cooking Time: 20 Minutes

Ingredients:
- 1 avocado, peeled, pitted, cubed
- 12 ounces asparagus
- ½-teaspoon ground black pepper
- 1-teaspoon garlic powder
- 1-teaspoon sea salt
- 2 tablespoons olive oil, divided
- 1/2 of a lemon, juiced
- 2 cups vegetable stock

Directions:
Switch on the air fryer, insert fryer basket, grease it with olive oil, then shut with its lid, set the fryer at 425 degrees F and preheat for 5 minutes.   Meanwhile, place asparagus in a shallow dish, drizzle with 1-tablespoon oil, sprinkle with garlic powder, salt, and black pepper and toss until well mixed.   Open the fryer, add asparagus in it, close with its lid and cook for 10 minutes until nicely golden and roasted, shaking halfway through the frying. When air fryer beeps, open its lid and transfer asparagus to a food processor.   Add remaining ingredients into a food processor and pulse until well combined and smooth.   Tip the soup in a saucepan, pour in water if the soup is too thick and heat it over medium-low heat for 5 minutes until thoroughly heated.   Ladle soup into bowls and serve.

Nutrition Info: Calories: 208 Cal Carbs: 2 g Fat: 11 g Protein: 4 g Fiber: 5 g

386. Roasted Broccoli With Garlic

Servings: 3   Cooking Time: 10 Minutes

Ingredients:
- 1 large broccoli cut 5
- 15 ml of olive oil
- 3g garlic powder
- 3g of salt
- 1g black pepper

Directions:
Preheat the air fryer for 5 minutes. Set it to 150°C. Sprinkle the broccoli pieces with olive oil and mix them until they are well covered.   Mix broccoli with seasonings.   Add the broccoli to the preheated air fryer at 150oC for 5 minutes.

Nutrition Info: Calories: 278 Fat: 4.2g Carbohydrate: 9g Protein: 1g

387. Roasted Asparagus And Red Peppers

Servings: 4   Cooking Time: 15 Minutes

Ingredients:
- 1 pound (454 g) asparagus, woody ends trimmed, cut into 2-inch segments
- 2 red bell peppers, seeded, cut into 1-inch pieces
- 1 small onion, quartered
- 2 tablespoons Italian dressing

Directions:
Preheat the oven to 400ºF (205ºC). Line a baking sheet with parchment paper and set aside.   Combine the asparagus with the peppers, onion, and dressing in a large bowl, and toss well.   Arrange the vegetables on the baking sheet and roast for about 15 minutes until softened. Flip the vegetables with a spatula once during cooking.   Transfer to a large platter and serve.

Nutrition Info:calories: 92   fat: 4.8g   protein: 2.9g   carbs: 10.7g   fiber: 4.0g   sugar: 5.7g   sodium: 31mg

388. Chopped Veggie Salad

Servings: 4   Cooking Time: 15 Minutes

Ingredients:
- 1 cucumber, chopped
- 1 pint cherry tomatoes, cut in half
- 3 radishes, chopped
- 1 yellow bell pepper chopped
- ½ cup fresh parsley, chopped
- What you'll need from store cupboard:
- 3 tbsp. lemon juice
- 1 tbsp. olive oil
- Salt to taste

Directions:
Place all Ingredients in a large bowl and toss to combine. Serve immediately, or cover and chill until ready to serve.
Nutrition Info: Calories 70 Total Carbs 9g Net Carbs 7g Protein 2g Fat 4g Sugar 5g Fiber 2g

389. Zucchini Fritters

Servings: 4   Cooking Time: 10 Minutes
Ingredients:
- 3 zucchini, grated
- 2 eggs
- 1 onion, diced
- ¾ cups feta cheese, crumbled
- ¼ cup fresh dill, chopped
- 1 tbsp. margarine
- What you'll need from store cupboard:
- ½ cup flour
- 1 tsp salt
- Pepper to taste
- Oil for frying

Directions:
Place zucchini in a large colander and sprinkle with the salt. Toss with fingers and let sit 30 minutes. Squeeze with back of spoon to remove the excess water. Place the zucchini between paper towels and squeeze again. Place in large bowl and let dry.   Melt margarine in a large skillet over med-high heat. Add onion and cook until soft, about 5 minutes. Add to zucchini along with the feta and dill and mix well.   In a small bowl, whisk together the flour and eggs. Pour over zucchini and mix well.   Add oil to the skillet to equal ½-inch and heat over med-high heat until very hot. Drop golf ball sized scoops of zucchini mixture into oil and flatten into a patty. Cook until golden brown on both sides. Transfer to paper towel line plate.   Serve with Garlic Dipping Sauce, (chapter 16), or sauce of your choice.
Nutrition Info: Calories 253   Total Carbs 21g Net Carbs 18g Protein 10g Fat 15g Sugar 5g Fiber 3g

390. Egg Stuffed Zucchini Balls

Servings: 4   Cooking Time: 45-60 Minutes
Ingredients:
- 2 zucchinis
- 1 onion
- 1 egg
- 120g of grated cheese
- 4 eggs
- Salt
- Ground pepper
- Flour

Directions:

Chop the zucchini and onion in the Thermo mix, 10 seconds speed 8, in the Cuisine with the kneader chopper at speed 10 about 15 seconds or we can chop the onion by hand and the zucchini grate. No matter how you do it, the important thing is that the zucchini and onion are as small as possible.   Put in a bowl and add the cheese and the egg. Pepper and bind well.   Incorporate the flour, until you have a very brown dough with which you can wrap the eggs without problems.   Cook the eggs and peel.   Cover the eggs with the zucchini dough and pass through the flour.   Place the four balls in the basket of the air fryer and paint with oil.   Select 1800C and leave for 45 to 60 minutes or until you see that the balls are crispy on the outside.
Nutrition Info: Calories: 23 Cal Carbs: 2 g Fat: 11 g Protein: 4 g Fiber: 15 g

391. Cauliflower "mac" And Cheese

Servings: 6   Cooking Time: 50 Minutes
Ingredients:
- 1 small head cauliflower, separated into small florets
- 1 ½ cup reduced-fat sharp cheddar cheese, grated
- 1 cup low-fat milk
- 1/2 cup chopped onion
- 2 tablespoons margarine, divided
- What you'll need:
- 2 tbsp. whole wheat flour
- 2 tbsp. whole wheat bread crumbs
- 1 tsp olive oil
- 1 tsp yellow mustard
- ½ tsp garlic powder
- ¼ tsp salt
- ¼ tsp black pepper
- Nonstick cooking spray

Directions:
Heat oven to 400 degrees. Coat a baking sheet with cooking spray.   In a medium bowl, combine oil, salt, pepper, onion, and cauliflower. Toss until cauliflower is coated evenly. Spread on baking sheet and cook 25-30 minutes until lightly browned.   In a medium saucepan, over medium heat, melt 1 ½ tablespoons margarine. Whisk in flour until no lumps remain.   Add milk and continue whisking until sauce thicken. Stir in mustard, garlic powder, and cheese until melted and smooth. Add cauliflower and mix well.   Pour into a 1 ½-quart baking dish.   In a small glass bowl, melt remaining margarine in microwave. Stir in bread crumbs until moistened. Sprinkle evenly over cauliflower.   Bake 20 minutes until bubbling and golden brown on top.
Nutrition Info: Calories 154 Total Carbs 15g Net Carbs 12g Protein 8g Fat 8g Sugar 4g Fiber 3g

392. Roasted Potatoes

Servings: 4   Cooking Time: 20 Minutes
Ingredients:
- 227g of small fresh potatoes, cleaned and halved
- 30 ml of olive oil
- 3g of salt
- 1g black pepper
- 2g garlic powder

- 1g dried thyme
- 1g dried rosemary

Directions:
Preheat the air fryer for a few minutes. Set it to 195°C. Cover the potatoes in half with olive oil and mix the seasonings.   Place the potatoes in the preheated air fryer. Set the time to 20 minutes. Be sure to shake the baskets in the middle of cooking.

Nutrition Info: Calories: 93 Fat: 0.2g Carbohydrate: 9g Protein: 1g

393. Roasted Brussels Sprouts With Wild Rice Bowl

Servings: 4   Cooking Time: 12 Minutes

Ingredients:
- 2 cups sliced Brussels sprouts
- 2 teaspoons plus 2 tablespoons extra-virgin olive oil
- 1 teaspoon Dijon mustard
- Juice of 1 lemon
- 1 garlic clove, minced
- ½ teaspoon salt
- ¼ teaspoon freshly ground black pepper
- 1 cup sliced radishes
- 1 cup cooked wild rice
- 1 avocado, sliced

Directions:
Preheat the oven to 400°F (205°C). Line a baking sheet with parchment paper and set aside.   Add 2 teaspoons of olive oil and Brussels sprouts to a medium bowl and toss to coat well.   Spread out the oiled Brussels sprouts on the prepared baking sheet. Roast in the preheated oven for 12 minutes, or until the Brussels sprouts are browned and crisp. Stir the Brussels sprouts once during cooking to ensure even cooking.   Meanwhile, make the dressing by whisking together the remaining olive oil, mustard, lemon juice, garlic, salt, and pepper in a small bowl.   Remove the Brussels sprouts from the oven to a large bowl. Add the radishes and cooked wild rice to the bowl. Drizzle with the prepared dressing and gently toss to coat everything evenly.   Divide the mixture into four bowls and scatter each bowl evenly with avocado slices. Serve immediately.

Nutrition Info:calories: 177   fat: 10.7g   protein: 2.3g   carbs: 17.6g   fiber: 5.1g   sugar: 2.0g   sodium: 297mg

394. Garlicky Mushrooms

Servings: 4   Cooking Time: 12 Minutes

Ingredients:
- 1 tablespoon butter
- 2 teaspoons extra-virgin olive oil
- 2 pounds (907 g) button mushrooms, halved
- 2 teaspoons minced fresh garlic
- 1 teaspoon chopped fresh thyme
- Sea salt and freshly ground black pepper, to taste

Directions:
Heat the butter and olive oil in a large skillet over medium-high heat.   Add the mushrooms and sauté for 10 minutes, stirring occasionally, or until the mushrooms are lightly browned and cooked through.

Stir in the garlic and thyme and cook for an additional 2 minutes.   Season with salt and pepper and serve on a plate.

Nutrition Info:calories: 96   fat: 6.1g   protein: 6.9g   carbs: 8.2g   fiber: 1.7g   sugar: 3.9g   sodium: 91mg

395. Tofu Salad Sandwiches

Servings: 4   Cooking Time: 20 Minutes

Ingredients:
- 1 pkg. silken firm tofu, pressed
- 4 lettuce leaves
- 2 green onions, diced
- ¼ cup celery, diced
- What you'll need from store cupboard:
- 8 slices bread, (chapter 14)
- ¼ cup lite mayonnaise
- 2 tbsp. sweet pickle relish
- 1 tbsp. Dijon mustard
- ¼ tsp turmeric
- ¼ tsp salt
- 1/8 tsp cayenne pepper

Directions:
Press tofu between layers of paper towels for 15 minutes to remove excess moisture. Cut into small cubes.   In a medium bowl, stir together remaining Ingredients. Fold in tofu. Spread over 4 slices of bread. Top with a lettuce leaf and another slice of bread. Serve.

Nutrition Info: Calories 378 Total Carbs 15g Net Carbs 13g Protein 24g Fat 20g Sugar 2g Fiber 2g

396. Roasted Tomato Brussels Sprouts

Servings: 4   Cooking Time: 20 Minutes

Ingredients:
- 1 pound (454 g) Brussels sprouts, trimmed and halved
- 1 tablespoon extra-virgin olive oil
- Sea salt and freshly ground black pepper, to taste
- ½ cup sun-dried tomatoes, chopped
- 2 tablespoons freshly squeezed lemon juice
- 1 teaspoon lemon zest

Directions:
Preheat the oven to 400°F (205°C). Line a large baking sheet with aluminum foil.   Toss the Brussels sprouts in the olive oil in a large bowl until well coated. Sprinkle with salt and pepper.   Spread out the seasoned Brussels sprouts on the prepared baking sheet in a single layer.   Roast in the preheated oven for 20 minutes, shaking the pan halfway through, or until the Brussels sprouts are crispy and browned on the outside. Remove from the oven to a serving bowl. Add the tomatoes, lemon juice, and lemon zest, and stir to incorporate. Serve immediately.

Nutrition Info:calories: 111   fat: 5.8g   protein: 5.0g   carbs: 13.7g   fiber: 4.9g   sugar: 2.7g   sodium: 103mg

397. Butternut Fritters

Servings: 6   Cooking Time: 15 Minutes

Ingredients:
- 5 cup butternut squash, grated
- 2 large eggs
- 1 tbsp. fresh sage, diced fine

- What you'll need from store cupboard:
- 2/3 cup flour
- 2 tbsp. olive oil
- Salt and pepper, to taste

Directions:
Heat oil in a large skillet over med-high heat. In a large bowl, combine squash, eggs, sage and salt and pepper to taste. Fold in flour. Drop ¼ cup mixture into skillet, keeping fritters at least 1 inch apart. Cook till golden brown on both sides, about 2 minutes per side. Transfer to paper towel lined plate. Repeat. Serve immediately with your favorite dipping sauce.
Nutrition Info: Calories 164 Total Carbs 24g Net Carbs 21g Protein 4g Fat 6g Sugar 3g Fiber 3g

398. Crock Pot Stroganoff

Servings: 2   Cooking Time: 2 Hours
Ingredients:
- 8 cups mushrooms, cut into quarters
- 1 onion, halved and sliced thin
- 4 tbsp. fresh parsley, chopped
- 1 ½ tbsp. low fat sour cream
- What you'll need from store cupboard:
- 1 cup low sodium vegetable broth
- 3 cloves garlic, diced fine
- 2 tsp smoked paprika
- Salt and pepper to taste

Directions:
Add all Ingredients, except sour cream and parsley to crock pot.cover and cook on high 2 hours. Stir in sour cream and serve garnished with parsley.
Nutrition Info: Calories 111 Total Carbs 18g Net Carbs 14g Protein 10g Fat 2g Sugar 8g Fiber 4g

399. Lobster Roll Salad With Bacon Vinaigrette

Servings: 6   Cooking Time: 35 Minutes
Ingredients:
- 6 slices bacon
- 2 whole grain ciabatta rolls, halved horizontally
- 3 medium tomatoes, cut into wedges
- 2 (8 oz.) spiny lobster tails, fresh or frozen (thawed)
- 2 cups fresh baby spinach
- 2 cups romaine lettuce, torn
- 1 cup seeded cucumber, diced
- 1 cup red sweet peppers, diced
- 2 tablespoons shallot, diced fine
- 2 tablespoons fresh chives, diced fine
- What you'll need from the store cupboard
- 2 cloves garlic, diced fine
- 3 tbsp. white wine vinegar
- 3 tbsp. olive oil, divided

Directions:
Heat a grill to medium heat, or medium heat charcoals. Rinse lobster and pat dry. Butterfly lobster tails. Place on the grill, cover and cook 25 – 30 minutes, or until meat is opaque. Remove lobster and let cool. In a small bowl, whisk together 2 tablespoons olive oil and garlic. Brush the cut sides of the rolls with oil mixture. Place on

grill, cut side down, and cook until crisp, about 2 minutes. Transfer to cutting board. While lobster is cooking, chop bacon and cook in a medium skillet until crisp. Transfer to paper towels. Reserve 1 tablespoon bacon grease. To make the vinaigrette: combine reserved bacon grease, vinegar, shallot, remaining 1 tablespoons oil and chives in a glass jar with an air-tight lid. Screw on the lid and shake to combine. Remove the lobster from the shells and cut into 1 ½-inch pieces. Cut rolls into 1-inch cubes. To assemble salad: in a large bowl, combine spinach, romaine, tomatoes, cucumber, peppers, lobster, and bread cubes. Toss to combine. Transfer to serving platter and drizzle with vinaigrette. Sprinkle bacon over top and serve.
Nutrition Info: Calories 255 Total Carbs 18g Net Carbs 16g Protein 20g Fat 11g Sugar 3g Fiber 2g

400. Orange Tofu

Servings: 4   Cooking Time: 2 Hours
Ingredients:
- 1 package extra firm tofu, pressed for at least 15 minutes, cut into cubes
- 2 cups broccoli florets, fresh
- 1 tbsp. margarine
- What you'll need from store cupboard:
- ¼ cup orange juice
- ¼ cup reduced sodium soy sauce
- ¼ cup honey
- 2 cloves garlic, diced fine

Directions:
Melt butter in a medium skillet, over medium high heat. Add tofu and garlic and cook, stirring occasionally until tofu starts to brown, about 5-10 minutes. Transfer to crock pot. Whisk the wet Ingredients together in a small bowl. Pour over tofu and add the broccoli. Cover and cook on high 90 minutes, or on low 2 hours. Serve over cauliflower rice (chapter13).
Nutrition Info: Calories 137 Total Carbs 24g Net Carbs 22g Protein 4g Fat 4g Sugar 20g Fiber 2g

401. Pomegranate & Brussels Sprouts Salad

Servings: 6   Cooking Time: 10 Minutes
Ingredients:
- 3 slices bacon, cooked crisp & crumbled
- 3 cup Brussels sprouts, shredded
- 3 cup kale, shredded
- 1 ½ cup pomegranate seeds
- What you'll need from store cupboard:
- ½ cup almonds, toasted & chopped
- ¼ cup reduced fat parmesan cheese, grated
- Citrus Vinaigrette, (chapter 16)

Directions:
Combine all Ingredients in a large bowl. Drizzle vinaigrette over salad, and toss to coat well. Serve garnished with more cheese if desired.
Nutrition Info: Calories 256 Total Carbs 15g Net Carbs 10g Protein 9g Fat 18g Sugar 5g Fiber 5g

402. Strawberry & Avocado Salad

Servings: 6   Cooking Time: 10 Minutes
Ingredients:
- 6 oz. baby spinach
- 2 avocados, chopped
- 1 cup strawberries, sliced
- ¼ cup feta cheese, crumbled
- What you'll need from store cupboard:
- Creamy Poppy Seed Dressing (chapter 16)
- ¼ cup almonds, sliced

Directions:
Add spinach, berries, avocado, nuts and cheese to a large bowl and toss to combine.   Pour ½ recipe of Creamy Poppy Seed Dressing over salad and toss to coat. Add more dressing if desired. Serve.
Nutrition Info: Calories 253 Total Carbs 19g Net Carbs 13g Protein 4g Fat 19g Sugar 9g Fiber 6g

403. Vegetables With Provolone

Servings: 4   Cooking Time: 30 Minutes
Ingredients:
- 1 bag of 400g of frozen tempura vegetables
- Extra virgin olive oil
- Salt
- 1 slice of provolone cheese

Directions:
Put the vegetables in the basket of the air fryer. Add some strands of extra virgin olive oil and close.   Select 20 minutes, 2000C.   Pass the vegetables to a clay pot and place the provolone cheese on top.   Take to the oven, 1800C, about 10 minutes or so or until you see that, the cheese has melted to your liking.
Nutrition Info: Calories: 104Cal Carbs: 2 g Fat: 11 g Protein: 4 g Fiber: 0 g

404. Potato Wedges

Servings: 4   Cooking Time: 20 Minutes
Ingredients:
- 2 large thick potatoes, rinsed and cut into wedges 102 mm long
- 23 ml of olive oil
- 3g garlic powder
- 1g onion powder
- 3g of salt
- 1g black pepper
- 5g grated Parmesan cheese
- Tomato sauce or ranch sauce, for server

Directions:
Cut the potatoes into 102 mm long pieces.   Preheat the air fryer for 5 minutes. Set it to 195°C.   Cover the potatoes with olive oil and mix the condiments and Parmesan cheese until they are well covered.   Add the potatoes to the preheated fryer. Set the time to 20 minutes.   Be sure to shake the baskets in the middle of cooking.
Nutrition Info: Calories: 156 Fat: 8.01g Carbohydrate: 20.33g Protein: 1.98gSugar: 0.33g Cholesterol: 0mg

405. Crispy Tofu With Chili Garlic Noodles

Servings: 8   Cooking Time: 15 Minutes

Ingredients:
- 1 lb. extra firm tofu, cut in 1-inch slices & press 30 minutes
- 3 green onions, slice & separate white part from green
- 1 bell pepper, sliced thin
- 1 medium carrot, sliced thin
- 4 tbsp. cilantro, diced
- What you'll need from store cupboard:
- 1 recipe Homemade Pasta, cook & drain (chapter 15)
- 12 cloves garlic, diced fine
- 3 tbsp. lite soy sauce
- 3 tbsp. oyster sauce
- 2 tbsp. red chili paste
- 2 tbsp. cornstarch, plus more as needed
- 2 tbsp. sunflower oil
- 1 tbsp. fish sauce
- 1 tsp Splenda
- Red chili flakes, to taste
- Sesame seeds, to top

Directions:
In a small bowl, stir together soy sauce, oyster sauce, chili paste, fish sauce, and Splenda.   Crumble tofu into a medium bowl. Add cornstarch and toss to coat well. Heat oil in a large skillet over med-high heat. Add tofu and cook until brown and crispy, break tofu up as it cooks. Transfer to a plate.   Add more oil, if needed, to the skillet and sauté carrot and bell pepper until they start to soften, about 3 minutes. Add to tofu.   Add the garlic and white parts of the onions and cook 30 seconds, stirring. Stir in sauce mixture and cook 2 minutes or until sauce coats the back of a spoon.   Add the pasta along with the tofu and vegetables. Stir to coat. Sprinkle with chili flakes. Serve garnished with green parts of onions, sesame seeds, and cilantro.
Nutrition Info: Calories 266 Total Carbs 26g Net Carbs 24g   Protein 23g Fat 12g Sugar 12g Fiber 4g

406. Asian Style Slaw

Servings: 8   Cooking Time: 2 Hours
Ingredients:
- 1 lb. bag coleslaw mix
- 5 scallions, sliced
- What you'll need from store cupboard:
- 1 cup sunflower seeds
- 1 cup almonds, sliced
- 3 oz. ramen noodles, broken into small pieces
- ¾ cup vegetable oil
- ½ cup Splenda
- 1/3 cup vinegar

Directions:
In a large bowl, combine coleslaw, sunflower seeds, almonds, and scallions.   Whisk together the oil, vinegar and Splenda in a large measuring cup. Pour over salad, and stir to combine.   Stir in ramen noodles, cover and chill 2 hours.
Nutrition Info: Calories 354 Total Carbs 24g Net Carbs 21g Protein 5g Fat 26g Sugar 10g Fiber 3g

407. Shrimp & Avocado Salad

Servings: 4   Cooking Time: 5 Minutes

Ingredients:
- ½ lb. raw shrimp, peeled and deveined
- 3 cups romaine lettuce, chopped
- 1 cup napa cabbage, chopped
- 1 avocado, pit removed and sliced
- ¼ cup red cabbage, chopped
- 1/4 cucumber, julienned
- 2 tbsp. green onions, diced fine
- 2 tbsp. fresh cilantro, diced
- 1 tsp fresh ginger, diced fine
- What you'll need from the store cupboard
- 2 tbsp. coconut oil
- 1 tbsp. sesame seeds
- 1 tsp Chinese five spice
- Fat-free Ranch dressing

Directions:
Toast sesame seeds in a medium skillet over medium heat. Shake the skillet to prevent them from burning. Cook until they start to brown, about 2 minutes. Set aside. Add the coconut oil to the skillet. Pat the shrimp dry and sprinkle with the five spice. Add to hot oil. Cook 2 minutes per side, or until they turn pink. Set aside. Arrange lettuce and cabbage on a serving platter. Top with green onions, cucumber, and cilantro. Add shrimp and avocado.   Drizzle with desired amount of dressing and sprinkle sesame seeds over top. Serve.

Nutrition Info: Calories 306 Total Carbs 20g Net Carbs 15g Protein 15g Fat 19g Sugar 4g Fiber 5g

408. Garden Vegetable Pasta

Servings: 6   Cooking Time: 30 Minutes

Ingredients:
- 2 lbs. fresh cherry tomatoes, halved
- 2 zucchini, chopped
- 2 ears corn, cut kernels off the cob
- 1 yellow squash, chopped
- ½ cup mozzarella cheese, grated
- ½ cup fresh basil, sliced thin
- What you'll need from store cupboard:
- Homemade Pasta, cook & drain, (chapter 15)
- 5 tbsp. olive oil, divided
- 2 cloves garlic crushed
- Crushed red pepper flakes, to taste
- Salt, to taste

Directions:
Heat 3 tablespoons oil in a large skillet over medium heat. Add garlic and tomatoes. Cover, reduce heat to low, and cook 15 minutes, stirring frequently.   In a separate skillet, heat remaining oil over med-high heat. Add zucchini, squash, and corn. Reduce heat to medium, and cook until vegetables are tender. Sprinkle with salt. Heat oven to 400 degrees.   In a large bowl combine tomato mixture, vegetables, and pasta, toss to mix. Pour into a 9x13-inch baking dish and top with cheese. Bake 10 minutes, or until cheese melts and begins to brown. Serve.

Nutrition Info: Calories 347 Total Carbs 31g Net Carbs 24g Protein 21g Fat 18g Sugar 13g Fiber 7g

409. Teriyaki Tofu Burger

Servings: 2   Cooking Time: 15 Minutes

Ingredients:
- 2 3 oz. tofu portions, extra firm, pressed between paper towels 15 minutes
- ¼ red onion, sliced
- 2 tbsp. carrot, grated
- 1 tsp margarine
- Butter leaf lettuce
- What you'll need from store cupboard:
- 2 100% whole wheat sandwich thins
- 1 tbsp. teriyaki marinade
- 1 tbsp. Sriracha
- 1 tsp red chili flakes

Directions:
Heat grill, or charcoal, to a medium heat.   Marinate tofu in teriyaki marinade, red chili flakes and Sriracha. Melt margarine in a small skillet over med-high heat. Add onions and cook until caramelized, about 5 minutes. Grill tofu for 3-4 minutes per side.   To assemble, place tofu on bottom roll. Top with lettuce, carrot, and onion. Add top of the roll and serve.

Nutrition Info: Calories 178 Total Carbs 27g Net Carbs 20g Protein 12g Fat 5g Sugar 5g Fiber 7g

410. Tofu Curry

Servings: 4   Cooking Time: 2 Hours

Ingredients:
- 2 cup green bell pepper, diced
- 1 cup firm tofu, cut into cubes
- 1 onion, peeled and diced
- What you'll need from store cupboard:
- 1 ½ cups canned coconut milk
- 1 cup tomato paste
- 2 cloves garlic, diced fine
- 2 tbsp. raw peanut butter
- 1 tbsp. garam masala
- 1 tbsp. curry powder
- 1 ½ tsp salt

Directions:
Add all Ingredients, except the tofu to a blender or food processor. Process until thoroughly combined.   Pour into a crock pot and add the tofu. Cover and cook on high 2 hours.   Stir well and serve over cauliflower rice.

Nutrition Info: Calories 389 Total Carbs 28g Net Carbs 20g   Protein 13g Fat 28g Sugar 16g Fiber 8g

411. Faux Chow Mein

Servings: 4   Cooking Time: 20 Minutes

Ingredients:
- 1 large spaghetti squash, halved and seeds removed
- 3 stalks celery, sliced diagonally
- 1 onion, diced fine
- 2 cup Cole slaw mix
- 2 tsp fresh ginger, grated
- What you'll need from store cupboard:
- ¼ cup Tamari
- 3 cloves garlic, diced fine
- 3-4 tbsp. water

- 2 tbsp. olive oil
- 1 tbsp. Splenda
- ¼ tsp pepper

Directions:
Place squash, cut side down, in shallow glass dish and add water. Microwave on high 8-10 minutes, or until squash is soft. Use a fork to scoop out the squash into a bowl.   In a small bowl, whisk together Tamari, garlic, sugar, ginger and pepper.   Heat oil in large skillet over med-high heat. Add onion and celery and cook, stirring frequently, 3-4 minutes. Add Cole slaw and cook until heated through, about 1 minute.   Add the squash and sauce mixture and stir well. Cook 2 minutes, stirring frequently. Serve.
Nutrition Info: Calories 129 Total Carbs 13g Net Carbs 11g Protein 3g Fat 7g Sugar 6g Fiber 2g

412. Roasted Tomato And Bell Pepper Soup

Servings: 6   Cooking Time: 35 Minutes
Ingredients:
- 2 tablespoons extra-virgin olive oil, plus more for coating the baking dish
- 16 plum tomatoes, cored and halved
- 4 celery stalks, coarsely chopped
- 4 red bell peppers, seeded, halved
- 4 garlic cloves, lightly crushed
- 1 sweet onion, cut into eighths
- Sea salt and freshly ground black pepper, to taste
- 6 cups low-sodium chicken broth
- 2 tablespoons chopped fresh basil
- 2 ounces (57 g) goat cheese, grated

Directions:
Preheat the oven to 400°F (205°C). Coat a large baking dish lightly with olive oil.   Put the tomatoes in the oiled dish, cut-side down. Scatter the celery, bell peppers, garlic, and onion on top of the tomatoes. Drizzle with 2 tablespoons of olive oil and season with salt and pepper. Roast in the preheated oven for about 30 minutes, or until the vegetables are fork-tender and slightly charred. Remove the vegetables from the oven. Let them rest for a few minutes until cooled slightly.   Transfer to a food processor, along with the chicken broth, and purée until fully mixed and smooth.   Pour the purée soup into a medium saucepan and bring it to a simmer over medium-high heat.   Sprinkle the basil and grated cheese on top before serving.
Nutrition Info:calories: 187   fat: 9.7g   protein: 7.8g   carbs: 21.3g   fiber: 6.1g   sugar: 14.0g   sodium: 825mg

413. Festive Holiday Salad

Servings: 8   Cooking Time: 1 Hour
Ingredients:
- 1 head broccoli, separated into florets
- 1 head cauliflower, separated into florets
- 1 red onion, sliced thin
- 2 cup cherry tomatoes, halved
- ½ cup fat free sour cream
- What you'll need from store cupboard:
- 1 cup lite mayonnaise
- 1 tbsp. Splenda

Directions:
In a large bowl combine vegetables.   In a small bowl, whisk together mayonnaise, sour cream and Splenda. Pour over vegetables and toss to mix.   Cover and refrigerate at least 1 hour before serving.
Nutrition Info: Calories 152 Total Carbs 12g Net Carbs 10g Protein 2g Fat 10g Sugar 5g Fiber 2g

414. Grilled Vegetable & Noodle Salad

Servings: 4   Cooking Time: 10 Minutes
Ingredients:
- 2 ears corn-on-the-cob, husked
- 1 red onion, cut in ½-inch thick slices
- 1 tomato, diced fine
- 1/3 cup fresh basil, diced
- 1/3 cup feta cheese, crumbled
- What you'll need from store cupboard:
- 1 recipe Homemade Noodles, (chapter 15) cook & drain
- 4 tbsp. Herb Vinaigrette, (chapter 16)
- Nonstick cooking spray

Directions:
Heat grill to medium heat. Spray rack with cooking spray. Place corn and onions on the grill and cook, turning when needed, until lightly charred and tender, about 10 minutes.   Cut corn off the cob and place in a medium bowl. Chop the onion and add to the corn.   Stir in noodles, tomatoes, basil, and vinaigrette, toss to mix. Sprinkle cheese over top and serve.
Nutrition Info: Calories 330 Total Carbs 19g Net Carbs 16g Protein 10g Fat 9g Sugar 5g Fiber 3g

415. Creamy Macaroni And Cheese

Servings: 6   Cooking Time: 25 Minutes
Ingredients:
- 1 cup fat-free evaporated milk
- ½ cup skim milk
- ½ cup low-fat Cheddar cheese
- ½ cup low-fat cottage cheese
- 1 teaspoon nutmeg
- Pinch cayenne pepper
- Sea salt and freshly ground black pepper, to taste
- 6 cups cooked whole-wheat elbow macaroni
- 2 tablespoons grated Parmesan cheese

Directions:
Preheat the oven to 350°F (180°C).   Heat the milk in a large saucepan over low heat until it steams.   Add the Cheddar cheese and cottage cheese to the milk, and keep whisking, or until the cheese is melted.   Add the nutmeg and cayenne pepper and stir well. Sprinkle the salt and pepper to season.   Remove from the heat. Add the cooked macaroni to the cheese mixture and stir until well combined. Transfer the macaroni and cheese to a large casserole dish and top with the grated Parmesan cheese.   Bake in the preheated oven for about 20 minutes, or until bubbly and lightly browned.   Divide the macaroni and cheese among six bowls and serve.
Nutrition Info:calories: 245   fat: 2.1g   protein: 15.7g   carbs: 43.8g   fiber: 3.8g   sugar: 6.8g   sodium: 186mg

416. Creamy Pasta With Peas

Servings: 4   Cooking Time: 10 Minutes

Ingredients:
- 4 tomatoes, deseeded & diced
- 4 oz. fat free cream cheese, cut in cubes
- 1 cup peas, thawed
- ½ cup skim milk
- 4 tbsp. fresh parsley, diced
- What you'll need from store cupboard:
- ½ recipe Homemade Pasta, cook & drain, (chapter 15)
- 4 cloves garlic, diced fine
- 3 tbsp. olive oil
- 1 tsp oregano
- 1 tsp basil
- ½ tsp garlic salt

Directions:
Heat oil in a large skillet over medium heat. Add garlic and tomatoes, cook 3-4 minutes, stirring frequently. Add peas, milk, cream cheese, and seasonings. Cook, stirring, 5 minutes, or until cream cheese has melted. Add pasta and toss to coat. Serve garnished with parsley.

Nutrition Info: Calories 332 Total Carbs 19g Net Carbs 14g Protein 14g Fat 23g Sugar 10g Fiber 5g

417. Sesame Bok Choy With Almonds

Servings: 4   Cooking Time: 7 Minutes

Ingredients:
- 2 teaspoons sesame oil
- 2 pounds (907 g) bok choy, cleaned and quartered
- 2 teaspoons low-sodium soy sauce
- Pinch red pepper flakes
- ½ cup toasted sliced almonds

Directions:
Heat the sesame oil in a large skillet over medium heat until hot.   Sauté the bok choy in the hot oil for about 5 minutes, stirring occasionally, or until tender but still crisp.   Add the soy sauce and red pepper flakes and stir to combine.   Continue sautéing for 2 minutes. Transfer to a plate and serve topped with sliced almonds.

Nutrition Info: calories: 118   fat: 7.8g   protein: 6.2g carbs: 7.9g   fiber: 4.1g   sugar: 3.0g   sodium: 293mg

418. Roasted Cauliflower With Tomatoes

Servings: 4   Cooking Time: 45 Minutes

Ingredients:
- 1 large head cauliflower, separated in florets
- 3 scallions, sliced
- 1 onion, diced fine
- What you'll need from store cupboard:
- 15 oz. can petite tomatoes, diced
- 4 cloves garlic, diced fine
- 4 tbsp. olive oil, divided
- 1 tbsp. red wine vinegar
- 1 tbsp. balsamic vinegar
- 3 tsp Splenda
- 1 tsp salt
- 1 tsp pepper
- ½ tsp chili powder

Directions:

Heat oven to 400 degrees.   Place cauliflower on a large baking sheet and drizzle with 2 tablespoons of oil. Sprinkle with salt and pepper, to taste. Use hands to rub oil and seasoning into florets then lay in single layer. Roast until fork tender.   Heat 1 tablespoon oil in a large skillet over med-low heat. Add onion and cook until soft. Stir in tomatoes, with juice, Splenda, both vinegars, and the teaspoon of salt. Bring to a boil, reduce heat and simmer 20-25 minutes. For a smooth sauce, use an immersion blender to process until smooth, or leave it chunky.   In a separate skillet, heat remaining oil over med-low heat and saute garlic 1-2 minutes. Stir in tomato sauce, and increase heat to medium. Cook, stirring frequently, 5 minutes. Add chili powder and cauliflower and toss to coat. Serve garnished with scallions.

Nutrition Info: Calories 107 Total Carbs 23g Net Carbs 16g Protein 6g Fat 0g Sugar 12g Fiber 7g

419. Fried Avocado

Servings: 2   Cooking Time: 10 Minutes

Ingredients:
- 2 avocados cut into wedges 25 mm thick
- 50g Pan crumbs bread
- 2g garlic powder
- 2g onion powder
- 1g smoked paprika
- 1g cayenne pepper
- Salt and pepper to taste
- 60g all-purpose flour
- 2 eggs, beaten
- Nonstick Spray Oil
- Tomato sauce or ranch sauce, to serve

Directions:
Cut the avocados into 25 mm thick pieces.   Combine the crumbs, garlic powder, onion powder, smoked paprika, cayenne pepper and salt in a bowl.   Separate each wedge of avocado in the flour, then dip the beaten eggs and stir in the breadcrumb mixture.   Preheat the air fryer.   Place the avocados in the preheated air fryer baskets, spray with oil spray and cook at 205°C for 10 minutes.   Turn the fried avocado halfway through cooking and sprinkle with cooking oil.

Nutrition Info: Calories: 123 Cal Carbs: 2 g Fat: 11 g Protein: 4 g Fiber: 0 g

420. French Toast

Servings: 8   Cooking Time: 15 Minutes

Ingredients:
- For the bread:
- 500g of flour
- 25g of oil
- 300 g of water
- 25g of fresh bread yeast
- 12g of salt
- For French toast:
- Milk and cinnamon or milk and sweet wine
- Eggs
- Honey

Directions:
The first thing is to make bread a day before. Put in the Master Chef Gourmet the ingredients of the bread and

knead 1 minute at speed   Let the dough rise 1 hour and knead 1 minute at speed 1 again. Remove the dough and divide into 4 portions. Make a ball and spread like a pizza. Roll up to make a small loaf of bread and let rise 1 hour or so.   Take to the oven and bake 40 minutes, 2000C. Let the bread cool on a rack and reserve for the next day. Cut the bread into slices and reserve.   Prepare the milk to wet the slices of bread.   To do so, put the milk to heat, like 500 ml or so with a cinnamon stick or the same milk with a glass of sweet wine, as you like.   When the milk has started to boil, remove from heat, and let cool. Beat the eggs.   Place a rack on a plate and we dip the slices of bread in the cold milk, then in the beaten egg and pass to the rack with the plate underneath to release the excess liquid.   Put the slices of bread in the bucket of the air fryer, in batches, not piled up, and we take the air fryer, 180 degrees, 10 minutes each batch.   When you have all the slices passed through the air fryer, put the honey in a casserole, like 500g, next to 1 small glass of water and 4 tablespoons of sugar. When the honey starts to boil, lower the heat, and pass the bread slices through the honey.   Place in a fountain and the rest of the honey we put it on top, bathing again the French toast. Ready our French toast, when they cool, they can already be eaten.

Nutrition Info: Calories: 224 Fat: 15.2g Carbohydrates: 17.39g Protein: 4.81g Sugar: 5.76g Cholesterol: 84mg

421. Butter-orange Yams

Servings: 8   Cooking Time: 45 Minutes
Ingredients:
- 2 medium jewel yams, cut into 2-inch dices
- 2 tablespoons unsalted butter
- Juice of 1 large orange
- 1½ teaspoons ground cinnamon
- ¼ teaspoon ground ginger
- ¾ teaspoon ground nutmeg
- ⅛ teaspoon ground cloves

Directions:
Preheat the oven to 350°F (180°C).   Arrange the yam dices on a rimmed baking sheet in a single layer. Set aside. Add the butter, orange juice, cinnamon, ginger, nutmeg, and garlic cloves to a medium saucepan over medium-low heat. Cook for 3 to 5 minutes, stirring continuously, or until the sauce begins to thicken and bubble.   Spoon the sauce over the yams and toss to coat well.   Bake in the preheated oven for 40 minutes until tender.   Let the yams cool for 8 minutes on the baking sheet before removing and serving.

Nutrition Info:calories: 129   fat: 2.8g   protein: 2.1g carbs: 24.7g   fiber: 5.0g   sugar: 2.9g   sodium: 28mg

422. Grilled Portobello & Zucchini Burger

Servings: 2   Cooking Time: 10 Minutes
Ingredients:
- 2 large portabella mushroom caps
- ½ small zucchini, sliced
- 2 slices low fat cheese
- Spinach
- What you'll need from store cupboard:
- 2 100% whole wheat sandwich thins
- 2 tsp roasted red bell peppers
- 2 tsp olive oil

Directions:
Heat grill, or charcoal, to med-high heat.   Lightly brush mushroom caps with olive oil. Grill mushroom caps and zucchini slices until tender, about 3-4 minutes per side.   Place on sandwich thin. Top with sliced cheese, roasted red bell pepper, and spinach. Serve.

Nutrition Info: Calories 177 Total Carbs 26g Protein 15g Fat 3g Sugar 3g Fiber 8g

423. Tarragon Spring Peas

Servings: 6   Cooking Time: 12 Minutes
Ingredients:
- 1 tablespoon unsalted butter
- ½ Vidalia onion, thinly sliced
- 1 cup low-sodium vegetable broth
- 3 cups fresh shelled peas
- 1 tablespoon minced fresh tarragon

Directions:
Melt the butter in a skillet over medium heat.   Sauté the onion in the melted butter for about 3 minutes until translucent, stirring occasionally.   Pour in the vegetable broth and whisk well. Add the peas and tarragon to the skillet and stir to combine.   Reduce the heat to low, cover, and cook for about 8 minutes more, or until the peas are tender.   Let the peas cool for 5 minutes and serve warm.

Nutrition Info:calories: 82   fat: 2.1g   protein: 4.2g carbs: 12.0g   fiber: 3.8g   sugar: 4.9g   sodium: 48mg

424. Potatoes With Provencal Herbs With Cheese

Servings: 4   Cooking Time: 20 Minutes
Ingredients:
- 1kg of potatoes
- Provencal herbs
- Extra virgin olive oil
- Salt
- Grated cheese

Directions:
Peel the potatoes and cut the cane salt and sprinkle with Provencal herbs.   Put in the basket and add some strands of extra virgin olive oil.   Take the air fryer and select 1800C, 20 minutes.   Take out and move on to a large plate.   Cover cheese.   Gratin in the microwave or in the oven, a few minutes until the cheese is melted.

Nutrition Info: Calories: 437 Fat: 0.6g Carbohydrates: 24.19g Protein: 1g Sugar: 5.g Cholesterol: 0mg

425. Spiced Potato Wedges

Servings: 4   Cooking Time: 40 Minutes
Ingredients:
- 8 medium potatoes
- Salt
- Ground pepper
- Garlic powder
- Aromatic herbs, the one we like the most
- 2 tbsp. extra virgin olive oil

- 4 tbsp. breadcrumbs or chickpea flour.

Directions:
Put the unpeeled potatoes in a pot with boiling water and a little salt. Let cook 5 minutes. Drain and let cool. Cut into thick segments, without peeling. Put the potatoes in a bowl and add salt, pepper, garlic powder, the aromatic herb that we have chosen oil and breadcrumbs or chickpea flour. Stir well and leave 15 minutes. Pass to the basket of the air fryer and select 20 minutes, 1800C. From time to time shake the basket so that the potatoes mix and change position. Check that they are tender.

Nutrition Info: Calories: 123 Cal Carbs: 2 g Fat: 11 g Protein: 4 g Fiber: 0 g

426. Roasted Delicata Squash With Thyme

Servings: 4   Cooking Time: 20 Minutes
Ingredients:
- 1 (1- to 1½-pound / 454- to 680-g) delicata squash, halved, seeded, and cut into ½-inch-thick strips
- 1 tablespoon extra-virgin olive oil
- ½ teaspoon dried thyme
- ¼ teaspoon salt
- ¼ teaspoon freshly ground black pepper

Directions:
Preheat the oven to 400ºF (205ºC). Line a baking sheet with parchment paper and set aside. Add the squash strips, olive oil, thyme, salt, and pepper in a large bowl, and toss until the squash strips are fully coated. Place the squash strips on the prepared baking sheet in a single layer. Roast for about 20 minutes until lightly browned, flipping the strips halfway through. Remove from the oven and serve on plates.

Nutrition Info:calories: 78 fat: 4.2g protein: 1.1g carbs: 11.8g fiber: 2.1g sugar: 2.9g sodium: 122mg

427. Scrambled Eggs With Beans, Zucchini, Potatoes And Onions

Servings: 4   Cooking Time: 35 Minutes
Ingredients:
- 300g of beans
- 2 onions
- 1 zucchini
- 4 potatoes
- 8 eggs
- Extra virgin olive oil
- Salt
- Ground pepper
- A splash of soy sauce

Directions:
Put the beans taken from their pod to cook in abundant saltwater. Drain when they are tender and reserve. Peel the potatoes and cut into dice. Season and put some threads of oil. Mix and take to the air fryer. Select 1800C, 15 minutes. After that time, add together with the potatoes, diced zucchini, and onion in julienne, mix and select 1800C, 20 minutes. From time to time, mix and stir. Pass the contents of the air fryer together with the beans to a pan. Add a little soy sauce and salt to taste. Sauté and peel the eggs. Do the scrambled.

Nutrition Info: Calories: 65 Cal Carbs: 2 g Fat: 11 g Protein: 4 g Fiber: 0 g

428. Cantaloupe & Prosciutto Salad

Servings: 4   Cooking Time: 15 Minutes
Ingredients:
- 6 mozzarella balls, quartered
- 1 medium cantaloupe, peeled and cut into small cubes
- 4 oz. prosciutto, chopped
- 1 tbsp. fresh lime juice
- 1 tbsp. fresh mint, chopped
- What you'll need from store cupboard
- 2 tbsp. extra virgin olive oil
- 1 tsp honey

Directions:
In a large bowl, whisk together oil, lime juice, honey, and mint. Season with salt and pepper to taste. Add the cantaloupe and mozzarella and toss to combine. Arrange the mixture on a serving plate and add prosciutto. Serve.

Nutrition Info: Calories 240 Total Carbs 6g Protein 18g Fat 16g Sugar 4g Fiber 0g

429. Green Beans

Servings: 4   Cooking Time: 13 Minutes
Ingredients:
- 1-pound green beans
- ¾-teaspoon garlic powder
- ¾-teaspoon ground black pepper
- 1 ¼-teaspoon salt
- ½-teaspoon paprika

Directions:
Switch on the air fryer, insert fryer basket, grease it with olive oil, then shut with its lid, set the fryer at 400 degrees F and preheat for 5 minutes. Meanwhile, place beans in a bowl, spray generously with olive oil, sprinkle with garlic powder, black pepper, salt, and paprika and toss until well coated. Open the fryer, add green beans in it, close with its lid and cook for 8 minutes until nicely golden and crispy, shaking halfway through the frying. When air fryer beeps, open its lid, transfer green beans onto a serving plate and serve.

Nutrition Info: Calories: 45Cal Carbs: 2 g Fat: 11 g Protein: 4 g Fiber: 3 g

430. Holiday Apple & Cranberry Salad

Servings: 10   Cooking Time: 15 Minutes
Ingredients:
- 12 oz. salad greens
- 3 Honeycrisp apples, sliced thin
- 1/2 lemon
- ½ cup blue cheese, crumbled
- What you'll need from store cupboard:
- Apple Cider Vinaigrette (chapter 16)
- 1 cup pecan halves, toasted
- ¾ cup dried cranberries

Directions:
Put the apple slices in a large plastic bag and squeeze the half lemon over them. Close the bag and shake to coat.

In a large bowl, layer greens, apples, pecans, cranberries, and blue cheese. Just before serving, drizzle with enough vinaigrette to dress the salad. Toss to coat all Ingredients evenly.

Nutrition Info: Calories 291 Total Carbs 19g Net Carbs 15g Protein 5g Fat 23g Sugar 13g Fiber 4g

431. Asparagus & Bacon Salad

Servings: 1   Cooking Time: 5 Minutes

Ingredients:
- 1 hard-boiled egg, peeled and sliced
- 1 2/3 cups asparagus, chopped
- 2 slices bacon, cooked crisp and crumbled
- What you'll need from store cupboard:
- 1 tsp extra virgin olive oil
- 1 tsp red wine vinegar
- ½ tsp Dijon mustard
- Pinch salt and pepper, to taste

Directions:
Bring a pot of water to a boil. Add the asparagus and cook 2-3 minutes or until tender-crisp. Drain and add cold water to stop the cooking process.   In a small bowl, whisk together, mustard, oil, vinegar, and salt and pepper to taste.   Place the asparagus on a plate, top with egg and bacon. Drizzle with vinaigrette and serve.

Nutrition Info: Calories 356 Total Carbs 10g Net Carbs 5g Protein 25g Fat 25g Sugar 5g Fiber 5g

432. Eggplant-zucchini Parmesan

Servings: 6   Cooking Time: 2 Hours

Ingredients:
- 1 medium eggplant, peeled and cut into 1-inch cubes
- 1 medium zucchini, cut into 1-inch pieces
- 1 medium onion, cut into thin wedges
- What you'll need from store cupboard:
- 1½ cups purchased light spaghetti sauce
- 2/3 cup reduced fat parmesan cheese, grated

Directions:
Place the vegetables, spaghetti sauce and 1/3 cup parmesan in the crock pot. Stir to combine. Cover and cook on high 2 – 2 1/2 hours, or on low 4-5 hours. Sprinkle remaining parmesan on top before serving.

Nutrition Info: Calories 81 Total Carbs 12g Net Carbs 7g Protein 5g Fat 2g Sugar 7g Fiber 5g

433. Southwest Chicken Salad

Servings: 6

Ingredients:
- 2 cups chicken, cooked and shredded
- 1 small red bell pepper, diced fine
- ¼ cup red onion, diced fine
- What you'll need from the store cupboard
- ¼ cup reduced-fat mayonnaise
- 1 ½ tsp ground cumin
- 1 tsp garlic powder
- 1/2 tsp coriander
- Salt and pepper to taste

Directions:

Combine all Ingredients in a large bowl and mix to thoroughly combine. Taste and adjust seasonings as desired. Cover and chill until ready to serve.

Nutrition Info: Calories 117 Total Carbs 4g Net Carbs 0g Protein 14g Fat 5g Sugar 2g Fiber 0g

434. Tempeh Lettuce Wraps

Servings: 2   Cooking Time: 5 Minutes

Ingredients:
- 1 pkg. tempeh, crumbled
- 1 head butter-leaf lettuce
- ½ red bell pepper, diced
- ½ onion, diced
- What you'll need from store cupboard:
- 1 tbsp. garlic, diced fine
- 1 tbsp. olive oil
- 1 tbsp. low-sodium soy sauce
- 1 tsp ginger,
- 1 tsp onion powder
- 1 tsp garlic powder

Directions:
Heat oil and garlic in a large skillet over medium heat. Add onion, tempeh, and bell pepper and sauté for 3 minutes.   Add soy sauce and spices and cook for another 2 minutes.   Spoon mixture into lettuce leaves.

Nutrition Info: Calories 130 Total Carbs 14g Net Carbs 10g Protein 8g Fat 5g Sugar 2g Fiber 4g

435. Crispy Rye Bread Snacks With Guacamole And Anchovies

Servings: 4   Cooking Time: 10 Minutes

Ingredients:
- 4 slices of rye bread
- Guacamole
- Anchovies in oil

Directions:
Cut each slice of bread into 3 strips of bread.   Place in the basket of the air fryer, without piling up, and we go in batches giving it the touch you want to give it. You can select 1800C, 10 minutes.   When you have all the crusty rye bread strips, put a layer of guacamole on top, whether homemade or commercial.   In each bread, place 2 anchovies on the guacamole.

Nutrition Info: Calories: 180Cal Carbs: 4 g Fat: 11 g Protein: 4 g Fiber: 09 g

436. Lime Asparagus With Cashews

Servings: 4   Cooking Time: 15 To 20 Minutes

Ingredients:
- 2 pounds (907 g) asparagus, woody ends trimmed
- 1 tablespoon extra-virgin olive oil
- Sea salt and freshly ground black pepper, to taste
- ½ cup chopped cashews
- Zest and juice of 1 lime

Directions:
Preheat the oven to 400ºF (205ºC). Line a baking sheet with aluminum foil.   Toss the asparagus with the olive oil in a medium bowl. Sprinkle the salt and pepper to season.   Arrange the asparagus on the baking sheet and bake for 15 to 20 minutes, or until lightly browned

and tender.   Remove the asparagus from the oven to a serving bowl. Add the cashews, lime zest and juice, and toss to coat well. Serve immediately.
Nutrition Info:calories: 173   fat: 11.8g   protein: 8.0g   carbs: 43.7g   fiber: 4.9g   sugar: 5.0g   sodium: 65mg

437. Cabbage Wedges

Servings: 6   Cooking Time: 29 Minutes
Ingredients:
- 1 small head of green cabbage
- 6 strips of bacon, thick-cut, pastured
- 1-teaspoon onion powder
- ½-teaspoon ground black pepper
- 1-teaspoon garlic powder
- ¾-teaspoon salt
- 1/4 teaspoon red chili flakes
- 1/2 teaspoon fennel seeds
- 3 tablespoons olive oil

Directions:
Switch on the air fryer, insert fryer basket, grease it with olive oil, then shut with its lid, set the fryer at 350 degrees F and preheat for 5 minutes.   Open the fryer, add bacon strips in it, close with its lid and cook for 10 minutes until nicely golden and crispy, turning the bacon halfway through the frying.   Meanwhile, prepare the cabbage, for this, remove the outer leaves of the cabbage, and then cut it into eight wedges, keeping the core intact. Prepare the spice mix and for this, place onion powder in a bowl, add black pepper, garlic powder, salt, red chili, and fennel and stir until mixed.   Drizzle cabbage wedges with oil and then sprinkle with spice mix until well coated.   When air fryer beeps, open its lid, transfer bacon strips to a cutting board and let it rest. Add seasoned cabbage wedges into the fryer basket, close with its lid, then cook for 8 minutes at 400 degrees F, flip the cabbage, spray with oil and continue air frying for 6 minutes until nicely golden and cooked.   When done, transfer cabbage wedges to a plate.   Chop the bacon, sprinkle it over cabbage and serve.
Nutrition Info: Calories: 123 Cal Carbs: 2 g Fat: 11 g Protein: 4 g Fiber: 0 g

438. Broccoli & Bacon Salad

Servings: 4
Ingredients:
- 2 cups broccoli, separated into florets
- 4 slices bacon, chopped and cooked crisp
- ½ cup cheddar cheese, cubed
- ¼ cup low-fat Greek yogurt
- 1/8 cup red onion, diced fine
- 1/8 cup almonds, sliced
- What you'll need from the store cupboard
- ¼ cup reduced-fat mayonnaise
- 1 tbsp. lemon juice
- 1 tbsp. apple cider vinegar
- 1 tbsp. granulated sugar substitute
- ¼ tsp salt
- ¼ tsp pepper

Directions:

In a large bowl, combine broccoli, onion, cheese, bacon, and almonds.   In a small bowl, whisk remaining Ingredients together till combined.   Pour dressing over broccoli mixture and stir. Cover and chill at least 1 hour before serving.
Nutrition Info: Calories 217 Total Carbs 12g Net Carbs 10g Protein 11g Fat 14g Sugar 6g Fiber 2g

439. Black Pepper & Garlic Tofu

Servings: 4   Cooking Time: 40 Minutes
Ingredients:
- 14 oz. pkg. extra firm tofu
- 1 lb. asparagus, trim & cut in 1-inch pieces
- 8 oz. kale, remove stems & slice leaves
- 3 oz. Shiitake mushrooms, sliced
- 1 onion, halved & slice in thin wedges
- 1 green bell pepper, sliced
- What you'll need from store cupboard:
- ½ cup low sodium vegetable broth
- 8 cloves garlic, pressed, divided
- 2 ½ tbsp. light soy sauce, divided
- 2 -4 tbsp. water
- 2 tsp cornstarch
- 2 tsp black pepper, freshly ground, divided
- 1 tsp rice vinegar
- 1 tsp sriracha

Directions:
Heat oven to 400 degrees. Line a baking sheet with parchment paper.   Cut tofu in ½-inch slices and press between paper towels to remove excess moisture. Cut each slice into smaller rectangles.   In a Ziploc bag combine, 1 tablespoon soy sauce, water, 2 tablespoons garlic, rice vinegar, and 1 teaspoon pepper. Add tofu and turn to coat. Let marinate 15 minutes.   Place the tofu on the prepared pan and bake 15 minutes. Flip over and bake 15 minutes more. Remove from oven.   Place a large nonstick skillet over med-high heat. Add onion and cook until translucent, stirring frequently. Add bell pepper and cook 1 minute more.   Add garlic and mushrooms and cook 2 minutes, add a little water if the vegetables start to stick.   Stir in the kale and 2 tablespoons water and cover. Let cook 1 minutes, then stir and add more water if needed. Cover and cook another minute before adding asparagus and cook, stirring, until asparagus is tender crisp.   In a small bowl, stir together remaining soy sauce, broth, Sriracha, cornstarch, and pepper. Pour over vegetables and cook until heated through.   To serve plate the vegetables and place tofu on top.
Nutrition Info: Calories 176 Total Carbs 33g Net Carbs 27g Protein 16g Fat 4g Sugar 12g Fiber 6g

440. Watermelon & Arugula Salad

Servings: 6   Cooking Time: 1 Hour
Ingredients:
- 4 cups watermelon, cut in 1-inch cubes
- 3 cup arugula
- 1 lemon, zested
- ½ cup feta cheese, crumbled
- ¼ cup fresh mint, chopped
- 1 tbsp. fresh lemon juice

- What you'll need from store cupboard:
- 3 tbsp. olive oil
- Fresh ground black pepper
- Salt to taste

Directions:
Combine oil, zest, juice and mint in a large bowl. Stir together.   Add watermelon and gently toss to coat. Add remaining Ingredients and toss to combine. Taste and adjust seasoning as desired.   Cover and chill at least 1 hour before serving.

Nutrition Info: Calories 148 Total Carbs 10g Net Carbs 9g Protein 4g Fat 11g Sugar 7g Fiber 1g

441. Broccoli & Mushroom Salad

Servings: 4   Cooking Time: 10 Minutes

Ingredients:
- 4 sun-dried tomatoes, cut in half
- 3 cup torn leaf lettuce
- 1 ½ cup broccoli florets
- 1 cup mushrooms, sliced
- 1/3 cup radishes, sliced
- What you'll need from store cupboard:
- 2 tbsp. water
- 1 tbsp. balsamic vinegar
- 1 tsp vegetable oil
- ¼ tsp chicken bouillon granules
- ¼ tsp parsley
- ¼ tsp dry mustard
- 1/8 tsp cayenne pepper

Directions:
Place tomatoes in a small bowl and pour boiling water over, just enough to cover. Let stand 5 minutes, drain. Chop tomatoes and place in a large bowl. Add lettuce, broccoli, mushrooms, and radishes.   In a jar with a tight fitting lid, add remaining Ingredients and shake well. Pour over salad and toss to coat. Serve.

Nutrition Info: Calories 54, Total Carbs 9g Net Carbs 7g Protein 3g Fat 2g Sugar 2g Fiber 2g

442. Crust Less Broccoli Quiche

Servings: 6   Cooking Time: 1 Hour

Ingredients:
- 3 large eggs
- 2 cups broccoli florets, chopped
- 1 small onion, diced
- 1 cup cheddar cheese, grated
- 2/3 cup unsweetened almond milk
- ½ cup feta cheese, crumbled
- What you'll need from store cupboard:
- 1 tbsp. extra virgin olive oil
- ½ tsp sea salt
- ¼ tsp black pepper
- Nonstick cooking spray

Directions:
Heat oven to 350 degrees. Spray a 9-inch baking dish with cooking spray.   Heat the oil in a large skillet over medium heat. Add onion and cook 4-5 minutes, until onions are translucent.   Add broccoli and stir to combine. Cook until broccoli turns a bright green, about 2 minutes. Transfer to a bowl.   In a small bowl, whisk together almond milk, egg, salt, and pepper. Pour over

the broccoli. Add the cheddar cheese and stir the Ingredients together. Pour into the prepared baking dish. Sprinkle the feta cheese over the top and bake 45 minutes to 1 hour, or until eggs are set in the middle and top is lightly browned. Serve.

Nutrition Info: Calories 182 Total Carbs 5g Net Carbs 4g Protein 10g Fat 14g Sugar 2g Fiber 1g

443. Zucchini "pasta" Salad

Servings: 5   Cooking Time: 1 Hour

Ingredients:
- 5 oz. zucchini, spiralized
- 1 avocado, peeled and sliced
- 1/3 cup feta cheese, crumbled
- ¼ cup tomatoes, diced
- ¼ cup black olives, diced
- What you'll need from the store cupboard
- 1/3 cup Green Goddess Salad Dressing
- 1 tsp olive oil
- 1 tsp basil
- Salt and pepper to taste

Directions:
Place zucchini on paper towel lined cutting board. Sprinkle with a little bit of salt and let sit for 30 minutes to remove excess water. Squeeze gently.   Add oil to medium skillet and heat over med-high heat. Add zucchini and cook, stirring frequently, until soft, about 3 – 4 minutes.   Transfer zucchini to a large bowl and add remaining Ingredients, except for the avocado. Cover and chill for 1 hour.   Serve topped with avocado.

Nutrition Info: Calories 200 Total Carbs 7g Net Carbs 4g Protein 3g Fat 18g Sugar 2g Fiber 3g

444. Homemade Vegetable Chili

Servings: 4   Cooking Time: 15 Minutes

Ingredients:
- 2 tablespoons extra-virgin olive oil
- 1 onion, finely chopped
- 1 green bell pepper, deseeded and chopped
- 1 (14-ounce / 397-g) can kidney beans, drained and rinsed
- 2 (14-ounce / 397-g) cans crushed tomatoes
- 2 cups veggie crumbles
- 1 teaspoon garlic powder
- 1 tablespoon chili powder
- ½ teaspoon sea salt

Directions:
Heat the olive oil in a large skillet over medium-high heat until shimmering.   Add the onion and bell pepper and sauté for 5 minutes, stirring occasionally.   Fold in the beans, tomatoes, veggie crumbles, garlic powder, chili powder, and salt. Stir to incorporate and bring them to a simmer.   Reduce the heat and cook for an additional 5 minutes, stirring occasionally, or until the mixture is heated through.   Allow the mixture to cool for 5 minutes and serve warm.

Nutrition Info:calories: 282   fat: 10.1g   protein: 16.7g   carbs: 38.2g   fiber: 12.9g   sugar: 7.2g sodium: 1128mg

445. Collard Greens With Tomato

Servings: 4   Cooking Time: 20 Minutes
Ingredients:
- 1 cup low-sodium vegetable broth, divided
- ½ onion, thinly sliced
- 2 garlic cloves, thinly sliced
- 1 medium tomato, chopped
- 1 large bunch collard greens including stems, roughly chopped
- 1 teaspoon ground cumin
- ½ teaspoon freshly ground black pepper

Directions:
Add ½ cup of vegetable broth to a Dutch oven over medium heat and bring to a simmer.   Stir in the onion and garlic and cook for about 4 minutes until tender. Add the remaining broth, tomato, greens, cumin, and pepper, and gently stir to combine.   Reduce the heat to low and simmer uncovered for 15 minutes. Serve warm.
Nutrition Info: calories: 68   fat: 2.1g   protein: 4.8g carbs: 13.8g   fiber: 7.1g   sugar: 2.0g   sodium: 67mg

446. Okra

Servings: 4   Cooking Time: 10 Minutes
Ingredients:
- 1-cup almond flour
- 8 ounces fresh okra
- 1/2 teaspoon sea salt
- 1-cup milk, reduced-fat
- 1 egg, pastured

Directions:
Crack the egg in a bowl, pour in the milk and whisk until blended.   Cut the stem from each okra, then cut it into ½-inch pieces, add them into egg and stir until well coated.   Mix flour and salt and add it into a large plastic bag.   Working on one okra piece at a time, drain the okra well by letting excess egg drip off, add it to the flour mixture, then seal the bag and shake well until okra is well coated.   Place the coated okra on a grease air fryer basket, coat remaining okra pieces in the same manner and place them into the basket.   Switch on the air fryer, insert fryer basket, spray okra with oil, then shut with its lid, set the fryer at 390 degrees F and cook for 10 minutes until nicely golden and cooked, stirring okra halfway through the frying.
Nutrition Info: Calories: 250Cal Carbs: 2 g Fat: 11 g Protein: 4 g Fiber: 2 g

447. Grilled Tofu & Veggie Skewers

Servings: 6   Cooking Time: 15 Minutes
Ingredients:
- 1 block tofu
- 2 small zucchini, sliced
- 1 red bell pepper, cut into 1-inch cubes
- 1 yellow bell pepper, cut into 1-inch cubes
- 1 red onion, cut into 1-inch cubes
- 2 cups cherry tomatoes
- What you'll need from store cupboard:
- 2 tbsp. lite soy sauce
- 3 tsp barbecue sauce (chapter 15)
- 2 tsp sesame seeds
- Salt & pepper, to taste
- Nonstick cooking spray

Directions:
Press tofu to extract liquid, for about half an hour. Then, cut tofu into cubes and marinate in soy sauce for at least 15 minutes.   Heat the grill to med-high heat. Spray the grill rack with cooking spray.   Assemble skewers with tofu alternating with vegetables.   Grill 2-3 minutes per side until vegetables start to soften, and tofu is golden brown. At the very end of cooking time, season with salt and pepper and brush with barbecue sauce. Serve garnished with sesame seeds.
Nutrition Info: Calories 64 Total Carbs 10g Net Carbs 7g Protein 5g Fat   2g Sugar 6g Fiber 3g

448. Tex Mex Veggie Bake

Servings: 8   Cooking Time: 35 Minutes
Ingredients:
- 2 cup cauliflower, grated
- 1 cup fat free sour cream
- 1 cup reduced fat cheddar cheese, grated
- 1 cup reduced fat Mexican cheese blend, grated
- ½ cup red onion, diced
- What you'll need from store cupboard:
- 11 oz. can Mexicorn, drain
- 10 oz. tomatoes & green chilies
- 2 ¼ oz. black olives, drain
- 1 cup black beans, rinsed
- 1 cup salsa
- ¼ tsp pepper
- Nonstick cooking spray

Directions:
Heat oven to 350 degrees. Spray a 2 ½-quart baking dish with cooking spray.   In a large bowl, combine beans, corn, tomatoes, salsa, sour cream, cheddar cheese, pepper, and cauliflower. Transfer to baking dish. Sprinkle with onion and olives.   Bake 30 minutes. Sprinkle with Mexican blend cheese and bake another 5-10 minutes, or until cheese is melted and casserole is heated through. Let rest 10 minutes before serving.
Nutrition Info: Calories 266 Total Carbs 33g Net Carbs 27g Protein 16g Fat 8g Sugar 8g Fiber 6g

449. Pad Thai

Servings: 6   Cooking Time: 30 Minutes
Ingredients:
- 12 oz. extra firm tofu organic, cut into 1-inch cubes
- 2 zucchini, shredded into long zoodles
- 1 carrot, grated
- 3 cups bean sprouts
- 2 Green onions sliced
- 1 cup red cabbage, shredded
- ¼ cup cilantro, chopped
- What you'll need from store cupboard:
- ¼ cup lime juice
- 2 cloves garlic, diced fine
- 2 tbsp. reduced fat peanut butter
- 2 tbsp. tamari
- 1 tbsp. sesame seeds
- ½ tbsp. sesame oil
- 2 tsp red chili flakes

Directions:

Heat half the oil in a saucepan over medium heat. Add tofu and cook until it starts to brown, about 5 minutes. Add garlic and stir until light brown. Add zucchini, carrot, cabbage, lime juice, peanut butter, tamari, and chili flakes. Stir to combine all Ingredients. Cook, stirring frequently, until vegetables are tender, about 5 minutes. Add bean sprouts and remove from heat. Serve topped with green onions, sesame seeds and cilantro.

Nutrition Info: Calories 134 Total Carbs 13g Net Carbs 11g Protein 12g Fat 6g Sugar 3g Fiber 2g

450. Pecan Pear Salad

Servings: 8   Cooking Time: 15 Minutes

Ingredients:
- 10 oz. mixed greens
- 3 pears, chopped
- ½ cup blue cheese, crumbled
- What you'll need from store cupboard:
- 2 cup pecan halves
- 1 cup dried cranberries
- ½ cup olive oil
- 6 tbsp. champagne vinegar
- 2 tbsp. Dijon mustard
- ¼ tsp salt

Directions:

In a large bowl combine greens, pears, cranberries and pecans. Whisk remaining Ingredients, except blue cheese, together in a small bowl Pour over salad and toss to coat. Serve topped with blue cheese crumbles.

Nutrition Info: Calories 325 Total Carbs 20g Net Carbs 14g Protein 5g Fat 26g Sugar 10g Fiber 6g

Other Favorite Recipes

451. Orange Marmalade

Servings: 48   Cooking Time: 30 Minutes

Ingredients:
- 4 navel oranges
- 1 lemon
- What you'll need from store cupboard:
- 2 ½ cup water
- ¼ cup warm water
- 4 tbsp. Splenda
- 1 oz. gelatin

Directions:
Quarter the oranges and remove all the pulp. Scrap the white part off the rind and cut it into thin 2-inch strips. Remove as much of the membrane between orange segments as you can and place the seeds in a small piece of cheesecloth, pull up the sides to make a "bag" and tie closed.   Repeat with the lemon but discard the seeds. Cut the lemon rind into smaller strips than the orange rind.   Chop the orange and lemon pulp and add it to a medium saucepan along with 2 ½ cups water. Bring to a rapid boil over med-high heat.   Reduce heat to med-low and add the bag of seeds. Boil gently for 30 minutes, or until the citrus fruit is soft. Remove and discard the seed bag.   Dissolve the gelatin in the warm water. Add it to the orange mixture with ½ the Splenda. Being careful not to burn yourself, taste the marmalade and adjust sweetener as desired.   Spoon the marmalade into 3 ½-pint jars with air-tight lids. Seal and chill.

Nutrition Info: Calories 15 Total Carbs 3g Protein 1g Fat 0g Sugar 3g Fiber 0g

452. Homemade Pasta

Servings: 8   Cooking Time: 5 Minutes

Ingredients:
- 1 egg + 2 egg yolks
- What you'll need from store cupboard:
- 1 ¾ cup soy flour
- ¼ cup ground wheat germ
- 3-4 tbsp. cold water
- 1 tsp light olive oil
- ½ tsp salt

Directions:
In a large bowl, whisk egg, egg yolks, oil and 3 tablespoons water until smooth.   In a separate bowl, combine flour, wheat germ, and salt. Stir into egg mixture until smooth. Use the last tablespoon of water if needed to make a smooth dough.   Turn out onto a lightly floured surface and knead 5-8 minutes or until smooth. Cover and let rest 10 minutes.   Divide dough into 4 equal pieces and roll out, one at a time, as thin as possible, or run it through a pasta machine until it reaches the thinnest setting.   Let dough dry out for 30 minutes. Cut into desired size with pasta machine or pizza cutter. It not using right away, let it dry overnight on a pasta or cooling rack. Fresh pasta should be used within 3 days.   It will store in the freezer, after drying for just an hour, in an airtight bag, 6-8 months. Pasta dried overnight can be stored in an airtight container for up to 1 week.   To cook it when fresh, add to a pot of boiling water for 4-5 minutes or until tender. Dried pasta will take a couple minutes longer.

Nutrition Info: Calories 152 Total Carbs 12g Net Carbs 9g Protein 16g Fat 5g Sugar 6g Fiber 3g

453. Pizza Sauce

Servings: 8   Cooking Time: 5 Minutes

Ingredients:
- ½ cup yellow onion, diced
- What you'll need from store cupboard:
- 15 oz. tomatoes, crushed, no sugar added
- 1/3 cup + 1 tbsp. olive oil
- 3 cloves garlic, diced
- 2 tsp parsley
- 1 tsp rosemary
- 1 tsp thyme
- 1 tsp smoked paprika
- Salt, to taste

Directions:
Heat 1 tablespoon oil in a small skillet over medium heat. Add onion and garlic and cook until onions are translucent.   In a medium saucepan, over medium heat, stir all Ingredients together, along with onions. Bring to a simmer and cook 2-3 minutes, stirring constantly.   Remove from heat and let cool completely. Store in a jar with an air tight lid in the refrigerator up to 2 weeks. Or in the freezer up to 6 months.

Nutrition Info: Calories 179 Total Carbs 8g Net carbs 6g Protein 2g Fat 17g Sugar 5g Fiber 2g

454. Beef Burgundy & Mushroom Stew

Servings: 4   Cooking Time: 8 Hours

Ingredients:
- 1 lb. sirloin steak, cut into bite size pieces
- 2 carrots, peeled and cut into 1-inch pieces
- 1 cup mushrooms, sliced
- ¾ cup pearl onions, thawed if frozen
- What you'll need from store cupboard:
- 1 cup Burgundy wine
- ½ cup low sodium beef broth
- 3 cloves garlic, diced
- 2 tbsp. olive oil
- 1 bay leaf
- 1 tsp marjoram
- ½ tsp salt
- ½ tsp thyme
- ¼ tsp pepper

Directions:
Heat the oil in a large skillet over med-high heat. Add steak and brown on all sides. Transfer to a crock pot. Add remaining Ingredients and stir to combine. Cover and cook on low 7-8 hours or until steak is tender and vegetables are cooked through. Discard the bay leaf before serving.

Nutrition Info:al Facts Per ServingCalories 353 Total Carbs 8g Net Carbs 7g Protein 36g Fat 14g Sugar 3g Fiber 1g

455. Kale Chips

Servings: 1   Cooking Time: 15 Minutes
Ingredients:
- ¼ teaspoon garlic powder
- Pinch cayenne, to taste
- 1 tablespoon extra-virgin olive oil
- ½ teaspoon sea salt, or to taste
- 1 (8-ounce / 227-g) bunch kale, trimmed and cut into 2-inch pieces, rinsed

Directions:
Preheat the oven to 350°F (180°C). Line two baking sheets with parchment paper.   Combine the garlic powder, cayenne pepper, olive oil, and salt in a large bowl, then dunk the kale in the bowl. Toss to coat well.   Place the kale in the single layer on one of the baking sheet. Arrange the sheet in the preheated oven and bake for 7 minutes. Remove the sheet from the oven and pour the kale in the single layer of the other baking sheet.   Move the sheet of kale back to the oven and bake for another 7 minutes or until the kale is crispy.   Serve immediately.
Nutrition Info:calories: 136   fat: 14.0g   protein: 1.0g carbs: 3.0g   fiber: 1.1g sugar: 0.6g sodium: 1170mg

456. Cucumber Ginger Detox

Servings: 2   Cooking Time: 5 Minutes
Ingredients:
- Spinach – 1 ½ oz.
- Orange – 1, peeled
- Ginger – ½ inch, peeled
- Water – 1 cup
- Cucumber – 1, chopped
- Avocado – ½ chopped
- Ice – 1 cup
- Rosehips – 1 tsp.

Directions:
Combine everything in the blender and blend until smooth.   Serve.
Nutrition Info:144 Fat: 4Carb: 46g Protein: 3g

457. Spicy Tomato Chicken Soup

Servings: 6   Cooking Time: 3 Hours
Ingredients:
- 1 ½ lbs. chicken breasts, boneless, skinless and cut into bite size pieces
- 1 onion, diced
- 2 cup tomatoes, diced
- ½ cup green chilies, diced
- What you'll need from store cupboard
- 4 cup low sodium chicken broth
- 3 cloves garlic, diced
- 1 ½ tbsp. chili powder
- 1 tbsp. olive oil
- 1 tbsp. cumin
- 2 tsp paprika
- 2 tsp salt

Directions:
Season chicken with salt. Heat oil in a large skillet over medium heat. Add chicken and cook until no longer pink. Remove from skillet and place in crock pot.   Add the tomatoes, onions, green chilies and garlic to a blender or food processor and pulse until smooth. Pour over chicken.   Add the broth and seasonings. Cover and cook on high 2-3 hours until chicken is cooked through and the soup has thickened slightly. Serve.
Nutrition Info: Calories 276 Total Carbs 7g Net Carbs 5g Protein 35g Fat 11g Sugar 4g Fiber 2g

458. Chicken And Zoodle Soup

Servings: 4   Cooking Time: 15 Minutes
Ingredients:
- 2 tablespoons extra-virgin olive oil
- 12 ounces (340 g) chicken breast, cut into bite-sized pieces
- 2 carrots, chopped
- 2 celery stalks, chopped
- 1 onion, chopped
- 2 garlic cloves
- 1 teaspoon dried thyme
- 6 cups low-sodium chicken broth
- 1 teaspoon sea salt
- 2 medium zucchinis, spiralized

Directions:
Heat the olive oil in a pot over medium-high heat until shimmering.   Add the chicken and sear for 5 minutes or until well browned. Remove the cooked chicken from the pot and set aside on a plate.   Add the carrots, celery, and onion to the pot and sauté for 5 minutes or until tender.   Add the garlic and sauté for 1 minutes or until fragrant.   Add the thyme, chicken broth, and salt. Bring to a boil, then reduce the heat to medium.   Put the chicken back to the pot and add the spiralized zucchini. Simmer for 2 minutes or until the zucchini is tender. Keep stirring during the simmering.   Pour the soup in a large bowl and serve immediately.
Nutrition Info:calories: 292   fat: 16.9g   protein: 25.8g carbs: 10.8g   fiber: 1.6g sugar: 3.2g sodium: 772mg

459. Beef And Mushroom Barley Soup

Servings: 6   Cooking Time: 10 Minutes
Ingredients:
- 1 pound beef stew meat, cubed
- ¼ teaspoon salt
- ¼ teaspoon freshly ground black pepper
- 1 tablespoon extra-virgin olive oil
- 8 ounces sliced mushrooms
- 1 onion, chopped
- 2 carrots, chopped
- 3 celery stalks, chopped
- 6 garlic cloves, minced
- ½ teaspoon dried thyme
- 4 cups low-sodium beef broth
- 1 cup water
- ½ cup pearl barley

Directions:
Season the meat with the salt and pepper.   In an Instant Pot, heat the oil over high heat. Add the meat and brown on all sides. Remove the meat from the pot and set aside.   Add the mushrooms to the pot and cook for 1 to 2 minutes, until they begin to soften. Remove the

mushrooms and set aside with the meat. Add the onion, carrots, and celery to the pot. Sauté for 3 to 4 minutes until the vegetables begin to soften. Add the garlic and continue to cook until fragrant, about 30 seconds longer. Return the meat and mushrooms to the pot, then add the thyme, beef broth, and water. Set the pressure to high and cook for 15 minutes. Let the pressure release naturally. Open the Instant Pot and add the barley. Use the slow cooker function on the Instant Pot, affix the lid (vent open), and continue to cook for 1 hour until the barley is cooked through and tender. Serve.
Nutrition Info: Calories: 245; Total Fat: 9g; Protein: 21g; Carbohydrates: 19g; Sugars: 3g; Fiber: 4g; Sodium: 516mg

460. Cinnamon Blueberry Sauce

Servings: 16   Cooking Time: 10 Minutes
Ingredients:
- 2 cup blueberries
- 2 tbsp. fresh lemon juice
- What you'll need from store cupboard:
- ¼ cup Splenda
- ¼ cup water
- 2 tsp corn starch
- ½ tsp cinnamon

Directions:
In a small saucepan, over medium heat, Splenda and cornstarch. Stir in remaining Ingredients and bring to a boil, stirring frequently. Reduce heat and simmer 5 minutes, until thickened. Let cool completely. Pour into a jar with an airtight lid and refrigerate until ready to use. Serving size is 1 tablespoon.
Nutrition Info: Calories 27 Total Carbs 6g Protein 0g Fat 0g Sugar 5g Fiber 0g

461. Bunless Sloppy Joes

Servings: 6   Cooking Time: 15 Minutes
Ingredients:
- 6 small sweet potatoes
- 1 pound lean ground beef
- 1 onion, finely chopped
- 1 carrot, finely chopped
- ¼ cup finely chopped mushrooms
- ¼ cup finely chopped red bell pepper
- 3 garlic cloves, minced
- 2 teaspoons Worcestershire sauce
- 1 tablespoon white wine vinegar
- 1 (15-ounce) can low-sodium tomato sauce
- 2 tablespoons tomato paste

Directions:
Preheat the oven to 400°F. Place the sweet potatoes in a single layer in a baking dish. Bake for 25 to 40 minutes, depending on the size, until they are soft and cooked through. While the sweet potatoes are baking, in a large skillet, cook the beef over medium heat until it's browned, breaking it apart into small pieces as you stir. Add the onion, carrot, mushrooms, bell pepper, and garlic, and sauté briefly for 1 minute. Stir in the Worcestershire sauce, vinegar, tomato sauce, and tomato paste. Bring to a simmer, reduce the heat, and

cook for 5 minutes for the flavors to meld. Scoop ½ cup of the meat mixture on top of each baked potato and serve.
Nutrition Info: Calories: 372; Total Fat: 19g; Protein: 16g; Carbohydrates: 34g; Sugars: 13g; Fiber: 6g; Sodium: 161mg

462. Cilantro Lime Quinoa

Servings: 6   Cooking Time: 25 Minutes
Ingredients:
- 1 cup uncooked quinoa
- 1-tablespoon olive oil
- 1 medium yellow onion, diced
- 2 cloves minced garlic
- 1 (4-ounce) can diced green chills, drained
- 1 ½ cups fat-free chicken broth
- ¾-cup fresh chopped cilantro
- ½ cup sliced green onion
- 2 tablespoons lime juice
- Salt and pepper

Directions:
Rinse the quinoa thoroughly in cool water using a fine mesh sieve. Heat the oil in a large saucepan over medium heat. Add the onion and sauté for 2 minutes then stir in the chili and garlic. Cook for 1 minute then stir in the quinoa and chicken broth. Bring to a boil then reduce heat and simmer, covered, until the quinoa absorbs the liquid – about 20 to 25 minutes. Remove from heat then stir in the cilantro, green onions, and limejuice. Season with salt and pepper to taste and serve hot.
Nutrition Info: Calories 150Total Fat 4.8gSaturated Fat 0.7gTotal Carbs 8.5gNet Carbs 4.6g Protein 2.1g Sugar 1.7g Fiber 3.9g Sodium 179mg

463. Almond Vanilla Fruit Dip

Servings: 10   Cooking Time: 10 Minutes
Ingredients:
- 2 ½ cup fat free half-n-half
- What you'll need from store cupboard:
- 4-serving size fat-free sugar-free vanilla instant pudding mix
- 1 tbsp. Splenda
- 1 tsp vanilla
- 1 tsp almond extract

Directions:
Place all Ingredients in a medium bowl, and beat on medium speed 2 minutes. Cover and chill until ready to serve. Serve with fruit for dipping. Serving size is ¼ cup.
Nutrition Info: Calories 87 Total Carbs 4g Protein 2g Fat 7g Sugar 1g Fiber 0g

464. Slow-cooked Simple Lamb And Vegetable Stew

Servings: 6   Cooking Time: 10 Minutes
Ingredients:
- 1 pound boneless lamb stew meat
- 1 pound turnips, peeled and chopped
- 1 fennel bulb, trimmed and thinly sliced
- 10 ounces mushrooms, sliced

- 1 onion, diced
- 3 garlic cloves, minced
- 2 cups low-sodium chicken broth
- 2 tablespoons tomato paste
- ¼ cup dry red wine (optional)
- 1 teaspoon chopped fresh thyme
- ½ teaspoon salt
- ¼ teaspoon freshly ground black pepper
- Chopped fresh parsley, for garnish

Directions:
In a slow cooker, combine the lamb, turnips, fennel, mushrooms, onion, garlic, chicken broth, tomato paste, red wine (if using), thyme, salt, and pepper.   Cover and cook on high for 3 hours or on low for 6 hours. When the meat is tender and falling apart, garnish with parsley and serve.   If you don't have a slow cooker, in a large pot, heat 2 teaspoons of olive oil over medium heat, and sear the lamb on all sides. Remove from the pot and set aside. Add the turnips, fennel, mushrooms, onion, and garlic to the pot, and cook for 3 to 4 minutes until the vegetables begin to soften. Add the chicken broth, tomato paste, red wine (if using), thyme, salt, pepper, and browned lamb. Bring to a boil, then reduce the heat to low. Simmer for 1½ to 2 hours until the meat is tender. Garnish with parsley and serve.

Nutrition Info: Calories: 303; Total Fat: 7g; Protein: 32g; Carbohydrates: 27g; Sugars: 7g; Fiber: 4g; Sodium: 310mg

465. Turkey, Barley And Vegetable Stock

Servings: 8   Cooking Time: 3 Hours 7 Minutes
Ingredients:
- 2 tablespoons avocado oil
- 1 pound (454 g) ground turkey
- 28 ounces (1.3 kg) tomatoes, diced
- 2 tablespoons sugar-free tomato paste
- 4 cups low-sodium chicken broth
- 1 (15-ounce / 425-g) package frozen peppers and onions (about 2½ cups)
- 1 (15-ounce / 425-g) package frozen chopped carrots (about 2½ cups)
- ⅓ cup dry barley
- 2 bay leaves
- 1 teaspoon kosher salt
- ¼ teaspoon freshly ground black pepper

Directions:
Heat the avocado oil in a pot over medium-high heat. Add the turkey and sauté for 7 minutes or until lightly browned.   Add the tomatoes, tomato paste, and chicken broth. Stir to mix well.   Add the peppers and onions, carrots, barley, bay leaves, salt, and pepper. Stir to mix well.   Bring to a boil. Reduce the heat to low, then cover the pot and simmer for 3 hours.   Once the simmering is finished, allow to cool for 20 minutes, then discard the bay leaves and pour the soup in a large bowl to serve.

Nutrition Info:(1¼ Cups)calories: 253   fat: 12.0g protein: 19.0g   carbs: 21.0g   fiber: 7.0g   sugar: 7.0g sodium: 560mg

466. Red Pepper, Goat Cheese, And Arugula Open-faced Grilled Sandwich

Servings: 1   Cooking Time: 5 Minutes
Ingredients:
- ½ red bell pepper, seeded
- Nonstick cooking spray
- 1 slice whole-wheat thin-sliced bread (I love Ezekiel sprouted bread and Dave's Killer Bread)
- 2 tablespoons crumbled goat cheese
- Pinch dried thyme
- ½ cup arugula

Directions:
Preheat the broiler to high. Line a baking sheet with parchment paper.   Cut the ½ bell pepper lengthwise into two pieces and arrange on the prepared baking sheet with the skin facing up.   Broil for 5 to 10 minutes until the skin is blackened. Transfer to a covered container to steam for 5 minutes, then remove the skin from the pepper using your fingers. Cut the pepper into strips. Heat a small skillet over medium-high heat. Spray it with nonstick cooking spray and place the bread in the skillet. Top with the goat cheese and sprinkle with the thyme. Pile the arugula on top, followed by the roasted red pepper strips. Press down with a spatula to hold in place. Cook for 2 to 3 minutes until the bread is crisp and browned and the cheese is warmed through. (If you prefer, you can make a half-closed sandwich instead: Cut the bread in half and place one half in the skillet. Top with the cheese, thyme, arugula, red pepper, and the other half slice of bread. Cook for 4 to 6 minutes, flipping once, until both sides are browned.)

Nutrition Info: Calories: 109; Total Fat: 2g; Protein: 4g; Carbohydrates: 21g; Sugars: 5g; Fiber: 6g; Sodium: 123mg

467. Roasted Salmon With Salsa Verde

Servings: 4   Cooking Time: 5 Minutes
Ingredients:
- Nonstick cooking spray
- 8 ounces tomatillos, husks removed
- ½ onion, quartered
- 1 jalapeño or serrano pepper, seeded
- 1 garlic clove, unpeeled
- 1 teaspoon extra-virgin olive oil
- ½ teaspoon salt, divided
- 4 (4-ounce) wild-caught salmon fillets
- ¼ teaspoon freshly ground black pepper
- ¼ cup chopped fresh cilantro
- Juice of 1 lime

Directions:
Preheat the oven to 425°F. Spray a baking sheet with nonstick cooking spray.   In a large bowl, toss the tomatillos, onion, jalapeño, garlic, olive oil, and ¼ teaspoon of salt to coat. Arrange in a single layer on the prepared baking sheet, and roast for about 10 minutes until just softened. Transfer to a dish or plate and set aside.   Arrange the salmon fillets skin-side down on the same baking sheet, and season with the remaining ¼ teaspoon of salt and the pepper. Bake for 12 to 15 minutes

until the fish is firm and flakes easily.   Meanwhile, peel the roasted garlic and place it and the roasted vegetables in a blender or food processor. Add a scant ¼ cup of water to the jar, and process until smooth.   Add the cilantro and lime juice and process until smooth. Serve the salmon topped with the salsa verde.

Nutrition Info: Calories: 199; Total Fat: 9g; Protein: 23g; Carbohydrates: 6g; Sugars: 3g; Fiber: 2g; Sodium: 295mg

468. Black Bean Enchilada Skillet Casserole

Servings: 6   Cooking Time: 15 Minutes
Ingredients:
- 1 tablespoon extra-virgin olive oil
- ½ onion, chopped
- ½ red bell pepper, seeded and chopped
- ½ green bell pepper, seeded and chopped
- 2 small zucchini, chopped
- 3 garlic cloves, minced
- 1 (15-ounce) can low-sodium black beans, drained and rinsed
- 1 (10-ounce) can low-sodium enchilada sauce
- 1 teaspoon ground cumin
- ¼ teaspoon salt
- ¼ teaspoon freshly ground black pepper
- ½ cup shredded cheddar cheese, divided
- 2 (6-inch) corn tortillas, cut into strips
- Chopped fresh cilantro, for garnish
- Plain yogurt, for serving

Directions:
Heat the broiler to high.   In a large oven-safe skillet, heat the oil over medium-high heat.   Add the onion, red bell pepper, green bell pepper, zucchini, and garlic to the skillet, and cook for 3 to 5 minutes until the onion softens.   Add the black beans, enchilada sauce, cumin, salt, pepper, ¼ cup of cheese, and tortilla strips, and mix together. Top with the remaining ¼ cup of cheese. Put the skillet under the broiler and broil for 5 to 8 minutes until the cheese is melted and bubbly. Garnish with cilantro and serve with yogurt on the side.

Nutrition Info: Calories: 171; Total Fat: 7g; Protein: 8g; Carbohydrates: 21g; Sugars: 3g; Fiber: 7g; Sodium: 565mg

469. Pear & Poppy Jam

Servings: 32   Cooking Time: 30 Minutes
Ingredients:
- 3 pears, peeled, seeded and chopped
- ½ lemon
- What you'll need from store cupboard:
- ¾ cup Splenda
- 1 tbsp. poppy seeds

Directions:
Place pears in a large bowl. Sprinkle with Splenda and toss to coat. Squeeze the lemon over the pears and toss again. Let sit for 2 hours so the fruit will release its juice. Place poppy seeds in a medium saucepan over medium heat. Cook, stirring, 1-2 minutes to lightly toast the. Transfer them to a bowl.   Add the pears, with the juice, to the saucepan and bring to a boil, stirring frequently. Reduce the heat and let boil 10 minutes or until

thickened.   Spoon ½ the pears into a blender and process until smooth. Add the puree back to the saucepan along with the poppy seeds. Continue cooking 5-10 minutes or the jam is thick.   Spoon into 2 pint sized jars with air tight lids. Let cool completely, screw on the lids and store in the refrigerator. Serving size is 1 tablespoon.

Nutrition Info: Calories 36 Total Carbs 8g Net Carbs 7g Protein 0g Fat 0g Sugar 6g Fiber 1g

470. White Bean & Chicken Soup

Servings: 12   Cooking Time: 2 Hours
Ingredients:
- 2 lbs. chicken breasts, boneless, skinless, cut in cubes
- 3 carrots, sliced
- 2 stalks celery, slice thin
- 1 onion, diced
- ¼ cup fresh parsley, diced
- What you'll need from store cupboard:
- ½ lb. baby lima beans, dried
- ½ lb. great northern beans, dried
- 4 cup low sodium chicken broth
- 2 cup water
- 1 clove garlic, diced
- 2 tbsp. sunflower oil, divided
- 1 tsp salt, divided
- ½ tsp pepper

Directions:
Sort the beans and discard any discolored ones. Rinse under cold water and add to a large pot. Add enough water to cover beans by 2 inches. Place over med-high heat and bring to a boil, cook 2 minutes. Remove from heat, cover, and let stand 2-4 hours or until beans have softened.   Drain and rinse beans, transfer to a large bowl.   Sprinkle chicken with ½ teaspoon salt. Heat 1 tablespoon oil in the large pot over med-high heat and add chicken. Cook until no longer pink. Transfer to a bowl and drain fat.   Heat remaining tablespoon of oil in the pot and add onion. Cook until tender. Add carrots and celery, and garlic and cook 1-2 minutes.   Stir in broth, water, pepper, beans and chicken and bring to a boil. Reduce heat, cover and simmer 2 hours, or until beans are tender. Stir in parsley and remaining salt and serve.

Nutrition Info: Calories 237 Total Carbs 18g Net Carbs 13g Protein 29g Fat 5g Sugar 2g Fiber 5g

471. Chocolate-zucchini Muffins

Servings: 12 (1 Muffin Each)   Cooking Time: 15 Minutes
Ingredients:
- 1½ cups grated zucchini
- 1½ cups rolled oats
- 1 teaspoon ground cinnamon
- 2 teaspoons baking powder
- ¼ teaspoon salt
- 1 large egg
- 1 teaspoon vanilla extract
- ¼ cup coconut oil, melted
- ½ cup unsweetened applesauce
- ¼ cup honey

119

- ¼ cup dark chocolate chips

Directions:
Preheat the oven to 350°F. Grease the cups of a 12-cup muffin tin or line with paper baking liners. Set aside. Place the zucchini in a colander over the sink to drain. In a blender jar, process the oats until they resemble flour. Transfer to a medium mixing bowl and add the cinnamon, baking powder, and salt. Mix well. In another large mixing bowl, combine the egg, vanilla, coconut oil, applesauce, and honey. Stir to combine. Press the zucchini into the colander, draining any liquids, and add to the wet mixture. Stir the dry mixture into the wet mixture, and mix until no dry spots remain. Fold in the chocolate chips. Transfer the batter to the muffin tin, filling each cup a little over halfway. Cook for 16 to 18 minutes until the muffins are lightly browned and a toothpick inserted in the center comes out clean. Store in an airtight container, refrigerated, for up to 5 days.

Nutrition Info: Calories: 121; Total Fat: 7g; Protein: 2g; Carbohydrates: 16g; Sugars: 7g; Fiber: 2g; Sodium: 106mg

472. Slow Cooker Poblano Soup

Servings: 8   Cooking Time: 35 Minutes

Ingredients:
- 1 ½ lbs. chicken breast, cut into large pieces
- 3 Poblano peppers, chopped
- 1 cup onion, diced
- 1 cup cauliflower, diced
- ¼ cup cilantro diced
- ¼ cup reduced fat cream cheese, cubed
- What you'll need from store cupboard:
- 2 ½ cups water
- ½ cup navy beans, soak in hot water 1 hour
- 5 cloves garlic, diced fine
- 1-2 tsp salt
- 1 tsp coriander
- 1 tsp cumin

Directions:
Place all Ingredients, except cream cheese, into a crock pot. Cover and cook on high 4-5 hours, or until chicken is cooked through. Remove chicken and let cool slightly. With an immersion blender, puree the soup until almost smooth. Add the cream cheese and stir until melted. Shred the chicken and add it back to the soup. Let cook just until heated through. Serve.

Nutrition Info: Calories 211 Total Carbs 13g Net Carbs 9g Protein 29g Fat 5g Sugar 3g Fiber 4g

473. Chicken & Pepper Stew

Servings: 4   Cooking Time: 4 Hours

Ingredients:
- 2 small onions, quartered
- 1 ½ cup chicken, cut into 1-inch pieces
- 1 cup broccoli florets
- ½ cup green bell pepper, diced
- ½ cup yellow pepper, diced
- ½ cup red pepper, diced
- ½ cup mushrooms, diced
- 2 tbsp. margarine

- What you'll need from store cupboard:
- 4 cup low sodium chicken broth
- 1/8 cup water
- 4 cloves garlic, diced fine
- 1 tsp rosemary
- 1 tsp corn starch
- ½ tsp thyme
- Salt and pepper to taste

Directions:
Heat 1 tablespoon margarine in large skillet over medium heat. Add chicken and cook till no longer pink. Remove from skillet and add to crock pot. Add remaining tablespoon of margarine to skillet along with onions and garlic. Sauté until onions begin to soften. Add to chicken. Add the broth, vegetables and seasonings to the crock pot. Cover and cook on high 2-3 hours till chicken is cooked through and vegetables are tender. Stir the corn starch into the 1/8 cup of water and stir into the stew. Cook another 60 minutes, or until thickened.

Nutrition Info: Calories 207 Total Carbs 15g Net Carbs 12g Protein 20g Fat 8g Sugar 6g Fiber 3g

474. Lemon Garlic Green Beans

Servings: 6   Cooking Time: 10 Minutes

Ingredients:
- 1 ½ pounds green beans, trimmed
- 2 tablespoons olive oil
- 1-tablespoon fresh lemon juice
- Two cloves minced garlic
- Salt and pepper

Directions:
Fill a large bowl with ice water and set aside. Bring a pot of salted water to boil then add the green beans. Cook for 3 minutes then drain and immediately place in the ice water. Cool the beans completely then drain them well. Heat the oil in a large skillet over medium-high heat. Add the green beans, tossing to coat, then add the lemon juice, garlic, salt, and pepper. Sauté for 3 minutes until the beans are tender-crisp then serve hot.

Nutrition Info: Calories 75Total Fat 4.8gSaturated Fat 0.7gTotal Carbs 8.5gNet Carbs 4.6g Protein 2.1g Sugar 1.7g Fiber 3.9g Sodium 7mg

475. "flour" Tortillas

Servings: 4   Cooking Time: 15 Minutes

Ingredients:
- ¾ cup egg whites
- What you'll need from store cupboard:
- 1/3 cup water
- ¼ cup coconut flour
- 1 tsp sunflower oil
- ½ tsp salt
- ½ tsp cumin
- ½ tsp chili powder

Directions:
Add all Ingredients, except oil, to a food processor and pulse until combined. Let rest 7-8 minutes. Heat oil in a large skillet over med-low heat. Pour ¼ cup batter into center and tilt to spread to 7-8-inch circle. When the top is no longer shiny, flip tortilla and cook another 1-2 minutes. Repeat with remaining batter. Place each

tortilla on parchment paper and slightly wipe off any access oil.

Nutrition Info: Calories 27 Total Carbs 1g Protein 5g Fat 0g Sugar 0g Fiber 0g

476. African Christmas Stew

Servings: 6   Cooking Time: 1 Hour 40 Minutes

Ingredients:
- 3 ½ lbs. chicken, whole pieces with bones in
- 6 Roma tomatoes
- 2 scallions, diced white and green parts
- 1 onion, sliced thin
- 1 cup carrots, sliced
- What you'll need from store cupboard:
- 2 cups water
- 1/8 cup vegetable oil
- 3 tbsp. parsley
- 2 cloves garlic, diced fine
- 1 tbsp. paprika
- 1 ½ tsp thyme
- ¼ tsp curry powder
- 1 bay leaf
- Salt and pepper, to taste

Directions:
Season chicken with salt and pepper on both sides. Place the tomatoes, onion, and scallions in a food processor and pulse until pureed.   In a large soup pot, heat the oil over medium heat. Add chicken and brown on both sides.   Pour the tomato mixture over the chicken and add the remaining Ingredients. Bring to a low boil.   Reduce heat to low, cover, and simmer 60-90 minutes until the chicken is cooked through and the carrots are tender. Discard bay leaf before serving. Serve as is or over cauliflower rice.

Nutrition Info: Calories 480 Total Carbs 9g Net Carbs 7g Protein 78g Fat 13g Sugar 5g Fiber 2g

477. Cauliflower Pizza Crust

Servings: 8   Cooking Time: 30 Minutes

Ingredients:
- 1 ½ lb. cauliflower, separated in florets
- 1 egg
- What you'll need from store cupboard:
- 1 ½ cup reduced fat parmesan cheese
- ½ tbsp. Italian seasoning
- ½ tsp garlic powder

Directions:
Heat oven to 400 degrees. Line a pizza pan, or stone, with parchment paper.   Place the cauliflower in a food processor and pulse until it resembles rice.   Cook the cauliflower in a skillet over medium heat, stirring frequently, until soft, about 10 minutes.   In a large bowl, whisk the egg, cheese and seasonings.   Place the cauliflower in a clean kitchen towel and squeeze out any excess moisture. Stir into cheese mixture to form a soft dough, press with a spatula if needed.   Spread the dough on the prepared pan about ¼-inch thick. Bake 20 minutes, or until top is dry and firm and edges are golden brown.   Let cool 5-10 minutes, the crust will firm up as it cools. Add desired toppings and bake 5-10 minutes more. Slice and serve.

Nutrition Info: Calories 158 Total Carbs 10g net Carbs 6g Protein 12g Fat 9g Sugar 4g Fiber 4g

478. Crispy Cowboy Black Bean Fritters

Servings: 20 Fritters   Cooking Time: 25 Minutes

Ingredients:
- 1¾ cups all-purpose flour
- ½ teaspoon cumin
- 2 teaspoons baking powder
- 2 teaspoons salt
- ½ teaspoon black pepper
- 4 egg whites, lightly beaten
- 1 cup salsa
- 2 (16-ounce / 454-g) cans no-salt-added black beans, rinsed and drained
- 1 tablespoon canola oil, plus extra if needed

Directions:
Combine the flour, cumin, baking powder, salt, and pepper in a large bowl, then mix in the egg whites and salsa. Add the black beans and stir to mix well.   Heat the canola oil in a nonstick skillet over medium-high heat. Spoon 1 teaspoon of the mixture into the skillet to make a fritter. Make more fritters to coat the bottom of the skillet. Keep a little space between each two fritters. You may need to work in batches to avoid overcrowding. Cook for 3 minutes or until the fritters are golden brown on both sides. Flip the fritters and flatten with a spatula halfway through the cooking time. Repeat with the remaining mixture. Add more oil as needed.   Serve immediately.

Nutrition Info:calories: 115   fat: 1.0g   protein: 6.0g carbs: 20.0g   fiber: 5.0g   sugar: 2.0g   sodium: 350mg

479. Simple Deviled Eggs

Servings: 12   Cooking Time: 8 Minutes

Ingredients:
- 6 large eggs
- ⅛ teaspoon mustard powder
- 2 tablespoons plus 1 teaspoon light mayonnaise
- Salt and freshly ground black pepper, to taste

Directions:
Sit the eggs in a saucepan, then pour in enough water to cover the egg. Bring to a boil, then boil the eggs for another 8 minutes. Turn off the heat and cover, then let sit for 15 minutes.   Transfer the boiled eggs in a pot of cold water and peel under the water.   Transfer the eggs on a large plate, then cut in half. Remove the egg yolks and place them in a bowl, then mash with a fork.   Add the mustard powder, mayo, salt, and pepper to the bowl of yolks, then stir to mix well.   Spoon the yolk mixture in the egg white on the plate. Serve immediately.

Nutrition Info:calories: 45   fat: 3.0g   protein: 3.0g carbs: 1.0g   fiber: 0g   sugar: 0g   sodium: 70mg

480. Seafood, Mango, And Avocado Salad

Servings: 4   Cooking Time: 20 Minutes

Ingredients:
- 1 cup quinoa, rinsed
- ½ pound (227 g) medium shrimps, peeled and deveined

- ½ pound (227 g) scallops
- 1 tablespoon olive oil
- ½ red bell pepper, chopped
- 1 roma plum tomatoes, deseeded and chopped
- 1 jalapeño pepper, stemmed and finely chopped
- ½ cup cooked black beans
- 1 mango, chopped
- 1 avocado, chopped
- 2 small scallions, chopped
- 2 tablespoons cilantro leaves, chopped
- Citrus Dressing:
- 2 tablespoons lime juice
- 2 tablespoons orange juice
- 1 teaspoon honey
- ¼ teaspoon cayenne pepper
- 1 tablespoon extra virgin olive oil
- Sea salt, to taste

Directions:
Pour the quinoa in a pot, then pour in enough water to cover. Bring to a boil, then reduce the heat to low and simmer to 10 to 15 minutes or until the liquid has been absorbed. Fluffy with a fork and let stand until ready to use.   Meanwhile, combine the ingredients for the citrus dressing in a small bowl. Stir to mix well. Set aside until ready to use.   Put the shrimps and scallops in a separate bowl, then drizzle with the olive oil. Toss to coat well.   Add the oiled shrimps and scallops in a nonstick skillet and grill over medium-high heat for 4 minutes or until opaque. Flip them halfway through. Remove them from the skillet and allow to cool.   Combine the cooked quinoa, shrimp and scallops with bell pepper, tomato, jalapeño, beans, mango, avocado, and scallions in a large salad bowl, then drizzle with the citrus dressing. Toss to combine well.   Garnish with cilantro leaves and serve immediately.

Nutrition Info:calories: 470   fat: 16.0g   protein: 30.0g   carbs: 56.0g   fiber: 10.0g   sugar: 16.0g   sodium: 320mg

481. Winter Chicken And Citrus Salad

Servings: 4   Cooking Time: 10 Minutes
Ingredients:
- 4 cups baby spinach
- 2 tablespoons extra-virgin olive oil
- 1 tablespoon freshly squeezed lemon juice
- ⅛ teaspoon salt
- Freshly ground black pepper
- 2 cups chopped cooked chicken
- 2 mandarin oranges, peeled and sectioned
- ½ peeled grapefruit, sectioned
- ¼ cup sliced almonds

Directions:
In a large mixing bowl, toss the spinach with the olive oil, lemon juice, salt, and pepper.   Add the chicken, oranges, grapefruit, and almonds to the bowl. Toss gently.   Arrange on 4 plates and serve.

Nutrition Info: Calories: 249; Total Fat: 12g; Protein: 24g; Carbohydrates: 11g; Sugars: 7g; Fiber: 3g; Sodium: 135mg

482. Blueberry Orange Dessert Sauce

Servings: 16   Cooking Time: 10 Minutes
Ingredients:
- 1 ½ cup orange segments
- 1 cup blueberries
- ¼ cup orange juice
- What you'll need from store cupboard:
- ¼ cup water
- 1/3 cup almonds, sliced
- 3 tbsp. Splenda
- 1 tbsp. cornstarch
- 1/8 tsp salt

Directions:
In a small saucepan, combine Splenda, cornstarch, and salt. Whisk in orange juice and water until smooth. Bring to a boil over med-high heat, cook, stirring frequently, 1-2 minutes or until thickened.   Reduce heat and stir in fruit. Cook 5 minutes. Remove from heat and let cool completely.   Store in an airtight jar in the refrigerator until ready to use. Serving size is 1 tablespoon.

Nutrition Info: Calories 46 Total Carbs 8g Protein 1g Fat 1g Sugar 6g Fiber 0g

483. Homemade Turkey Breakfast Sausage

Servings: 8 (1 Patty Each)   Cooking Time: 10 Minutes
Ingredients:
- 1 pound lean ground turkey
- ½ teaspoon salt
- ½ teaspoon dried sage
- ½ teaspoon dried thyme
- ½ teaspoon freshly ground black pepper
- ¼ teaspoon ground fennel seeds
- 1 teaspoon extra-virgin olive oil

Directions:
In a large mixing bowl, combine the ground turkey, salt, sage, thyme, pepper, and fennel. Mix well.   Shape the meat into 8 small, round patties.   Heat the olive oil in a skillet over medium-high heat. Cook the patties in the skillet for 3 to 4 minutes on each side until browned and cooked through.   Serve warm, or store in an airtight container in the refrigerator for up to 3 days or in the freezer for up to 1 month.

Nutrition Info: Calories: 92; Total Fat: 5g; Protein: 11g; Carbohydrates: 0g; Sugars: 0g; Fiber: 0g; Sodium: 156mg

484. Almond Banana Smoothie

Servings: 2   Cooking Time: 5 Munutes
Ingredients:
- Baby spinach – 1 ½ oz.
- Rolled oats – 3 Tbsps.
- Cinnamon – 1 tsp.
- Ice – 1 cup
- Bananas – 2, peeled
- Walnuts – 3 Tbsps.
- Almond milk – 1 cup

Directions:

Except for the cinnamon and walnuts, blend everything in the blender.   Top with cinnamon and walnuts and serve.

Nutrition Info:266Fat: 10Carb: 47g Protein: 5g

485. Roasted Mushroom & Cauliflower Soup

Servings: 4   Cooking Time: 30 Minutes

Ingredients:
- 1 small (600g) cauliflower, trimmed, chopped
- 5 cup mushrooms, sliced
- 1 leek, halved lengthways, thinly sliced
- ½ cup flat-leaf parsley, chopped
- What you'll need from store cupboard:
- 4 cup low sodium chicken broth
- 4 tbsp. olive oil
- 3 tsp curry powder
- Nonstick cooking spray

Directions:
Heat oven to 425 degrees.   Spray two large baking sheets with cooking spray. Place cauliflower in one pan and mushrooms in the other. Drizzle each with 1 ½ tablespoons oil and sprinkle with 1 ½ teaspoons curry powder.   Place cauliflower on the top rack of oven and mushrooms below, cook 20-25 minutes or until vegetables are tender.   In a large saucepan, heat remaining oil over medium heat. Add leek, cook 5 minutes, stirring occasionally, until soft. Add broth and bring to a boil. Add roasted vegetables and return to boil. Remove from heat, use an immersion blender, and process until almost smooth. Stir in parsley and adjust seasonings to taste. Serve.

Nutrition Info: Calories 187 Total Carbs 11g Net Carbs 8g Protein 7g Fat 15g Sugar 4g Fiber 3g

486. Spicy Sweet Dipping Sauce

Servings: 16   Cooking Time: 5 Minutes

Ingredients:
- ¼ tsp habanero pepper, diced fine
- 1 tbsp. lime juice
- What you'll need from store cupboard:
- 1 cup sugar free orange marmalade
- 1 tbsp. fish sauce
- ½ tsp red pepper flakes
- ¼ tsp sesame oil
- Pinch of salt

Directions:
Mix all Ingredients together in a small bowl. Spoon into a jar with an air tight lid and store in the refrigerator. Serving size is 1 tablespoon. Will last up to one week in the refrigerator.

Nutrition Info: Calories 12 Total Carbs 5g Protein 0g Fat 0g Sugar 0g Fiber 0g

487. Healthy Loaf Of Bread

Servings: 20   Cooking Time: 30 Minutes

Ingredients:
- 6 eggs, separated
- 4 tbsp. butter, melted
- What you'll need from store cupboard:
- 1 ½ cup almond flour, sifted
- 3 tsp baking powder
- ¼ tsp cream of tartar
- 1/8 tsp salt
- Butter flavored cooking spray

Directions:
Heat oven to 375 degrees. Spray an 8-inch loaf pan with cooking spray.   In a large bowl, beat egg whites and cream of tartar until soft peaks form   Add the yolks, 1/3 of egg whites, butter, flour, baking powder, and salt to a food processor and pulse until combined.   Add remaining egg whites and pulse until thoroughly combined, being careful not to over mix the dough. Pour into prepared pan and bake 30 minutes, or until bread passes the toothpick test. Cool 10 minutes in the pan then invert and cool completely before slicing.

Nutrition Info: Calories 81 Total Carbs 2g Net Carbs 1g Protein 3g Fat 7g Sugar 0g Fiber 1g

488. Oat And Walnut Granola

Servings: 16 (⅓ Cup Each)   Cooking Time: 10 Minutes

Ingredients:
- 4 cups rolled oats
- 1 cup walnut pieces
- ½ cup pepitas
- ¼ teaspoon salt
- 1 teaspoon ground cinnamon
- 1 teaspoon ground ginger
- ½ cup coconut oil, melted
- ½ cup unsweetened applesauce
- 1 teaspoon vanilla extract
- ½ cup dried cherries

Directions:
Preheat the oven to 350°F. Line a baking sheet with parchment paper.   In a large bowl, toss the oats, walnuts, pepitas, salt, cinnamon, and ginger.   In a large measuring cup, combine the coconut oil, applesauce, and vanilla. Pour over the dry mixture and mix well.   Transfer the mixture to the prepared baking sheet. Cook for 30 minutes, stirring about halfway through. Remove from the oven and let the granola sit undisturbed until completely cool. Break the granola into pieces, and stir in the dried cherries.   Transfer to an airtight container, and store at room temperature for up to 2 weeks.

Nutrition Info: Calories: 224; Total Fat: 15g; Protein: 5g; Carbohydrates: 20g; Sugars: 5g; Fiber: 3g; Sodium: 30mg

489. Ginger-glazed Salmon And Broccoli

Servings: 4   Cooking Time: 10 Minutes

Ingredients:
- Nonstick cooking spray
- 1 tablespoon low-sodium tamari or gluten-free soy sauce
- Juice of 1 lemon
- 1 tablespoon honey
- 1 (1-inch) piece fresh ginger, grated
- 1 garlic clove, minced
- 1 pound salmon fillet
- ¼ teaspoon salt, divided

- ⅛ teaspoon freshly ground black pepper
- 2 broccoli heads, cut into florets
- 1 tablespoon extra-virgin olive oil

Directions:
Preheat the oven to 400°F. Spray a baking sheet with nonstick cooking spray.   In a small bowl, mix the tamari, lemon juice, honey, ginger, and garlic. Set aside. Place the salmon skin-side down on the prepared baking sheet. Season with ⅛ teaspoon of salt and the pepper. In a large mixing bowl, toss the broccoli and olive oil. Season with the remaining ⅛ teaspoon of salt. Arrange in a single layer on the baking sheet next to the salmon. Bake for 15 to 20 minutes until the salmon flakes easily with a fork and the broccoli is fork-tender.   In a small pan over medium heat, bring the tamari-ginger mixture to a simmer and cook for 1 to 2 minutes until it just begins to thicken.   Drizzle the sauce over the salmon and serve.

Nutrition Info: Calories: 238; Total Fat: 11g; Protein: 25g; Carbohydrates: 11g; Sugars: 6g; Fiber: 2g; Sodium: 334mg

490. Tomato And Kale Soup

Servings: 4   Cooking Time: 10 Minutes

Ingredients:
- 1 tablespoon extra-virgin olive oil
- 1 medium onion, chopped
- 2 carrots, finely chopped
- 3 garlic cloves, minced
- 4 cups low-sodium vegetable broth
- 1 (28-ounce) can crushed tomatoes
- ½ teaspoon dried oregano
- ¼ teaspoon dried basil
- 4 cups chopped baby kale leaves
- ¼ teaspoon salt

Directions:
In a large pot, heat the oil over medium heat. Add the onion and carrots to the pan. Sauté for 3 to 5 minutes until they begin to soften. Add the garlic and sauté for 30 seconds more, until fragrant.   Add the vegetable broth, tomatoes, oregano, and basil to the pot and bring to a boil. Reduce the heat to low and simmer for 5 minutes. Using an immersion blender, purée the soup.   Add the kale and simmer for 3 more minutes. Season with the salt. Serve immediately.

Nutrition Info: Calories: 170; Total Fat: 5g; Protein: 6g; Carbohydrates: 31g; Sugars: 13g; Fiber: 9g; Sodium: 600mg

491. Blackened Tilapia With Mango Salsa

Servings: 2   Cooking Time: 15 Minutes

Ingredients:
- FOR THE SALSA
- 1 cup chopped mango
- 2 tablespoons chopped red onion
- 2 tablespoons chopped fresh cilantro
- 2 tablespoons freshly squeezed lime juice
- ½ jalapeño pepper, seeded and minced
- Pinch salt
- FOR THE TILAPIA
- 1 tablespoon paprika

- 1 teaspoon onion powder
- ½ teaspoon freshly ground black pepper
- ½ teaspoon dried thyme
- ½ teaspoon garlic powder
- ¼ teaspoon cayenne pepper
- ¼ teaspoon salt
- ½ pound boneless tilapia fillets
- 2 teaspoons extra-virgin olive oil
- 1 lime, cut into wedges, for serving

Directions:
TO MAKE THE SALSA   In a medium bowl, toss together the mango, onion, cilantro, lime juice, jalapeño, and salt. Set aside.   TO MAKE THE TILAPIA   In a small bowl, mix the paprika, onion powder, pepper, thyme, garlic powder, cayenne, and salt. Rub the mixture on both sides of the tilapia fillets.   In a large skillet, heat the oil over medium heat, and cook the fish for 3 to 5 minutes on each side until the outer coating is crisp and the fish is cooked through.   Spoon half of the salsa over each fillet and serve with lime wedges on the side.

Nutrition Info: Calories: 240; Total Fat: 8g; Protein: 25g; Carbohydrates: 22g; Sugars: 13g; Fiber: 4g; Sodium: 417mg

492. Scallops And Asparagus Skillet

Servings: 4   Cooking Time: 10 Minutes

Ingredients:
- 3 teaspoons extra-virgin olive oil, divided
- 1 pound asparagus, trimmed and cut into 2-inch segments
- 1 tablespoon butter
- 1 pound sea scallops
- ¼ cup dry white wine
- Juice of 1 lemon
- 2 garlic cloves, minced
- ¼ teaspoon freshly ground black pepper

Directions:
In a large skillet, heat 1½ teaspoons of oil over medium heat.   Add the asparagus and sauté for 5 to 6 minutes until just tender, stirring regularly. Remove from the skillet and cover with aluminum foil to keep warm. Add the remaining 1½ teaspoons of oil and the butter to the skillet. When the butter is melted and sizzling, place the scallops in a single layer in the skillet. Cook for about 3 minutes on one side until nicely browned. Use tongs to gently loosen and flip the scallops, and cook on the other side for another 3 minutes until browned and cooked through. Remove and cover with foil to keep warm.   In the same skillet, combine the wine, lemon juice, garlic, and pepper. Bring to a simmer for 1 to 2 minutes, stirring to mix in any browned pieces left in the pan.   Return the asparagus and the cooked scallops to the skillet to coat with the sauce. Serve warm.

Nutrition Info: Calories: 252; Total Fat: 7g; Protein: 26g; Carbohydrates: 15g; Sugars: 3g; Fiber: 2g; Sodium: 493mg

493. Crab & Cauliflower Bisque

Servings: 8   Cooking Time: 30 Minutes

Ingredients:
- 1 lb. lump crabmeat, cooked and shells removed

- 1 medium head cauliflower, separated into very small florets
- 1 white onion, diced fine
- 1 cup celery, diced fine
- 1 cup carrots, diced fine
- 1 cup half-n-half
- 1 tbsp. sherry
- 4 tbsp. margarine
- What you'll need from store cupboard:
- 6 cup chicken broth
- 1½ tsp coarse salt
- 1 tsp white pepper

Directions:
In a large saucepan, over med-high heat, melt margarine. Add celery, onion, and carrot. Cook, stirring frequently, until vegetables are tender. Add in cauliflower, broth, salt, and pepper, and cook until soup starts to boil. Reduce heat to medium and cook 15 minutes, or until cauliflower is tender. Pour into a blender and add cream and sherry. Process until combined and soup is smooth. Pour back into the saucepan. Fold in crab and heat through. Serve.

Nutrition Info: Calories 201 Total Carbs 10g Net Carbs 7g Protein 14g Fat 11g Sugar 4g Fiber 3g

494. Peanut Chicken Satay

Servings: 8   Cooking Time: 20 Minutes, Plus 2 Hours To Marinate
Ingredients:
- FOR THE PEANUT SAUCE
- 1 cup natural peanut butter
- 2 tablespoons low-sodium tamari or gluten-free soy sauce
- 1 teaspoon red chili paste
- 1 tablespoon honey
- Juice of 2 limes
- ½ cup hot water
- FOR THE CHICKEN
- 2 pounds boneless, skinless chicken thighs, trimmed of fat and cut into 1-inch pieces
- ½ cup plain nonfat Greek yogurt
- 2 garlic cloves, minced
- 1 teaspoon minced fresh ginger
- ½ onion, coarsely chopped
- 1½ teaspoons ground coriander
- 2 teaspoons ground cumin
- ½ teaspoon salt
- 1 teaspoon extra-virgin olive oil
- Lettuce leaves, for serving

Directions:
TO MAKE THE PEANUT SAUCE   In a medium mixing bowl, combine the peanut butter, tamari, chili paste, honey, lime juice, and hot water. Mix until smooth. Set aside.   TO MAKE THE CHICKEN   In a large mixing bowl, combine the chicken, yogurt, garlic, ginger, onion, coriander, cumin, and salt, and mix well.   Cover and marinate in the refrigerator for at least 2 hours. Thread the chicken pieces onto bamboo skewers.   In a grill pan or large skillet, heat the oil. Cook the skewers for 3 to 5 minutes on each side until the pieces are cooked through.   Remove the chicken from the skewers and

place a few pieces on each lettuce leaf. Drizzle with the peanut sauce and serve.
Nutrition Info: Calories: 386; Total Fat: 26g; Protein: 30g; Carbohydrates: 14g; Sugars: 6g; Fiber: 2g; Sodium: 442mg

495. Lamb Chops With Cherry Glaze

Servings: 4   Cooking Time: 10 Minutes
Ingredients:
- 4 (4-ounce) lamb chops
- 1½ teaspoons chopped fresh rosemary
- ¼ teaspoon salt
- ¼ teaspoon freshly ground black pepper
- 1 cup frozen cherries, thawed
- ¼ cup dry red wine
- 2 tablespoons orange juice
- 1 teaspoon extra-virgin olive oil

Directions:
Season the lamb chops with the rosemary, salt, and pepper.   In a small saucepan over medium-low heat, combine the cherries, red wine, and orange juice, and simmer, stirring regularly, until the sauce thickens, 8 to 10 minutes.   Heat a large skillet over medium-high heat. When the pan is hot, add the olive oil to lightly coat the bottom.   Cook the lamb chops for 3 to 4 minutes on each side until well-browned yet medium rare. Serve, topped with the cherry glaze.
Nutrition Info: Calories: 356; Total Fat: 27g; Protein: 20g; Carbohydrates: 6g; Sugars: 4g; Fiber: 1g; Sodium: 199mg

496. Garlic Dipping Sauce

Servings: 4   Cooking Time: 5 Minutes
Ingredients:
- 1 cup Greek yogurt
- 1 tbsp. fresh dill, diced fine
- What you'll need from store cupboard:
- 2 cloves garlic, diced fine

Directions:
In a small bowl, whisk all Ingredients together.   Serve warm or cover and chill until ready to use.
Nutrition Info: Calories 40 Total Carbs 2g Protein 5g Fat 1g Sugar 2g Fiber 0g

497. Teriyaki Sauce

Servings: 16   Cooking Time: 10 Minutes
Ingredients:
- What you'll need from store cupboard:
- 1 ¼ cup water, divided
- ¼ cup lite soy sauce
- 2 tbsp. + ½ tsp liquid stevia
- 1 ½ tbsp. corn starch
- ½ tsp ginger
- ¼ tsp garlic powder

Directions:
Combine soy sauce, 1 cup water, ginger, garlic powder, and stevia in a small saucepan. Place over med-low heat and bring to a simmer.   Whisk the corn starch with the ¼ cup water until smooth. Add it to the sauce in the pan and mix thoroughly. Let sauce simmer until it starts to thicken, about 1 minute.   Remove from heat and cool

completely. Sauce will continue to thicken as it cools. Use as a marinade or dipping sauce. Serving size is 1 tablespoon.

Nutrition Info: Calories 5 Total Carbs 1g Protein 0g Fat 0g Sugar 0g Fiber 0g

498. Clam & Bacon Soup

Servings: 8   Cooking Time: 20 Minutes
Ingredients:
- 10-12 large clams, in the shell
- 4 slices bacon, chopped and cooked almost crisp
- 3 cups cauliflower, separated into florets
- ½ cup onion, diced
- What you'll need from store cupboard:
- 6 cup water
- 1 tsp Worcestershire sauce

Directions:
Scrub clams and rinse under cold running water. Place in a large pot and add water. Bring to a simmer over med-high heat. Cover and cook until clams open, about 8-10 minutes. Transfer clams to bowl to cool.   Cook onion in the same pan used for the bacon, 2-3 minutes. Stir to scrape up the brown bits on the bottom of the pan. When clams are cool enough to touch, remove the meat from the shells and chop it.   Bring the clam liquid to a boil. Add cauliflower and cook until almost tender, about 5 minutes.   Stir in the bacon, Worcestershire sauce and clams. Season with salt and pepper to taste and cook until everything is heated through. Serve immediately.

Nutrition Info: Calories 105 Total Carbs 4g Protein 7g Fat 7g Sugar 2g Fiber 1g

499. Spinach, Artichoke, And Goat Cheese Breakfast Bake

Servings: 8   Cooking Time: 10 Minutes
Ingredients:
- Nonstick cooking spray
- 1 (10-ounce) package frozen spinach, thawed and drained
- 1 (14-ounce) can artichoke hearts, drained
- ¼ cup finely chopped red bell pepper
- 2 garlic cloves, minced
- 8 eggs, lightly beaten
- ¼ cup unsweetened plain almond milk
- ½ teaspoon salt
- ½ teaspoon freshly ground black pepper
- ½ cup crumbled goat cheese

Directions:
Preheat the oven to 375°F. Spray an 8-by-8-inch baking dish with nonstick cooking spray.   In a large mixing bowl, combine the spinach, artichoke hearts, bell pepper, garlic, eggs, almond milk, salt, and pepper. Stir well to combine.   Transfer the mixture to the baking dish. Sprinkle with the goat cheese.   Bake for 35 minutes until the eggs are set. Serve warm.

Nutrition Info: Calories: 104; Total Fat: 5g; Protein: 9g; Carbohydrates: 6g; Sugars: 1g; Fiber: 2g; Sodium: 488mg

500. Pizza Crust

Servings: 4   Cooking Time: 40 Minutes
Ingredients:
- 1 ½ cup mozzarella cheese, grated
- 2 oz. cream cheese
- 1 egg, beaten
- What you'll need from store cupboard:
- ¾ cup almond flour
- ½ tsp Italian seasoning
- ½ tsp salt
- ½ tsp garlic powder
- ½ tsp onion powder

Directions:
Heat oven to 400 degrees. Line a large baking sheet with parchment paper.   In large bowl, microwave cream cheese and mozzarella for 60 seconds. Remove from microwave and stir. Return to microwave and cook another 30 seconds. Stir until well combined.   Add flour, salt, onion powder, garlic powder, and egg. Stir until almond flour is well incorporated into cheese. If mixture becomes too sticky, microwave another 10-15 seconds to warm up.   Place dough on parchment paper and roll out thin. Poke holes in crust with fork. Bake 10 minutes.   Remove from oven and turn over. Bake another 10 minutes.   Remove from oven and top with desired pizza toppings.   Return to oven and bake another 10 minutes, until toppings are hot and cheese is melted.

Nutrition Info: Calories 198 Total Carbs 5g Net Carbs 3g Protein 9g Fat 17g Sugar 1g Fiber 2g

501. Cream Cheese Swirl Brownies

Servings: 12 (1 Brownie Each)   Cooking Time: 10 Minutes
Ingredients:
- 2 eggs
- ¼ cup unsweetened applesauce
- ¼ cup coconut oil, melted
- 3 tablespoons pure maple syrup, divided
- ¼ cup unsweetened cocoa powder
- ¼ cup coconut flour
- ¼ teaspoon salt
- 1 teaspoon baking powder
- 2 tablespoons low-fat cream cheese

Directions:
Preheat the oven to 350°F. Grease an 8-by-8-inch baking dish.   In a large mixing bowl, beat the eggs with the applesauce, coconut oil, and 2 tablespoons of maple syrup.   Stir in the cocoa powder and coconut flour, and mix well. Sprinkle the salt and baking powder evenly over the surface and mix well to incorporate. Transfer the mixture to the prepared baking dish.   In a small, microwave-safe bowl, microwave the cream cheese for 10 to 20 seconds until softened. Add the remaining 1 tablespoon of maple syrup and mix to combine.   Drop the cream cheese onto the batter, and use a toothpick or chopstick to swirl it on the surface. Bake for 20 minutes, until a toothpick inserted in the center comes out clean. Cool and cut into 12 squares.   Store refrigerated in a covered container for up to 5 days.

Nutrition Info: Calories: 84; Total Fat: 6g; Protein: 2g; Carbohydrates: 6g; Sugars: 4g; Fiber: 2g; Sodium: 93mg

502. Citrus Vinaigrette

Servings: 6   Cooking Time: 10 Minutes

Ingredients:
- 1 orange, zested and juiced
- 1 lemon, zested and juiced
- What you'll need from store cupboard:
- ¼ cup extra virgin olive oil
- 1 tsp Dijon mustard
- 1 tsp honey
- 1 clove garlic, crushed
- Salt & pepper, to taste

Directions:
Place the zest and juices, mustard, honey, garlic, salt and pepper in a food processor. Pulse to combine.   With the machine running, slowly pour in the olive oil and process until combined.   Use right away, or store in a jar with an airtight lid in the refrigerator.

Nutrition Info: Calories 94   Total Carbs 6g Net Carbs 5g Protein 0g Fat 8g Sugar 4g Fiber 1g

503. Salmon Dill Soup

Servings: 4   Cooking Time: 30 Minutes

Ingredients:
- 4 skinless salmon fillets, cut into pieces
- 1 green onion, diced fine
- 1 daikon radish, peeled and diced
- ½ cup heavy cream
- 2 tbsp. fresh dill, diced
- 2 tbsp. margarine
- What you'll need from store cupboard:
- 4 cups seafood stock or vegetable broth
- ½ cup white wine
- Salt and black pepper

Directions:
In a large saucepan, melt margarine over med-high heat. Add onions and sauté for 1-2 minutes.   Add wine and cook until liquid is reduced by half.   Add the radish and broth. Cook until radish is tender, about 15 minutes. Add salmon, cream and dill and cook another 5-8 minutes until salmon is flaky. Salt and pepper to taste.

Nutrition Info: Calories 537 Total Carbs 8g Net Carbs 7g Protein 46g Fat 33g Sugar 2g Fiber 1g

504. Smoky Pumpkin Soup

Servings: 6   Cooking Time: 40 Minutes

Ingredients:
- 10 slices bacon, diced
- 2 lb. fresh pumpkin, peel, remove seeds & cube
- 1 onion, diced
- ½ cup half-n-half
- 1 tsp margarine
- What you'll need from store cupboard:
- 2 pint low sodium chicken broth
- 1 tbsp. tomato puree

Directions:
Melt the margarine in large heavy pot over med-high heat. Add onion, bacon and pumpkin. Cook 2-3 minutes, stirring occasionally. Reduce heat and cook 6-8 minutes. Transfer about 2 tablespoons of bacon to a paper towel line plate for later.   Stir in tomato puree, broth and cream. Bring to a simmer. Reduce heat to low and cook 30 minutes, or until pumpkin is soft.   Use an immersion blender to process soup until smooth. Taste and season as needed. Ladle into bowls and sprinkle with reserved bacon. Serve.

Nutrition Info: Calories 260 Total Carbs 16g Net Carbs 11g Protein 15g Fat 15g Sugar 6g Fiber 5g

505. Sesame-ginger Chicken Soba

Servings: 6   Cooking Time: 10 Minutes

Ingredients:
- 8 ounces soba noodles
- 2 boneless, skinless chicken breasts, halved lengthwise
- ¼ cup tahini
- 2 tablespoons rice vinegar
- 1 tablespoon reduced-sodium gluten-free soy sauce or tamari
- 1 teaspoon toasted sesame oil
- 1 (1-inch) piece fresh ginger, finely grated
- ⅓ cup water
- 1 large cucumber, seeded and diced
- 1 scallions bunch, green parts only, cut into 1-inch segments
- 1 tablespoon sesame seeds

Directions:
Preheat the broiler to high.   Bring a large pot of water to a boil. Add the noodles and cook until tender, according to the package directions. Drain and rinse the noodles in cool water.   On a baking sheet, arrange the chicken in a single layer. Broil for 5 to 7 minutes on each side, depending on the thickness, until the chicken is cooked through and its juices run clear. Use two forks to shred the chicken.   In a small bowl, combine the tahini, rice vinegar, soy sauce, sesame oil, ginger, and water. Whisk to combine.   In a large bowl, toss the shredded chicken, noodles, cucumber, and scallions. Pour the tahini sauce over the noodles and toss to combine. Served sprinkled with the sesame seeds.

Nutrition Info: Calories: 251; Total Fat: 8g; Protein: 16g; Carbohydrates: 35g; Sugars: 2g; Fiber: 2g; Sodium: 482mg

506. Apple Cider Vinaigrette

Servings: 8   Cooking Time: 5 Minutes

Ingredients:
- What you'll need from store cupboard:
- ½ cup sunflower oil
- ¼ cup apple cider vinegar
- ¼ cup apple juice, unsweetened
- 2 tbsp. honey
- 1 tbsp. lemon juice
- ½ tsp salt
- Freshly ground black pepper, to taste

Directions:
Place all Ingredients in a mason jar. Screw on lid and shake until everything is thoroughly combined. Store in refrigerator until ready to use. Shake well before using.

Nutrition Info: Calories 138 Total Carbs 4g Protein 0g Fat 13g Sugar 4g Fiber 0g

507. Ginger Detox Twist

Servings: 2   Cooking Time: 5 Minutes
Ingredients:
- Collard greens – 1 ½ oz.
- Apple – One chopped
- Ginger – ½ inch
- Water – 1 cup
- Persian cucumbers – 2, chopped
- Meyer lemon – 1, peeled
- Chlorella – ½ tsp.
- Ice – 1 cup

Directions:
Blend everything in a blender and serve.
Nutrition Info: 114 Fat: 1Carb: 22g Protein: 5g

508. Cranberry Orange Compote

Servings: 8   Cooking Time: 10 Minutes
Ingredients:
- 1 lb. fresh cranberries, rinsed and drained
- 1 large orange, halved
- What you'll need from store cupboard:
- 1 tsp vanilla
- 1 tsp cinnamon

Directions:
Add cranberries to a medium saucepan and place over medium heat. Squeeze both halves of the orange, with pulp, into the berries. Stir in vanilla and cinnamon. Cook, stirring frequently, until berries start to open. Reduce heat and continue cooking for 10 minutes, or until mixture starts to thicken.   Let cool 15 minutes, then spoon into a jar with an airtight lid. Refrigerate until ready to use.
Nutrition Info: Calories 43 Total Carbs 8g Net Carbs 5g Protein 0g Fat 0g Sugar 4g Fiber 3g

509. Crispy Parmesan Cups With White Beans And Veggies

Servings: 4 (2 Cups Each)   Cooking Time: 10 Minutes
Ingredients:
- 1 cup grated Parmesan cheese, divided
- 1 (15-ounce) can low-sodium white beans, drained and rinsed
- 1 cucumber, peeled and finely diced
- ½ cup finely diced red onion
- ¼ cup thinly sliced fresh basil
- 1 garlic clove, minced
- ½ jalapeño pepper, diced
- 1 tablespoon extra-virgin olive oil
- 1 tablespoon balsamic vinegar
- ¼ teaspoon salt
- Freshly ground black pepper

Directions:
Heat a medium nonstick skillet over medium heat. Sprinkle 2 tablespoons of cheese in a thin circle in the center of the pan, flattening it with a spatula.   When the cheese melts, use a spatula to flip the cheese and lightly brown the other side.   Remove the cheese

"pancake" from the pan and place into the cup of a muffin tin, bending it gently with your hands to fit in the muffin cup.   Repeat with the remaining cheese until you have 8 cups.   In a mixing bowl, combine the beans, cucumber, onion, basil, garlic, jalapeño, olive oil, and vinegar, and season with the salt and pepper.   Fill each cup with the bean mixture just before serving.
Nutrition Info: Calories: 259; Total Fat: 12g; Protein: 15g; Carbohydrates: 24g; Sugars: 4g; Fiber: 8g; Sodium: 551mg

510. Saffron-spiced Chicken Breasts

Servings: 4   Cooking Time: 10 Minutes, Plus 1 Hour To Marinate
Ingredients:
- Pinch saffron (3 or 4 threads)
- ½ cup plain nonfat yogurt
- 2 tablespoons water
- ½ onion, chopped
- 3 garlic cloves, minced
- 2 tablespoons chopped fresh cilantro
- Juice of ½ lemon
- ½ teaspoon salt
- 1 pound boneless, skinless chicken breasts, cut into 2-inch strips
- 1 tablespoon extra-virgin olive oil

Directions:
In a blender jar, combine the saffron, yogurt, water, onion, garlic, cilantro, lemon juice, and salt. Pulse to blend.   In a large mixing bowl, combine the chicken and the yogurt sauce, and stir to coat. Cover and refrigerate for at least 1 hour or up to overnight.   In a large skillet, heat the oil over medium heat. Add the chicken pieces, shaking off any excess marinade. Discard the marinade. Cook the chicken pieces on each side for 5 minutes, flipping once, until cooked through and golden brown.
Nutrition Info: Calories: 155; Total Fat: 5g; Protein: 26g; Carbohydrates: 3g; Sugars: 1g; Fiber: 0g; Sodium: 501mg

511. Beef Vegetable Soup

Servings: 6   Cooking Time: 7 Hours
Ingredients:
- 1 lb. lean ground beef, cooked and drained
- 2 stalks celery, sliced
- 1 large head of cauliflower, separated medium sized florets
- 1 tomato, diced
- ½ onion, diced
- 1 cup carrots, sliced thick
- 1 cup corn kernels
- What you'll need from store cupboard:
- 4 cup water
- 1 ¾ cup low sodium beef broth
- 1 ½ cup tomato sauce
- ½ cup white cooking wine
- 1 tbsp. parsley

Directions:
Place everything but the cauliflower in a crock pot. Cover and cook on low 5-6 hours or until vegetables are almost

tender.   Add the cauliflower and cook another 60 minutes. Serve.
Nutrition Info: Calories 254 Total Carbs 20g Net Carbs 14g Protein 29g Fat 6g Sugar 9g Fiber 6g

512. Peaches And Cream Oatmeal Smoothie

Servings: 1   Cooking Time: 5 Minutes
Ingredients:
- Frozen peach slices – 1 cup
- Greek yogurt – 1 cup
- Oatmeal – ¼ cup
- Vanilla extract – ¼ tsp.
- Almond milk – 1 cup

Directions:
Combine everything in a blender and blend until smooth.
Nutrition Info:331 Fat: 4Carb: 46g Protein: 29g

513. Roasted Tomato Salsa

Servings: 8   Cooking Time: 30 Minutes
Ingredients:
- 6 plum tomatoes
- 1 ¼ cup cilantro
- What you'll need from store cupboard:
- 2 tsp olive oil
- 1 tsp adobo sauce
- ½ tsp salt, divided
- Nonstick cooking spray

Directions:
Heat oven to 425 degrees. Spray a broiler pan with cooking spray.   Cut tomatoes in half and remove seeds. Place, cut side up, on broiler pan. Brush with oil and sprinkle with ¼ teaspoon salt. Turn tomatoes cut side down and bake 30-40 minutes or until edges are browned.   Place cilantro in food processor and pulse until coarsely chopped. Add tomatoes, adobo, and remaining salt. Process until chunky. Store in jar with air tight lid and refrigerate until ready to use. Serving size is 2 tablespoons.
Nutrition Info: Calories 33 Total Carbs 5g Net Carbs 4g Protein 1g Fat 1g Sugar 4g Fiber 1g

514. Creamy Chicken & Cauliflower Rice Soup

Servings: 6   Cooking Time: 5 Hours
Ingredients:
- 2 carrots, peeled and diced
- 2 stalks celery, peeled and diced
- 1/2 onion, diced
- 2 cup skim milk
- 2 cups cauliflower, riced
- 1 cup chicken, cooked and shredded
- 3 tbsp. Margarine
- What you'll need from store cupboard:
- 4 cup low sodium chicken broth
- 5 cloves garlic, diced
- ½ tsp rosemary
- ½ tsp thyme
- ½ tsp parsley
- 1 bay leaf

Directions:
Melt margarine in a large skillet over medium heat. Add carrots, celery, onion and garlic. Cook, stirring frequently, about 5 minutes. Place in crock pot.   Add chicken broth and seasonings. Cover and cook on low 4 hours. Add in the chicken, milk and cauliflower rice. Cook another 60 minutes or until cauliflower is tender. Discard bay leaf before serving.
Nutrition Info: Calories 151 Total Carbs 10g Net Carbs 8g Protein 12g Fat 6g Sugar 6g Fiber 2g

515. Italian Salad Dressing

Servings: 8   Cooking Time: 5 Minutes
Ingredients:
- 2 tbsp. lemon juice
- What you'll need from store cupboard:
- ¾ cup olive oil
- ¼ cup red wine vinegar
- 2 cloves of garlic, diced
- 2 tsp Italian seasoning
- 1 tsp oregano
- ½ tsp honey
- ½ tsp salt
- ¼ tsp black pepper
- ¼ tsp red pepper flakes

Directions:
Combine all Ingredients in a measuring cup or jar. Whisk well.   Store in jar or bottle with an air tight lid for up to 1 week. Serving size is 1 tablespoon.
Nutrition Info: Calories 167 Total Carbs 1g Protein 0g Fat 18g Sugar 0g Fiber 0g

516. Rainbow Black Bean Salad

Servings: 5   Cooking Time: 15 Minutes
Ingredients:
- 1 (15-ounce) can low-sodium black beans, drained and rinsed
- 1 avocado, diced
- 1 cup cherry tomatoes, halved
- 1 cup chopped baby spinach
- ½ cup finely chopped red bell pepper
- ¼ cup finely chopped jicama
- ½ cup chopped scallions, both white and green parts
- ¼ cup chopped fresh cilantro
- 2 tablespoons freshly squeezed lime juice
- 1 tablespoon extra-virgin olive oil
- 2 garlic cloves, minced
- 1 teaspoon honey
- ¼ teaspoon salt
- ¼ teaspoon freshly ground black pepper

Directions:
In a large bowl, combine the black beans, avocado, tomatoes, spinach, bell pepper, jicama, scallions, and cilantro.   In a small bowl, mix the lime juice, oil, garlic, honey, salt, and pepper. Add to the salad and toss. Chill for 1 hour before serving.
Nutrition Info: Calories: 169; Total Fat: 7g; Protein: 6g; Carbohydrates: 22g; Sugars: 3g; Fiber: 9g; Sodium: 235mg

517. Mango-glazed Pork Tenderloin Roast

Servings: 4   Cooking Time: 10 Minutes
Ingredients:
- 1 pound boneless pork tenderloin, trimmed of fat
- 1 teaspoon chopped fresh rosemary
- 1 teaspoon chopped fresh thyme
- ¼ teaspoon salt, divided
- ¼ teaspoon freshly ground black pepper, divided
- 1 teaspoon extra-virgin olive oil
- 1 tablespoon honey
- 2 tablespoons white wine vinegar
- 2 tablespoons dry cooking wine
- 1 tablespoon minced fresh ginger
- 1 cup diced mango

Directions:
Preheat the oven to 400°F.   Season the tenderloin with the rosemary, thyme, ⅛ teaspoon of salt, and ⅛ teaspoon of pepper.   Heat the olive oil in an oven-safe skillet over medium-high heat, and sear the tenderloin until browned on all sides, about 5 minutes total. Transfer the skillet to the oven and roast for 12 to 15 minutes until the pork is cooked through, the juices run clear, and the internal temperature reaches 145°F. Transfer to a cutting board to rest for 5 minutes.   In a small bowl, combine the honey, vinegar, cooking wine, and ginger. Into the same skillet, pour the honey mixture and simmer for 1 minute. Add the mango and toss to coat. Transfer to a blender and purée until smooth. Season with the remaining ⅛ teaspoon of salt and ⅛ teaspoon of pepper.   Slice the pork into rounds and serve with the mango sauce.
Nutrition Info: Calories: 182; Total Fat: 4g; Protein: 24g; Carbohydrates: 12g; Sugars: 10g; Fiber: 1g; Sodium: 240mg

518. Herb Vinaigrette

Servings: 12   Cooking Time: 5 Minutes
Ingredients:
- 2 tbsp. shallot, diced fine
- 1 tbsp. fresh basil, diced
- 1 tbsp. fresh oregano, diced
- 1 tbsp. fresh tarragon, diced
- What you'll need from store cupboard:
- ¼ cup extra virgin olive oil
- ¼ cup low sodium chicken broth
- ¼ cup red-wine vinegar
- ¼ teaspoon salt
- ¼ teaspoon freshly ground pepper

Directions:
Place all Ingredients in a jar with an air tight lid. Secure lid and shake vigorously to combine.   Refrigerate until ready to use. Will keep up to 2 days. Serving size is 1 tablespoon.
Nutrition Info: Calories 39 Total Carbs 0 Protein 0g Fat 4g Sugar 0g Fiber 0g

519. Low-carb No-cook Tomato Ketchup

Servings: 32 (2 Tablespoons Each)   Cooking Time: 10 Minutes
Ingredients:
- 1 (28-ounce) can whole tomatoes, drained
- 2 (6-ounce) cans tomato paste
- 1 tablespoon olive oil
- 2 garlic cloves, peeled
- ⅓ cup apple cider vinegar
- 1 tablespoon dried minced onion
- ½ teaspoon ground cloves
- 1 teaspoon salt
- ¼ cup honey

Directions:
In a blender jar, combine the tomatoes, tomato paste, olive oil, garlic, vinegar, onion, cloves, salt, and honey. Process until smooth. Taste and adjust the spices and seasonings as needed.   Transfer to airtight storage jars, cover tightly, and refrigerate for up to 3 weeks.
Nutrition Info: Calories: 29; Total Fat: 1g; Protein: 1g; Carbohydrates: 6g; Sugars: 5g; Fiber: 1g; Sodium: 104mg

520. Sprig Of Parsley

Servings: 3   Cooking Time: 2 Minutes
Ingredients:
- Fresh parsley -1/4 cup
- Watercress – ½ cup
- Frozen strawberries – ½ cup
- Frozen banana – ½
- Chia seeds – 1 tsp.
- Plant-based protein powder – 1 scoop
- Water to blend

Directions:
Blend everything in a blender.   Serve.
Nutrition Info:214 Fat: 4Carb: 46g Protein: 29g

521. Easy Thai Peanut Sauce

Servings: ²/₃ Cup   Cooking Time: 0 Minutes
Ingredients:
- ½ cup natural peanut butter
- 2 tablespoons rice vinegar
- 4 teaspoons sesame oil
- 2 to 4 teaspoons freshly squeezed lime juice, to your liking
- 2 to 2½ teaspoons hot sauce (optional)
- 1 teaspoon low-sodium soy sauce
- 1 teaspoon chopped peeled fresh ginger
- 1 teaspoon honey

Directions:
Mix together the peanut butter, rice vinegar, sesame oil, lime juice, hot sauce (if desired), soy sauce, ginger, and honey in a small bowl, and whisk to combine well. You can store it in an airtight container in the fridge for up to 2 weeks.
Nutrition Info:(2½ Tablespoons)calories: 206 fat: 16.7g protein: 7.9g carbs: 8.2g fiber: 3.1g sugar: 3.0g sodium: 113mg

522. Tomato Tuna Melts

Servings: 2   Cooking Time: 5 Minutes
Ingredients:
- 1 (5-ounce) can chunk light tuna packed in water, drained
- 2 tablespoons plain nonfat Greek yogurt

- 2 teaspoons freshly squeezed lemon juice
- 2 tablespoons finely chopped celery
- 1 tablespoon finely chopped red onion
- Pinch cayenne pepper
- 1 large tomato, cut into ¾-inch-thick rounds
- ½ cup shredded cheddar cheese

Directions:
Preheat the broiler to high.   In a medium bowl, combine the tuna, yogurt, lemon juice, celery, red onion, and cayenne pepper. Stir well.   Arrange the tomato slices on a baking sheet. Top each with some tuna salad and cheddar cheese.   Broil for 3 to 4 minutes until the cheese is melted and bubbly. Serve.

Nutrition Info: Calories: 243; Total Fat: 10g; Protein: 30g; Carbohydrates: 7g; Sugars: 2g; Fiber: 1g; Sodium: 444mg

523. Sweet Potato, Chickpea, And Kale Bowl With Creamy Tahini Sauce

Servings: 2   Cooking Time: 10 Minutes
Ingredients:
- FOR THE SAUCE
- 2 tablespoons plain nonfat Greek yogurt
- 1 tablespoon tahini
- 2 tablespoons hemp seeds
- 1 garlic clove, minced
- Pinch salt
- Freshly ground black pepper
- FOR THE BOWL
- 1 small sweet potato, peeled and finely diced
- 1 teaspoon extra-virgin olive oil
- 1 cup from 1 (15-ounce) can low-sodium chickpeas, drained and rinsed
- 2 cups baby kale

Directions:
TO MAKE THE SAUCE   In a small bowl, whisk together the yogurt and tahini.   Stir in the hemp seeds, garlic, and salt. Season with pepper. Add 2 to 3 tablespoons water to create a creamy yet pourable consistency. Set aside.   TO MAKE THE BOWL Preheat the oven to 425°F. Line a baking sheet with parchment paper.   Arrange the sweet potato on the prepared baking sheet and drizzle with the olive oil. Toss. Roast for 10 to 15 minutes, stirring once, until tender and browned.   In each of 2 bowls, arrange ½ cup of chickpeas, 1 cup of kale, and half of the cooked sweet potato. Drizzle with half the creamy tahini sauce and serve.

Nutrition Info: Calories: 322; Total Fat: 14g; Protein: 17g; Carbohydrates: 36g; Sugars: 7g; Fiber: 8g; Sodium: 305mg

524. Spice-rubbed Crispy Roast Chicken

Servings: 6   Cooking Time: 10 Minutes
Ingredients:
- 1 teaspoon ground paprika
- 1 teaspoon garlic powder
- ½ teaspoon ground coriander
- ½ teaspoon ground cumin
- ½ teaspoon salt

- ¼ teaspoon ground cayenne pepper
- 6 chicken legs
- 1 teaspoon extra-virgin olive oil

Directions:
Preheat the oven to 400°F.   In a small bowl, combine the paprika, garlic powder, coriander, cumin, salt, and cayenne pepper. Rub the chicken legs all over with the spices.   In an ovenproof skillet, heat the oil over medium heat. Sear the chicken for 8 to 10 minutes on each side until the skin browns and becomes crisp. Transfer the skillet to the oven and continue to cook for 10 to 15 minutes until the chicken is cooked through and its juices run clear.

Nutrition Info: Calories: 276; Total Fat: 16g; Protein: 30g; Carbohydrates: 1g; Sugars: 0g; Fiber: 0g; Sodium: 256mg

525. Cheesy Jalapeno Dip

Servings: 10   Cooking Time: 3 Hours
Ingredients:
- 4 pkgs. cream cheese, soft
- 1 ½ cups low fat cheddar cheese, grated
- 1 cup bacon, cooked and crumbled
- 1 cup fat free sour cream
- 1 fresh jalapeño, sliced
- What you'll need from store cupboard
- 2 cans jalapenos, diced
- 1 packet ranch dressing mix

Directions:
In a large bowl, mix cream cheese, 2/3 cup bacon, diced jalapenos, 1 cup cheddar cheese, sour cream and dressing.   Spread in crock pot. Top with remaining bacon and cheese. Arrange sliced jalapeno across the top. Cover and cook on low 3 hours. Serve warm.

Nutrition Info: Calories 233 Total Carbs 12g Protein 24g Fat 9g Sugar 2g Fiber 0g

526. Mashed Butternut Squash

Servings: 6   Cooking Time: 25 Minutes
Ingredients:
- 3 pounds whole butternut squash (about 2 medium)
- 2 tablespoons olive oil
- Salt and pepper

Directions:
Preheat the oven to 400°F and line a baking sheet with parchment.   Cut the squash in half and remove the seeds.   Cut the squash into cubes and toss with oil then spread on the baking sheet.   Roast for 25 minutes until tender then place in a food processor.   Blend smooth then season with salt and pepper to taste.

Nutrition Info: Calories 90 Total Fat 4.8g Saturated Fat 0.7g Total Carbs 8.5g Net Carbs 4.6g Protein 2.1g Sugar 1.7g Fiber 3.9g Sodium 4mg

527. Beef & Lentil Soup

Servings: 8   Cooking Time: 7 Hours
Ingredients:
- 1 ½ lbs. beef stew meat
- 1 cup onion, diced
- ½ cup celery, diced

- What you'll need from store cupboard:
- 6 cup water
- ½ cup lentils
- 2 cloves garlic, diced
- 2 bay leaves
- 2 tsp salt
- 1 tsp olive oil
- Fresh ground black pepper

Directions:
In a large skillet over med-high heat, heat oil. Add beef and brown on all sides. Use a slotted spoon to transfer the meat to a crock pot.   Add remaining Ingredients, cover and cook on low 6-7 hours or until beef is tender. Discard bay leaves before serving.
Nutrition Info:al Facts Per ServingCalories 213 Total Carbs 9g Net Carbs 5g Protein 29g Fat 6g Sugar 1g Fiber 4g

528. Easy Coconut Chicken Tenders

Servings: 6 (2 Tenders Each)   Cooking Time: 10 Minutes
Ingredients:
- 4 chicken breasts, each cut lengthwise into 3 strips
- ½ teaspoon salt
- ¼ teaspoon freshly ground black pepper
- ½ cup coconut flour
- 2 eggs, beaten
- 2 tablespoons unsweetened plain almond milk
- 1 cup unsweetened coconut flakes

Directions:
Preheat the oven to 400°F. Line a baking sheet with parchment paper.   Season the chicken pieces with the salt and pepper.   Place the coconut flour in a small bowl. In another bowl, mix the eggs with the almond milk. Spread the coconut flakes on a plate.   One by one, roll the chicken pieces in the flour, then dip the floured chicken in the egg mixture and shake off any excess. Roll in the coconut flakes and transfer to the prepared baking sheet.   Bake for 15 to 20 minutes, flipping once halfway through, until cooked through and browned.
Nutrition Info: Calories: 216; Total Fat: 13g; Protein: 20g; Carbohydrates: 9g; Sugars: 2g; Fiber: 6g; Sodium: 346mg

529. Sweet Potato, Onion, And Turkey Sausage Hash

Servings: 4   Cooking Time: 10 Minutes
Ingredients:
- 1 tablespoon extra-virgin oil
- 2 medium sweet potatoes, cut into ½-inch dice
- ½ recipe Homemade Turkey Breakfast Sausage (here)
- 1 small onion, chopped
- ½ red bell pepper, seeded and chopped
- 2 garlic cloves, minced
- Chopped fresh parsley, for garnish

Directions:
In a large skillet, heat the oil over medium-high heat. Add the sweet potatoes and cook, stirring occasionally, for 12 to 15 minutes until they brown and begin to soften.

Add the turkey sausage in bulk, onion, bell pepper, and garlic. Cook for 5 to 6 minutes until the turkey sausage is cooked through and the vegetables soften.   Garnish with parsley and serve warm.
Nutrition Info: Calories: 190; Total Fat: 9g; Protein: 12g; Carbohydrates: 16g; Sugars: 7g; Fiber: 3g; Sodium: 197mg

530. Greek Yogurt Sundae

Servings: 1   Cooking Time: 5 Minutes
Ingredients:
- ¾ cup plain nonfat Greek yogurt
- ¼ cup mixed berries (blueberries, strawberries, blackberries)
- 2 tablespoons cashew, walnut, or almond pieces
- 1 tablespoon ground flaxseed
- 2 fresh mint leaves, shredded

Directions:
Spoon the yogurt into a small bowl. Top with the berries, nuts, and flaxseed.   Garnish with the mint and serve.
Nutrition Info: Calories: 237; Total Fat: 11g; Protein: 21g; Carbohydrates: 16g; Sugars: 9g; Fiber: 4g; Sodium: 64mg

531. Smoky Lentil & Leek Soup

Servings: 4   Cooking Time: 2 Hours
Ingredients:
- 4 slices bacon, chopped
- 1 leek, discard dark green part, wash and chop
- What you'll need from store cupboard
- 3 cup low sodium chicken broth
- 1 cup red lentils
- 2 cloves garlic, diced

Directions:
Place a medium saucepan over med-high heat and add bacon. Cook until almost crisp, 2-3 minutes. Add leek and garlic and cook until leek starts to get soft, 3 minutes. Transfer to crock pot.   Add remaining Ingredients and stir to combine. Cover and cook on high 2 hours. When the lentils are soft, the soup is done. Serve.
Nutrition Info: Calories 299 Total Carbs 33g   Net Carbs 18g Protein 21g Fat 8g Sugar 2g Fiber 15g

532. "cornbread" Stuffing

Servings: 6   Cooking Time: 40 Minutes
Ingredients:
- 1 strip bacon, diced
- 1 egg
- 1 cup onion, diced
- 1 cup celery, diced
- 2 tbsp. margarine, divided
- What you'll need from store cupboard:
- 1 cup almond flour
- ¼ cup low sodium chicken broth
- 3 cloves garlic, diced fine
- 2 tbsp. stone-ground cornmeal
- 1 tsp thyme
- 1 tsp sage
- ¾ tsp salt
- Fresh ground black pepper, to taste

Directions:

Heat the oven to 375 degrees.   Melt 1 tablespoon margarine in a skillet over low heat. Add onions and celery and cook, stirring, until soft, about 10 minutes. Add garlic and seasonings and cook 1-2 minutes more. Remove from heat and let cool.   Place the almond flour, cornmeal and bacon in a food processor and pulse until combined. Add the broth and egg and pulse just to combine. Add the onion mixture and pulse just until mixed.   Place remaining tablespoon of margarine in a cast iron skillet, or baking dish, and melt in the oven until hot. Swirl the pan to coat with melted margarine. Spread the dressing in the pan and bake 30 minutes or until top is nicely browned and center is cooked through. Serve.

Nutrition Info: Calories 177 Total Carbs 9g Net Carbs 6g Protein 6g Fat 14g Sugar 2g Fiber 3g

533. Caramel Sauce

Servings: 12   Cooking Time: 10 Minutes
Ingredients:
- 2/3 cup heavy cream
- 1/3 cup margarine
- What you'll need from store cupboard:
- 3 tbsp. Splenda
- 1 tsp vanilla

Directions:
Add the margarine and Splenda to a medium saucepan and place over low heat. Once the margarine melts, cook 3-4 minutes, stirring occasionally, until golden brown. Stir in the cream and bring to a low boil. Reduce heat and simmer 7-10 minutes, stirring occasionally, until mixture is a caramel color and coats the back of a spoon. Remove from heat and whisk in the vanilla. Cool completely and pour into a jar with an air tight lid. Store in the refrigerator. Serving size is 1 tablespoon.

Nutrition Info: Calories 84 Total Carbs 3g Protein 0g Fat 7g Sugar 3g Fiber 0g

534. Chunky Chicken Noodle Soup

Servings: 8   Cooking Time: 35 Minutes
Ingredients:
- 2 lbs. chicken thighs, boneless and skinless
- 2 carrots, sliced
- 2 celery stalks, sliced
- 2 tsp fresh ginger, grated
- What you'll need from store cupboard:
- 8 cup low sodium chicken broth
- 2 cup homemade pasta, (chapter 15)
- 1 tbsp. garlic, diced fine
- 1 tbsp. chicken bouillon
- Salt and pepper, to taste

Directions:
Place chicken and 1 cup broth in a large soup pot over medium heat. Bring to a simmer and cook until chicken is done, about 20 minutes. Transfer chicken to a bowl and shred using 2 forks.   Add the carrots, celery, garlic, ginger, and bouillon to the pot and stir well. Add in remaining broth and bring back to a boil. Reduce heat and simmer until vegetables are tender, about 15 minutes.   Add pasta and cook another 5 minutes for

fresh pasta, or 7 for dried. Add the chicken to the soup and salt and pepper to taste. Serve.
Nutrition Info: Calories 210 Total Carbs 15g Net Carbs 12g Protein 23g Fat 7g Sugar 7g Fiber 3g

535. Light Beer Bread

Servings: 14   Cooking Time: 55 Minutes
Ingredients:
- ¼ cup butter, soft
- What you'll need from store cupboard:
- 12 oz. light beer
- 3 cup low carb baking mix
- 1/3 cup Splenda

Directions:
Heat oven to 375 degrees. Use 1 tablespoon butter to grease the bottom of a 9x5-inch loaf pan.   In a large bowl, whisk together beer, baking mix, and Splenda. Pour into prepared pan.   Bake 45-55 minutes or until golden brown. Cool in pan 10 minutes, remove from pan and cool on wire rack.   In a small glass bowl, melt remaining butter in a microwave and brush over warm loaf. Cool 15 minutes before slicing.
Nutrition Info: Calories 162 Total Carbs 16g Net Carbs 12g Protein 9g Fat 5g Sugar 5g Fiber 4g

536. Curried Carrot Soup

Servings: 6   Cooking Time: 10 Minutes
Ingredients:
- 1 tablespoon extra-virgin olive oil
- 1 small onion, coarsely chopped
- 2 celery stalks, coarsely chopped
- 1½ teaspoons curry powder
- 1 teaspoon ground cumin
- 1 teaspoon minced fresh ginger
- 6 medium carrots, roughly chopped
- 4 cups low-sodium vegetable broth
- ¼ teaspoon salt
- 1 cup canned coconut milk
- ¼ teaspoon freshly ground black pepper
- 1 tablespoon chopped fresh cilantro

Directions:
Heat an Instant Pot to high and add the olive oil.   Sauté the onion and celery for 2 to 3 minutes. Add the curry powder, cumin, and ginger to the pot and cook until fragrant, about 30 seconds.   Add the carrots, vegetable broth, and salt to the pot. Close and seal, and set for 5 minutes on high. Allow the pressure to release naturally. In a blender jar, carefully purée the soup in batches and transfer back to the pot.   Stir in the coconut milk and pepper, and heat through. Top with the cilantro and serve.
Nutrition Info: Calories: 145; Total Fat: 11g; Protein: 2g; Carbohydrates: 13g; Sugars: 4g; Fiber: 3g; Sodium: 238mg

537. Marinara Sauce

Servings: 6   Cooking Time: 30 Minutes
Ingredients:
- What you'll need from store cupboard:
- 28 oz. can diced tomatoes, undrained
- 4–6 cloves garlic, diced fine

- 4 tbsp. extra virgin olive oil
- 2 tbsp. tomato paste
- 1 tbsp. basil,
- 1 tsp Splenda
- 1 tsp salt

Directions:
Heat oil in saucepan over medium heat. Add the garlic and cook 1 minute. Stir in the tomato paste and cook 1 minute more. Add the tomatoes and basil and simmer 10-15 minutes, breaking up the tomatoes as they cook. Stir in Splenda and salt. Use an immersion blender and process to desired consistency. Let cool and store in a jar with an airtight lid in the refrigerator up to 7 days. Or use right away.
Nutrition Info: Calories 179 Total Carbs 13g Net Carbs 10g Protein 2g Fat 14g Sugar 8g Fiber 3g

538. Quick Coconut Flour Buns

Servings: 4   Cooking Time: 20 Minutes
Ingredients:
- 3 eggs, room temperature
- 2 tbsp. coconut milk, room temperature
- What you'll need from store cupboard:
- ¼ cup coconut flour
- 2 tablespoons coconut oil, soft
- 1 tbsp. honey
- ½ tsp baking powder
- ½ tsp salt

Directions:
Heat oven to 375 degrees. Line a cookie sheet with parchment paper. In a small bowl, sift together flour, baking powder and salt. In a medium bowl, combine eggs, coconut oil, milk, and honey, mix well. Slowly add dry Ingredients to the egg mixture. Batter will be thick but make sure there is no lumps. Form into 4 balls and place on prepared pan. Press down into rounds ½-inch thick. Bake 15-20 minutes or until buns pass the toothpick test.
Nutrition Info: Calories 143 Total Carbs 6g Protein 4g Fat 12g Sugar 5g Fiber 0g

539. Harvest Vegetable Soup

Servings: 12   Cooking Time: 50 Minutes
Ingredients:
- 3 carrots, halved and slice thin
- 2 green onions, slice thin
- 2 tart apples, peeled and diced
- 2 turnips, peeled and diced
- 2 parsnips, peeled and sliced
- 1 onion, diced
- 3 cup potato, peeled and cubed
- 2 cup butternut squash, peeled and cubed
- 1 tbsp. margarine
- What you'll need from store cupboard:
- 7 cup low sodium vegetable broth
- 1 tbsp. olive oil
- 1 clove garlic, diced
- 1 bay leaf
- ½ tsp basil
- ¼ tsp thyme
- ¼ tsp pepper

Directions:
Heat margarine and oil in a large soup pot over medium heat. Add carrots, celery, and onion and cook until tender, about 10 minutes. Add garlic and cook 1 minute more. Add broth, potatoes, squash, apple, turnips, parsnips, and bay leaf, stir to combine. Bring to a boil. Reduce heat and simmer 20 minutes. Stir in seasonings and cook 15 minutes, or until all the vegetables are tender. Discard bay leaf and serve.
Nutrition Info: Calories 118 Total Carbs 24g Net Carbs 20g Protein 2g Fat 2g Sugar 9g Fiber 4g

540. French Onion Soup

Servings: 6-8   Cooking Time: 4 Hours
Ingredients:
- 2 large white onions, thinly sliced
- 2 cups gruyere cheese, grated
- 1 tbsp. margarine
- What you'll need from store cupboard:
- 6 cups low-sodium beef broth
- 1 clove garlic, diced fine
- 1 bay leaf
- ½ tsp salt
- ½ tsp thyme
- ¼ tsp pepper

Directions:
Place all Ingredients, except cheese, in the crock pot. Stir well to mix. Cover and cook on high 3-4 hours, or low 6-8 hours. Remove bay leaf. Heat broiler. Ladle soup into ovenproof bowls and top with cheese. Place bowls on baking sheet and broil until cheese is melted and starting to brown. Serve immediately.
Nutrition Info: Calories 219 Total Carbs 5g Protein 16g Fat 15g Sugar 2g Fiber 0g

541. Cheesy Vegetable And Hummus Pitas

Servings: 4   Cooking Time: 0 Minutes
Ingredients:
- 4 whole wheat pitas, sliced into pockets
- 2 tablespoons light mayonnaise
- ½ cup hummus
- 2¼ ounces (64 g) reduced-fat Swiss cheese, cut into 4 slices
- ¼ cup sunflower seeds
- 1 large tomato, cut into 4 equal slices
- 1 medium cucumber, sliced
- 1 medium red onion, thinly sliced
- 4 romaine lettuce leaves

Directions:
Smear the insides of the pita pockets with mayo. Divide the hummus on each cheese slice and smear to spread evenly, then sprinkle with sunflower seeds. Sit the tomato slices, cucumber slices, onion slices, and lettuce leaves on top of the hummus alternatively. Then stuff the pitas with these slices and serve immediately.
Nutrition Info:calories: 170   fat: 6.0g   protein: 8.0g carbs: 23.0g   fiber: 4.0g   sugar: 7.0g   sodium: 280mg

542. Ginger-garlic Cod Cooked In Paper

Servings: 4   Cooking Time: 10 Minutes
Ingredients:
- 1 chard bunch, stemmed, leaves and stems cut into thin strips
- 1 red bell pepper, seeded and cut into strips
- 1 pound cod fillets cut into 4 pieces
- 1 tablespoon grated fresh ginger
- 3 garlic cloves, minced
- 2 tablespoons white wine vinegar
- 2 tablespoons low-sodium tamari or gluten-free soy sauce
- 1 tablespoon honey

Directions:
Preheat the oven to 425°F.   Cut four pieces of parchment paper, each about 16 inches wide. Lay the four pieces out on a large workspace.   On each piece of paper, arrange a small pile of chard leaves and stems, topped by several strips of bell pepper. Top with a piece of cod.   In a small bowl, mix the ginger, garlic, vinegar, tamari, and honey. Top each piece of fish with one-fourth of the mixture.   Fold the parchment paper over so the edges overlap. Fold the edges over several times to secure the fish in the packets. Carefully place the packets on a large baking sheet.   Bake for 12 minutes. Carefully open the packets, allowing steam to escape, and serve.
Nutrition Info: Calories: 118; Total Fat: 1g; Protein: 19g; Carbohydrates: 9g; Sugars: 6g; Fiber: 1g; Sodium: 715mg

543. Chipotle Chicken & Corn Soup

Servings: 8   Cooking Time: 30 Minutes
Ingredients:
- 1 onion, diced
- 2 chipotle peppers in adobo sauce, diced
- 3 cup corn kernels
- 2 cup chicken breast, cooked and cut in cubes
- ½ cup fat free sour cream
- ¼ cup cilantro, diced
- What you'll need from store cupboard:
- 2 14 ½ oz. cans fire roasted tomatoes, diced
- 4 cup low sodium chicken broth
- 4 cloves garlic, diced
- 1 tbsp. sunflower oil
- 2 tsp adobo sauce
- 1 tsp cumin
- ¼ tsp pepper

Directions:
Heat oil in a large pot over med-high heat. Add onion and cook until tender, about 3-5 minutes. Add garlic and cook 1 minute more.   Add broth, tomatoes, corn, chipotle peppers, adobo sauce, and seasonings. Bring to a boil. Reduce heat and simmer 20 minutes.   Stir in chicken and cook until heated through. Serve garnished with sour cream and cilantro.
Nutrition Info: Calories 145 Total Carbs 20g Net Carbs 16g Protein 10g Fat 3g Sugar 6g Fiber 4g

544. Sautéed Spinach And Tomatoes

Servings: 4   Cooking Time: 5 Minutes

Ingredients:
- 1 tablespoon extra-virgin olive oil
- 1 cup cherry tomatoes, halved
- 3 spinach bunches, trimmed
- 2 garlic cloves, minced
- ¼ teaspoon salt

Directions:
In a large skillet, heat the oil over medium heat.   Add the tomatoes, and cook until the skins begin to blister and split, about 2 minutes.   Add the spinach in batches, waiting for each batch to wilt slightly before adding the next batch. Stir continuously for 3 to 4 minutes until the spinach is tender.   Add the garlic to the skillet, and toss until fragrant, about 30 seconds.   Drain the excess liquid from the pan. Add the salt. Stir well and serve.
Nutrition Info: Calories: 52; Total Fat: 4g; Protein: 2g; Carbohydrates: 4g; Sugars: 1g; Fiber: 2g; Sodium: 183mg

545. Quick Tomato Marinara

Servings: 8 (¼ Cup Each)   Cooking Time: 5 Minutes
Ingredients:
- 1 (28-ounce) can whole tomatoes
- 2 tablespoons extra-virgin olive oil
- 4 garlic cloves, minced
- ½ teaspoon salt
- ¼ teaspoon dried oregano

Directions:
Discard about half of the liquid from the can of tomatoes, and transfer the tomatoes and remaining liquid to a large bowl. Use clean hands or a large spoon to break the tomatoes apart.   In a large skillet, heat the olive oil over medium heat. Add the garlic and salt, and cook until the garlic just begins to sizzle, without letting it brown. Add the tomatoes and their liquid to the skillet. Simmer the sauce for about 15 minutes until the oil begins to separate and become dark orange and the sauce thickens. Add the oregano, stir, and remove from the heat.   After the marinara has cooled to room temperature, store in glass containers in the refrigerator for up to 3 or 4 days, or in zip-top freezer bags for up to 4 months.
Nutrition Info: Calories: 48; Total Fat: 4g; Protein: 1g; Carbohydrates: 4g; Sugars: 2g; Fiber: 1g; Sodium: 145mg

546. Baked Oysters

Servings: 2   Cooking Time: 30 Minutes
Ingredients:
- 2 cups coarse salt, for holding the oysters
- 1 dozen fresh oysters, scrubbed
- 1 tablespoon butter
- ½ cup finely chopped artichoke hearts
- ¼ cup finely chopped scallions, both white and green parts
- ¼ cup finely chopped red bell pepper
- 1 garlic clove, minced
- 1 tablespoon finely chopped fresh parsley
- Zest and juice of ½ lemon
- Pinch salt
- Freshly ground black pepper

Directions:
Pour the coarse salt into an 8-by-8-inch baking dish and spread to evenly fill the bottom of the dish.   Prepare a clean surface to shuck the oysters. Using a shucking knife, insert the blade at the joint of the shell, where it hinges open and shut. Firmly apply pressure to pop the blade in, and work the knife around the shell to open. Discard the empty half of the shell. Use the knife to gently loosen the oyster, and remove any shell particles. Set the oysters in their shells on the salt, being careful not to spill the juices. Preheat the oven to 425°F.   In a large skillet, melt the butter over medium heat. Add the artichoke hearts, scallions, and bell pepper, and cook for 5 to 7 minutes. Add the garlic and cook an additional minute. Remove from the heat and mix in the parsley, lemon zest and juice, and season with salt and pepper.   Divide the vegetable mixture evenly among the oysters and bake for 10 to 12 minutes until the vegetables are lightly browned.
Nutrition Info: Calories: 134; Total Fat: 7g; Protein: 6g; Carbohydrates: 11g; Sugars: 7g; Fiber: 2g; Sodium: 281mg

547. Macaroni And Vegetable Pie

Servings: 6   Cooking Time: 30 Minutes
Ingredients:
- 1 (1-pound / 454-g) package whole-wheat macaroni
- 2 celery stalks, thinly sliced
- 1 small yellow onion, chopped
- 2 garlic cloves, minced
- Salt, to taste
- ¼ teaspoon freshly ground black pepper
- 2 tablespoons chickpea flour
- 2 cups grated reduced-fat sharp Cheddar cheese
- 1 cup fat-free milk
- 2 large zucchini, finely grated and squeezed dry
- 2 roasted red peppers, chopped into ¼-inch pieces

Directions:
Preheat the oven to 350°F (180°C).   Bring a pot of water to a boil, then add the macaroni and cook for 4 minutes or until al dente.   Drain the macaroni and transfer to a large bowl. Reserve 1 cup of the macaroni water.   Pour the macaroni water in an oven-safe skillet and heat over medium heat.   Add the celery, onion, garlic, salt, and black pepper to the skillet and sauté for 4 minutes or until tender.   Gently mix in the chickpea flour, then fold in the cheese and milk. Keep stirring until the mixture is thick and smooth.   Add the cooked macaroni, zucchini, and red peppers. Stir to combine well.   Cover the skillet with aluminum foil and transfer it to the preheated oven.   Bake for 15 minutes or until the cheese melts, then remove the foil and bake for 5 more minutes or until lightly browned.   Remove the pie from the oven and serve immediately.
Nutrition Info:calories: 378   fat: 4.0g protein: 24.0g carbs: 67.0g fiber: 8.0g sugar: 6.0g sodium: 332mg

548. South American Fish Stew

Servings: 6   Cooking Time: 25 Minutes

Ingredients:
- 2 lbs. tilapia fillets, cut into bite-sized pieces
- 3 bell peppers, cut into 2-inch strips
- 1 large onion, diced
- 1/8 cup fresh cilantro, diced
- 4 tbsp. fresh lime juice
- What you'll need from store cupboard:
- 14 oz. can tomatoes, diced and drained
- 14 oz. can coconut milk
- 3-4 cloves garlic, diced fine
- 1 ½ tbsp. cumin
- 1 ½ tbsp. paprika
- 1 tbsp. olive oil
- 1 ½ tsp salt
- 1 ½ tsp pepper

Directions:
In a large bowl combine lime juice, cumin, paprika, garlic, salt and pepper. Add fish and stir to coat. Cover and refrigerate at least 20 minutes, or overnight.   Heat oil in a large sauce pot over med-high heat. Add onion and cook until they start to soften, about 3 minutes. Add peppers, tomatoes, and fish and stir to combine. Add coconut milk and stir in.   Reduce heat to low, cover, and cook 20 minutes, stirring occasionally. Stir in the cilantro for the last 5 minutes of cooking time. Serve.
Nutrition Info: Calories 347 Total Carbs 15g Net Carbs 12g Protein 31g Fat 19g Sugar 8g Fiber 3g

549. Oven-roasted Veggies

Servings: 6   Cooking Time: 25 Minutes
Ingredients:
- 1-pound cauliflower florets
- ½-pound broccoli florets
- 1 large yellow onion, cut into chunks
- 1 large red pepper, cored and chopped
- 2 medium carrots, peeled and sliced
- 2 tablespoons olive oil
- 2 tablespoons apple cider vinegar
- Salt and pepper

Directions:
Preheat the oven to 425°F and line a large rimmed baking sheet with parchment.   Spread the veggies on the baking sheet and drizzle with oil and vinegar.   Toss well and season with salt and pepper.   Spread the veggies in a single layer then roast for 20 to 25 minutes, stirring every 10 minutes, until tender.   Adjust seasoning to taste and serve hot.
Nutrition Info: Calories 100Total Fat 4.8gSaturated Fat 0.7gTotal Carbs 8.5gNet Carbs 4.6g Protein 2.1g Sugar 1.7g Fiber 3.9g Sodium 7mg

550. Pork Posole

Servings: 6   Cooking Time: 25 Minutes
Ingredients:
- 1 yellow onion, diced fine
- 1 ½ cup pork, cook & shred
- 1 fresh lime, cut in wedges
- ½ bunch cilantro, chopped
- What you'll need from store cupboard:
- 15 oz. can hominy, drain
- 4 oz. can green chilies, diced

- 3 oz. tomato paste
- 3 cup low sodium chicken broth
- 2 cup water
- 2 tbsp. vegetable oil
- 2 tbsp. flour
- 2 tbsp. chili powder
- ¾ tsp salt
- ½ tsp cumin
- ½ tsp garlic powder
- ¼ tsp cayenne pepper

Directions:
Heat oil in a large pot over medium heat. Add onion and cook 3-5 minutes, or until it softens.   Add the flour and chili powder and cook 2 minutes more, stirring continuously.   Add water, tomato paste, and seasonings. Whisk mixture until tomato paste dissolves. Bring to a simmer and let thicken, about 2-3 minutes. Stir in broth, pork, chilies, and hominy and cook until heated through, about 10 minutes.   Ladle into bowls and garnish with a lime wedge and chopped cilantro.
Nutrition Info: Calories 234 Total Carbs 33g Net Carbs 24g Protein 11g Fat 8g Sugar 12g Fiber 9g

551. Spaghetti Sauce

Servings: 6   Cooking Time: 30 Minutes
Ingredients:
- 1 onion, diced
- 1 carrot, grated
- 1 stalk celery, diced
- 1 zucchini, grated
- What you'll need from store cupboard:
- 1 (28 oz.) Italian-style tomatoes, in puree
- 1 (14 ½ oz.) diced tomatoes, with juice
- ½ cup water
- 2 cloves garlic, diced fine
- ½ tbsp. oregano
- 1 tsp olive oil
- 1 tsp basil
- 1 tsp thyme
- 1 tsp salt
- ¼ tsp red pepper flakes

Directions:
Heat oil in a large saucepan over medium heat. Add vegetables and garlic. Cook, stirring frequently, until vegetables get soft, about 5 minutes.   Add remaining Ingredients, use the back of a spoon to break up tomatoes. Bring to a simmer and cook, partially covered, over med-low heat 30 minutes, stirring frequently. Store sauce in an air-tight container in the refrigerator up to 3 days, or in the freezer up to 3 months.
Nutrition Info: Calories 47 Total Carbs 8g Net Carbs 6g Protein 2g Fat 1g Sugar 3g Fiber 2g

552. Dry Rub For Pork

Servings: 16   Cooking Time: 5 Minutes
Ingredients:
- What you'll need from store cupboard:
- 2 tbsp. ground coffee, extra fine ground
- 2 tbsp. chipotle powder
- 1 tbsp. smoked paprika
- 1 tbsp. Splenda brown sugar

- 1 tbsp. salt
- 1 tsp ginger
- 1 tsp mustard powder
- 1 tsp coriander

Directions:
Mix all Ingredients together.   Store in airtight container in cool, dry place for up to 1 month.
Nutrition Info: Calories 5 Total Carbs 1g Protein 0g Fat 0g Sugar 1g Fiber 0g

553. Mexican "rice"

Servings: 6   Cooking Time: 10 Minutes
Ingredients:
- 2 cups cauliflower rice, cooked
- 1 small jalapeño, seeded and diced fine
- ½ white onion, diced
- What you'll need from store cupboard:
- ½ cup water
- ½ cup tomato paste
- 3 cloves garlic, diced fine
- 2 tsp salt
- 2 tsp olive oil

Directions:
Heat oil in skillet over medium heat. Add onion, garlic, jalapeno, and salt and cook 3-4 min, stirring frequently. In a small bowl, whisk water and tomato paste together. Add to skillet. Cook, stirring frequently, 3-5 minutes. Stir in cauliflower, and cook just until heated through and most of the liquid is absorbed. Serve.
Nutrition Info: Calories 46 Total Carbs 7g Net Carbs 5g Protein 2g Fat 2g Sugar 4g Fiber 2g

554. Korean Beef Soup

Servings: 8   Cooking Time: 4 Hours
Ingredients:
- 1 pound of beef, cut into cubes
- 1 Korean white radish, peeled and diced
- 1 cup green onions, diced
- What you'll need from store cupboard:
- 1 gallon water
- 3 tbsp. soy sauce
- 1 tbsp. oil
- 1 tbsp. Sesame seeds, toasted
- 2 cloves garlic, diced fine
- 1 tsp salt
- 1 tsp pepper

Directions:
Set crock pot to high and pour the water in to start heating.   In a small bowl, combine green onions, soy sauce, oil, sesame seeds, garlic, salt, and pepper. Divide evenly between two Ziploc bags.   Place the meat in one bag and the radish in the other. Let set for 1 hour. Turn the crock pot down to low and add the contents of the meat bag. Let cook 1 hour, then add the contents of the radish bag. Cook another 3-4 hours.
Nutrition Info: Calories 120 Total Carbs 3g Net Carbs 2g Protein 18g Fat 4g Sugar 0g Fiber 1g

555. Beef & Sweet Potato Stew

Servings: 6   Cooking Time: 1 Hour 10 Minutes
Ingredients:

- 2 lb. top sirloin steak, diced
- 1 ½ lbs. sweet potato, peeled and cut in ½-inch cubes
- ½ lb. cremini mushrooms, quartered
- 2 stalks celery, diced
- 1 red onion, diced
- 1 carrot, peeled and diced
- 2 tbsp. fresh parsley, chopped
- 4 sprigs fresh thyme
- What you'll need from store cupboard:
- 4 cup low sodium beef broth
- ½ cup dry red wine
- ¼ cup flour
- 3 cloves garlic, diced
- 2 tbsp. tomato paste
- 2 tbsp. olive oil
- 2 bay leaves
- Salt and pepper, to taste

Directions:
Heat oil in a large stockpot over medium heat. Season steak with salt and pepper and add to pot. Cook, stirring occasionally, until brown on all sides. Remove from pot and set aside.   Add onion, carrot, and celery. Cook, stirring occasionally, 3-4 minutes or until tender.   Add garlic and mushrooms and cook another 3-4 minutes. Whisk in flour and tomato paste and cook until lightly browned, about 1 minute.   Stir in wine, scraping up any browned bits from the bottom of the pot. Add the broth, thyme, bay leaves and steak. Bring to a boil, reduce heat and simmer about 30 minutes, or until steak is tender.   Add sweet potato and cook 20 minutes or until potatoes are tender and stew has thickened. Discard bay leaves and thyme sprigs. Stir in parsley and serve.

Nutrition Info: Calories 421 Total Carbs 14g Net Carbs 12g Protein 51g Fat 15g Sugar 4g Fiber 2g

556. Simple Buttercup Squash Soup

Servings: 6   Cooking Time: 33 Minutes
Ingredients:
- 2 tablespoons extra-virgin olive oil
- 1 medium onion, chopped
- 1½ pounds (680 g) buttercup squash, peeled, deseeded, and cut into 1-inch chunks
- 4 cups vegetable broth
- ½ teaspoon kosher salt
- ¼ teaspoon ground white pepper
- Ground nutmeg, to taste

Directions:
Heat the olive oil in a pot over medium-high heat until shimmering.   Add the onion and sauté for 3 minutes or until translucent.   Add the buttercup squash, vegetable broth, salt, and pepper. Stir to mix well. Bring to a boil.   Reduce the heat to low and simmer for 30 minutes or until the buttercup squash is soft.   Pour the soup in a food processor, then pulse to purée until creamy and smooth.   Pour the soup in a large serving bowl, then sprinkle with ground nutmeg and serve.

Nutrition Info:(1⅓ Cups)calories: 110   fat: 5.0g   protein: 1.0g   carbs: 18.0g   fiber: 4.0g   sugar: 4.0g   sodium: 166mg

557. Herbed Chicken Meatball Wraps

Servings: 6 (2 Wraps Each)   Cooking Time: 10 Minutes
Ingredients:
- 1 pound ground chicken
- 3 scallions, both white and green parts, finely chopped
- 2 garlic cloves, minced
- 2 tablespoons chopped fresh mint
- ½ teaspoon dried oregano
- 1 egg, lightly beaten
- 12 large lettuce leaves
- 1 medium red bell pepper, seeded and cut into strips
- 1 carrot, cut into strips
- 1 recipe Cucumber-Yogurt Dip (here)

Directions:
Preheat the oven to 400°F. Line a baking sheet with parchment paper.   In a large mixing bowl, combine the chicken, scallions, garlic, mint, oregano, and egg. Stir well.   Using your hands, form the meat mixture into balls about the size of a tablespoon, making about 24 balls. Arrange on the prepared baking sheet.   Bake for 10 minutes, flip with a spatula, and continue baking for an additional 10 minutes until the meatballs are cooked through.   In each lettuce leaf, place two meatballs and several bell pepper and carrot strips. Top with 2 tablespoons of Cucumber-Yogurt Dip. Wrap the leaves around the filling and serve with the dip.

Nutrition Info: Calories: 220; Total Fat: 12g; Protein: 23g; Carbohydrates: 6g; Sugars: 3g; Fiber: 2g; Sodium: 199mg

558. Cheesy Broccoli Bites

Servings: 6   Cooking Time: 25 Minutes
Ingredients:
- 2 tablespoons olive oil
- 2 heads broccoli, trimmed
- 1 eggs
- ⅓ cup reduced-fat shredded Cheddar cheese
- 1 egg white
- ½ cup onion, chopped
- ⅓ cup bread crumbs
- ¼ teaspoon salt
- ¼ teaspoon black pepper

Directions:
Preheat the oven to 400°F (205°C). Coat a large baking sheet with olive oil.   Arrange a colander in a saucepan, then place the broccoli in the colander. Pour the water in the saucepan to cover the bottom. Bring to a boil, then reduce the heat to low. Cover and simmer for 6 minutes or until the broccoli is fork-tender. Allow to cool for 10 minutes.   Put the broccoli and remaining ingredients in a food processor. Process to combine until lightly chunky. Let sit for 10 minutes.   Make the bites: Drop 1 tablespoon of the mixture on the baking sheet. Repeat with the remaining mixture.   Bake in the preheated oven for 25 minutes or until lightly browned. Flip the bites halfway through the cooking time.   Serve immediately.

Nutrition Info:calories: 100   fat: 3.0g   protein: 7.0g   carbs: 13.0g   fiber: 3.0g   sugar: 3.0g   sodium: 250mg

559. Sausage & Pepper Soup

Servings: 6   Cooking Time: 1 Hour

Ingredients:
- 2 lbs. pork sausage
- 10 oz. raw spinach
- 1 medium bell pepper, diced
- What you'll need from store cupboard:
- 4 cups low sodium beef broth
- 1 can tomatoes w/ jalapenos
- 1 tbsp. olive oil
- 1 tbsp. chili powder
- 1 tbsp. cumin
- 1 tsp onion powder
- 1 tsp garlic powder
- 1 tsp Italian seasoning
- 3/4 tsp kosher salt

Directions:
In a large pot, over medium heat, heat oil until hot. Add sausage and cook until browned. Drain fat.   Add bell pepper and stir. Season with salt and pepper.   Add tomatoes and stir. Place spinach on top and cover. Once spinach wilts, add spices and broth and stir to combine. Reduce heat to medium-low. Cover and cook 30 minutes, stirring occasionally.   Remove lid and let simmer another 15 minutes. Serve.

Nutrition Info: Calories 580 Total Carbs 5g Net Carbs 3g Protein 34g Fat 46g Sugar 2g Fiber 2g

560. Walnut Vinaigrette

Servings: 4   Cooking Time: 5 Minutes

Ingredients:
- What you'll need from store cupboard:
- ½ cup water
- ¼ cup balsamic vinegar
- ¼ cup walnuts
- ¼ cup raisins
- 1 clove garlic
- 1 tsp Dijon mustard
- ¼ tsp thyme

Directions:
Place all Ingredients in a blender or food processor and pulse until smooth. Store in a jar with an air tight lid in the refrigerator.

Nutrition Info: Calories 53 Total Carbs 2g Net Carbs 1g Protein 2g Fat 5g Sugar 0g Fiber 1g

561. Easy Chicken Cacciatore

Servings: 6   Cooking Time: 10 Minutes

Ingredients:
- 3 teaspoons extra-virgin olive oil, divided
- 6 chicken legs
- 8 ounces brown mushrooms
- 1 large onion, sliced
- 1 red bell pepper, seeded and cut into strips
- 3 garlic cloves, minced
- ½ cup dry red wine
- 1 (28-ounce) can whole tomatoes, drained

- 1 thyme sprig
- 1 rosemary sprig
- ½ teaspoon salt
- ¼ teaspoon freshly ground black pepper
- ¼ cup water

Directions:
Preheat the oven to 350°F.   In a Dutch oven (or any oven-safe covered pot), heat 2 teaspoons of oil over medium-high heat. Sear the chicken on all sides until browned. Remove and set aside.   Heat the remaining 1 teaspoon of oil in the Dutch oven and sauté the mushrooms for 3 to 5 minutes until they brown and begin to release their water. Add the onion, bell pepper, and garlic, and mix together with the mushrooms. Cook an additional 3 to 5 minutes until the onion begins to soften.   Add the red wine and deglaze the pot. Bring to a simmer. Add the tomatoes, breaking them into pieces with a spoon. Add the thyme, rosemary, salt, and pepper to the pot and mix well.   Add the water, then nestle the cooked chicken, along with any juices that have accumulated, in the vegetables.   Transfer the pot to the oven. Cook for 30 minutes until the chicken is cooked through and its juices run clear. Remove the thyme and rosemary sprigs and serve.

Nutrition Info: Calories: 257; Total Fat: 11g; Protein: 28g; Carbohydrates: 11g; Sugars: 6g; Fiber: 2g; Sodium: 398mg

562. Beet, Goat Cheese, And Walnut Pesto With Zoodles

Servings: 2   Cooking Time: 15 Minutes

Ingredients:
- 1 medium red beet, peeled, chopped
- ½ cup walnut pieces
- 3 garlic cloves
- ½ cup crumbled goat cheese
- 2 tablespoons extra-virgin olive oil, plus 2 teaspoons
- 2 tablespoons freshly squeezed lemon juice
- ¼ teaspoon salt
- 4 small zucchini

Directions:
Preheat the oven to 375°F.   Wrap the chopped beet in a piece of aluminum foil and seal well. Roast for 30 to 40 minutes until fork-tender.   Meanwhile, heat a dry skillet over medium-high heat. Toast the walnuts for 5 to 7 minutes until lightly browned and fragrant. Transfer the cooked beets to the bowl of a food processor. Add the toasted walnuts, garlic, goat cheese, 2 tablespoons of olive oil, lemon juice, and salt. Process until smooth.   Using a spiralizer or sharp knife, cut the zucchini into thin "noodles."   In a large skillet, heat the remaining 2 teaspoons of oil over medium heat. Add the zucchini and toss in the oil. Cook, stirring gently, for 2 to 3 minutes, until the zucchini softens. Toss with the beet pesto and serve warm.

Nutrition Info: Calories: 422; Total Fat: 39g; Protein: 8g; Carbohydrates: 17g; Sugars: 10g; Fiber: 6g; Sodium: 339mg

563. Bacon Cheeseburger Dip

Servings: 8   Cooking Time: 30 Minutes

Ingredients:
- 1 lb. lean ground beef
- 1 pkg. cream cheese, soft
- 2 cups low fat cheddar cheese, grated
- 1 cup fat free sour cream
- 2/3 cup bacon, cooked crisp and crumbled
- What you'll need from store cupboard:
- 10 oz. can tomatoes with green chilies

Directions:
Heat oven to 350 degrees.   Place a large skillet over med-high heat and cook beef, breaking it up with a wooden spoon, until no longer pink. Drain off the fat. In a large bowl, combine remaining Ingredients until mixed well. Stir in beef.   Pour into a small baking dish. Bake 20-25 minutes or until mixture is hot and bubbly. Serve warm.

Nutrition Info: Calories 268 Total Carbs 9g Protein 33g Fat 10g Sugar 2g Fiber 0g

564. Spicy Asian Dipping Sauce

Servings: ½ Cup   Cooking Time: 0 Minutes

Ingredients:
- ⅓ cup low-fat mayonnaise
- 1 to 2 teaspoons hot sauce, to your liking
- 2 teaspoons rice vinegar
- 1 teaspoon sesame oil

Directions:
Stir together the mayo, hot sauce, rice vinegar, and oil in a small bowl until thoroughly smooth.   Chill for at least 30 minutes to blend the flavors.

Nutrition Info:(2 Tablespoons)calories: 54   fat: 4.7g protein: 0g   carbs: 1.7g   fiber: 0g   sugar: 1.0g sodium: 190mg

565. Tuscan Sausage Soup

Servings: 8   Cooking Time: 15 Minutes

Ingredients:
- 1 lb. pork sausage, cooked
- 2 cup half-n-half
- 1 ½ cup cauliflower, grated and cooked
- ½ cup onion, diced
- ¼ cup margarine
- What you'll need from store cupboard:
- 1 cup chicken broth
- 4 cloves garlic, diced fine
- 1 tsp salt
- ½ tsp black pepper

Directions:
In a large saucepan, over medium heat, melt margarine. Add onion and garlic, cook, stirring occasionally, 1-2 minutes.   Pour in the broth and cream. Bring to a boil stirring constantly.   Add sausage and cauliflower and season with salt and pepper. Heat through and serve.

Nutrition Info: Calories 336 Total Carbs 5g Net Carbs 4g Protein 14g Fat 29g Sugar 1g Fiber 1g

566. Blueberry And Chicken Salad On A Bed Of Greens

Servings: 4   Cooking Time: 10 Minutes

Ingredients:
- 2 cups chopped cooked chicken
- 1 cup fresh blueberries
- ¼ cup finely chopped almonds
- 1 celery stalk, finely chopped
- ¼ cup finely chopped red onion
- 1 tablespoon chopped fresh basil
- 1 tablespoon chopped fresh cilantro
- ½ cup plain, nonfat Greek yogurt or vegan mayonnaise
- ¼ teaspoon salt
- ¼ teaspoon freshly ground black pepper
- 8 cups salad greens (baby spinach, spicy greens, romaine)

Directions:
In a large mixing bowl, combine the chicken, blueberries, almonds, celery, onion, basil, and cilantro. Toss gently to mix.   In a small bowl, combine the yogurt, salt, and pepper. Add to the chicken salad and stir to combine. Arrange 2 cups of salad greens on each of 4 plates and divide the chicken salad among the plates to serve.

Nutrition Info: Calories: 207; Total Fat: 6g; Protein: 28g; Carbohydrates: 11g; Sugars: 6g; Fiber: 3g; Sodium: 235mg

567. Grilled Tofu With Sesame Seeds

Servings: 6   Cooking Time: 20 Minutes

Ingredients:
- 1½ tablespoons brown rice vinegar
- 1 scallion, green and white parts, minced
- 1 tablespoon ginger root, freshly grated
- 1 tablespoon no-sugar-added applesauce
- 2 tablespoons naturally brewed soy sauce
- ¼ teaspoon dried red pepper flakes, crushed
- 2 teaspoons sesame oil, toasted
- 1 (14-ounce / 397-g) package extra-firm tofu, drained and squeezed of excess liquid, cut into 18 pieces
- 2 tablespoons fresh cilantro
- 1 teaspoon toasted black or white sesame seeds

Directions:
Combine the vinegar, scallion, ginger, applesauce, soy sauce, red pepper flakes, and sesame oil in a large bowl. Stir to mix well.   Dunk the tofu pieces in the bowl, then refrigerate to marinate for 30 minutes.   Preheat a grill pan over medium-high heat.   Place the tofu on the grill pan with tongs and reserve the marinade, then grill for 8 minutes or until the tofu is golden brown and has deep grilled marks on both sides. Flip the tofu halfway through the cooking time. You may need to work in batches to avoid overcrowding.   Transfer the tofu on a large plate and sprinkle with cilantro leaves and sesame seeds. Serve with the marinade alongside.

Nutrition Info:calories: 90   fat: 6.0g   protein: 7.0g carbs: 3.0g   fiber: 1.0g   sugar: 1.0g   sodium: 310mg

568. Roasted Asparagus, Onions, And Red Peppers

Servings: 4   Cooking Time: 5 Minutes
Ingredients:
- 1 pound asparagus, woody ends trimmed, cut into 2-inch segments
- 1 small onion, quartered
- 2 red bell peppers, seeded, cut into 1-inch pieces
- 2 tablespoons Easy Italian Dressing (here)

Directions:
Preheat the oven to 400°F. Line a baking sheet with parchment paper.   In a large mixing bowl, toss the asparagus, onion, and peppers with the dressing. Transfer to the prepared baking sheet.   Roast for 10 minutes, then, using a spatula, flip the vegetables. Roast for 5 to 10 more minutes until the vegetables are tender. Stir well and serve.
Nutrition Info: Calories: 93; Total Fat: 5g; Protein: 3g; Carbohydrates: 11g; Sugars: 6g; Fiber: 4g; Sodium: 32mg

569. Chinese Hot Mustard

Servings: 4   Cooking Time: 15 Minutes
Ingredients:
- What you'll need from store cupboard:
- 1 tbsp. mustard powder
- 1½ tsp hot water
- ½ tsp vegetable oil
- ½ tsp rice vinegar
- ⅛ tsp salt
- ⅛ tsp white pepper

Directions:
In a small bowl, mix together the dry Ingredients. Add water and stir until mixture resembles liquid paste and dry Ingredients are absorbed.   Stir in oil and vinegar until thoroughly combined. Cover and let rest 10 minutes. Stir again. Taste and adjust any seasonings if desired. Cover and refrigerate until ready to use.
Nutrition Info: Calories 19 Total Carbs 1g Protein 1g Fat 1g Sugar 0g Fiber 0g

570. Roasted Halibut With Red Peppers, Green Beans, And Onions

Servings: 4   Cooking Time: 10 Minutes
Ingredients:
- 1 pound green beans, trimmed
- 2 red bell peppers, seeded and cut into strips
- 1 onion, sliced
- Zest and juice of 2 lemons
- 3 garlic cloves, minced
- 2 tablespoons extra-virgin olive oil
- 1 teaspoon dried dill
- 1 teaspoon dried oregano
- 4 (4-ounce) halibut fillets
- ½ teaspoon salt
- ¼ teaspoon freshly ground black pepper

Directions:
Preheat the oven to 400°F. Line a baking sheet with parchment paper.   In a large bowl, toss the green beans, bell peppers, onion, lemon zest and juice, garlic, olive oil, dill, and oregano.   Use a slotted spoon to transfer the vegetables to the prepared baking sheet in a single layer, leaving the juice behind in the bowl. Gently place the halibut fillets in the bowl, and coat in the juice. Transfer the fillets to the baking sheet, nestled between the vegetables, and drizzle them with any juice left in the bowl. Sprinkle the vegetables and halibut with the salt and pepper.   Bake for 15 to 20 minutes until the vegetables are just tender and the fish flakes apart easily.
Nutrition Info: Calories: 234; Total Fat: 9g; Protein: 24g; Carbohydrates: 16g; Sugars: 8g; Fiber: 5g; Sodium: 349mg

571. Comforting Summer Squash Soup With Crispy Chickpeas

Servings: 4   Cooking Time: 10 Minutes
Ingredients:
- 1 (15-ounce) can low-sodium chickpeas, drained and rinsed
- 1 teaspoon extra-virgin olive oil, plus 1 tablespoon
- ¼ teaspoon smoked paprika
- Pinch salt, plus ½ teaspoon
- 3 medium zucchini, coarsely chopped
- 3 cups low-sodium vegetable broth
- ½ onion, diced
- 3 garlic cloves, minced
- 2 tablespoons plain low-fat Greek yogurt
- Freshly ground black pepper

Directions:
Preheat the oven to 425°F. Line a baking sheet with parchment paper.   In a medium mixing bowl, toss the chickpeas with 1 teaspoon of olive oil, the smoked paprika, and a pinch salt. Transfer to the prepared baking sheet and roast until crispy, about 20 minutes, stirring once. Set aside.   Meanwhile, in a medium pot, heat the remaining 1 tablespoon of oil over medium heat. Add the zucchini, broth, onion, and garlic to the pot, and bring to a boil. Reduce the heat to a simmer, and cook until the zucchini and onion are tender, about 20 minutes.   In a blender jar, or using an immersion blender, purée the soup. Return to the pot.   Add the yogurt, remaining ½ teaspoon of salt, and pepper, and stir well. Serve topped with the roasted chickpeas.
Nutrition Info: Calories: 188; Total Fat: 7g; Protein: 8g; Carbohydrates: 24g; Sugars: 7g; Fiber: 7g; Sodium: 528mg

572. Beer Cheese & Chicken Soup

Servings: 6-8   Cooking Time: 5 Hours 30 Minutes
Ingredients:
- 6 slices bacon, cut into 1 inch pieces
- 1 lb. chicken breast, cut into bite size pieces
- 2 cup half-and-half
- 1 cup cheddar cheese, grated
- 1 cup light beer
- 4 tbsp. margarine
- What you'll need from store cupboard
- 1 cup low sodium chicken broth

- ¼ cup flour
- 2 tsp garlic powder
- 1 tsp cayenne pepper
- 1 tsp smoked paprika
- 1 tsp salt
- 1 tsp black pepper, coarsely ground
- 1 tsp Worcestershire sauce

Directions:
Cook bacon in a medium skillet, over med-high heat until almost crisp. Remove with a slotted spoon and add to crock pot.   Add chicken to the skillet and cook until no longer pink. Add it to the bacon along with the broth, beer, and Worcestershire. Cover and cook on low 4 hours. Melt margarine in a small saucepan over medium heat. Add flour and spices and whisk until smooth. Whisk in half-n-half and continue stirring until thoroughly combined. Stir into chicken mixture in crock pot.   Add the cheese and stir well. Cook another 60-90 minutes or until cheese has completely melted and soup has thickened. Serve.
Nutrition Info: Calories 453 Total Carbs 9g Protein 32g Fat 30g Sugar 0g Fiber 0g

573. Curried Chicken Soup

Servings: 12   Cooking Time: 20 Minutes
Ingredients:
- 2 carrots, diced
- 2 stalks celery, diced
- 1 onion, diced
- 3 cup chicken, cooked and cut in cubes
- 2 cups cauliflower, grated
- 1 cup half-n-half
- ¼ cup margarine, cubed
- What you'll need from store cupboard:
- 4 ½ cup low sodium vegetable broth
- 2 12 oz. can fat free evaporated milk
- ¾ cup + 2 tbsp. flour
- 1 tsp salt
- 1 tsp curry powder

Directions:
Melt butter in a large pot over medium heat. Add carrots, celery, and onion and cook 2 minutes.   Stir in flour until well blended. Stir in seasonings. Slowly add milk and half-n-half. Bring to a boil, cook, stirring, 2 minutes or until thickened.   Slowly stir in broth. Add chicken and cauliflower and bring back to boil. Reduce heat and simmer 10 minutes, or until vegetable are tender. Serve.
Nutrition Info: Calories 204 Total Carbs 17g Protein 17g Fat 7g Sugar 8g Fiber 1g

574. Horseradish Mustard Sauce

Servings: 8   Cooking Time: 5 Minutes
Ingredients:
- ¼ cup fat free sour cream
- What you'll need from store cupboard:
- ¼ cup lite mayonnaise
- 1 ½ tsp lemon juice
- 1 tsp Splenda
- ½ tsp ground mustard
- ½ tsp Dijon mustard
- ½ tsp horseradish

Directions:
In a small bowl, combine all Ingredients until thoroughly combined.   Store in an air tight jar in the refrigerator until ready to use. Serving size is 1 tablespoon.
Nutrition Info: Calories 36 Total Carbs 2g Protein 0g Fat 2g Sugar 1g Fiber 0g

575. Brown Rice With Carrot, And Scrambled Egg

Servings: 4   Cooking Time: 20 Minutes
Ingredients:
- 1 tablespoon extra-virgin olive oil
- 1 bunch collard greens, stemmed and cut into chiffonade
- 1 carrot, cut into 2-inch matchsticks
- 1 red onion, thinly sliced
- ½ cup low-sodium vegetable broth
- 2 tablespoons coconut aminos
- 1 garlic clove, minced
- 1 cup cooked brown rice
- 1 large egg
- 1 teaspoon red pepper flakes
- 1 teaspoon paprika
- Salt, to taste

Directions:
Heat the olive oil in a Dutch oven or a nonstick skillet over medium heat until shimmering.   Add the collard greens and sauté for 4 minutes or until wilted.   Add the carrot, onion, broth, coconut aminos, and garlic to the Dutch oven, then cover and cook 6 minutes or until the carrot is tender.   Add the brown rice and cook for 4 minutes. Keep stirring during the cooking.   Break the egg over them, then cook and scramble the egg for 4 minutes or until the egg is set.   Turn off the heat and sprinkle with red pepper flakes, paprika, and salt before serving.
Nutrition Info:calories: 154   fat: 6.0g   protein: 6.0g carbs: 22.0g   fiber: 6.0g   sugar: 2.0g   sodium: 78mg

576. Mozzarella And Artichoke Stuffed Spaghetti Squash

Servings: 4   Cooking Time: 10 Minutes
Ingredients:
- 1 small spaghetti squash, halved and seeded
- ½ cup low-fat cottage cheese
- ¼ cup shredded mozzarella cheese, divided
- 2 garlic cloves, minced
- 1 cup artichoke hearts, chopped
- 1 cup thinly sliced kale
- ⅛ teaspoon salt
- Pinch freshly ground black pepper

Directions:
Preheat the oven to 400°F. Line a baking sheet with parchment paper.   Place the cut squash halves on the prepared baking sheet cut-side down, and roast for 30 to 40 minutes, depending on the size and thickness of the squash, until they are fork-tender. Set aside to cool slightly.   In a large bowl, mix the cottage cheese, 2 tablespoons of mozzarella cheese, garlic, artichoke hearts, kale, salt, and pepper.   Preheat the broiler to

high.   Using a fork, break apart the flesh of the spaghetti squash into strands, being careful to leave the skin intact. Add the strands to the cheese and vegetable mixture. Toss gently to combine.   Divide the mixture between the two hollowed-out squash halves and top with the remaining 2 tablespoons of cheese.   Broil for 5 to 7 minutes until browned and heated through.   Cut each piece of stuffed squash in half to serve.
Nutrition Info: Calories: 142; Total Fat: 4g; Protein: 9g; Carbohydrates: 19g; Sugars: 10g; Fiber: 4g; Sodium: 312mg

577. Turkey Divan Casserole

Servings: 6   Cooking Time: 10 Minutes
Ingredients:
- Nonstick cooking spray
- 3 teaspoons extra-virgin olive oil, divided
- 1 pound turkey cutlets
- Pinch salt
- ¼ teaspoon freshly ground black pepper, divided
- ¼ cup chopped onion
- 2 garlic cloves, minced
- 2 tablespoons whole-wheat flour
- 1 cup unsweetened plain almond milk
- 1 cup low-sodium chicken broth
- ½ cup shredded Swiss cheese, divided
- ½ teaspoon dried thyme
- 4 cups chopped broccoli
- ¼ cup coarsely ground almonds

Directions:
Preheat the oven to 375°F. Spray a baking dish with nonstick cooking spray.   In a skillet, heat 1 teaspoon of oil over medium heat. Season the turkey with the salt and ⅛ teaspoon of pepper. Sauté the turkey cutlets for 5 to 7 minutes on each side until cooked through. Transfer to a cutting board, cool briefly, and cut into bite-size pieces. In the same pan, heat the remaining 2 teaspoons of oil over medium-high heat. Sauté the onion for 3 minutes until it begins to soften. Add the garlic and continue cooking for another minute. Stir in the flour and mix well. Whisk in the almond milk, broth, and remaining ⅛ teaspoon of pepper, and continue whisking until smooth. Add ¼ cup of cheese and the thyme, and continue stirring until the cheese is melted.   In the prepared baking dish, arrange the broccoli on the bottom. Cover with half the sauce. Place the turkey pieces on top of the broccoli, and cover with the remaining sauce. Sprinkle with the remaining ¼ cup of cheese and the ground almonds.   Bake for 35 minutes until the sauce is bubbly and the top is browned.
Nutrition Info: Calories: 207; Total Fat: 8g; Protein: 25g; Carbohydrates: 9g; Sugars: 2g; Fiber: 3g; Sodium: 128mg

578. Easy Italian Dressing

Servings: 12 (1 Tablespoon Each)   Cooking Time: 5 Minutes
Ingredients:
- ¼ cup red wine vinegar
- ½ cup extra-virgin olive oil
- ¼ teaspoon salt
- ¼ teaspoon freshly ground black pepper
- 1 teaspoon dried Italian seasoning
- 1 teaspoon Dijon mustard
- 1 garlic clove, minced

Directions:
In a small jar, combine the vinegar, olive oil, salt, pepper, Italian seasoning, mustard, and garlic. Close with a tight-fitting lid and shake vigorously for 1 minute. Refrigerate for up to 1 week.
Nutrition Info: Calories: 81; Total Fat: 9g; Protein: 0g; Carbohydrates: 0g; Sugars: 0g; Fiber: 0g; Sodium: 52mg

579. Coconut-berry Sunrise Smoothie

Servings: 2   Cooking Time: 5 Minutes
Ingredients:
- ½ cup mixed berries (blueberries, strawberries, blackberries)
- 1 tablespoon ground flaxseed
- 2 tablespoons unsweetened coconut flakes
- ½ cup unsweetened plain coconut milk
- ½ cup leafy greens (kale, spinach)
- ¼ cup unsweetened vanilla nonfat yogurt
- ½ cup ice

Directions:
In a blender jar, combine the berries, flaxseed, coconut flakes, coconut milk, greens, yogurt, and ice.   Process until smooth. Serve.
Nutrition Info: Calories: 181; Total Fat: 15g; Protein: 6g; Carbohydrates: 8g; Sugars: 3g; Fiber: 4g; Sodium: 24mg

580. Tomato Soup With Seafood

Servings: 8   Cooking Time: 45 Minutes
Ingredients:
- 1 lb. medium shrimp, peel and devein
- ½ lb. cod, cut in pieces
- 1 onions, diced
- 1 red bell pepper, diced
- 1 green pepper, diced
- 1 cup cauliflower, separated into small florets
- 3 tbsp. fresh parsley, diced fine
- What you'll need from store cupboard:
- 15 oz. tomato sauce
- 14 ½ oz. can tomatoes, diced and juice
- 1 quart vegetable broth
- 3 cloves garlic, diced fine
- 1 tbsp. olive oil
- ½ tsp oregano
- ¼ tsp basil
- ¼ tsp pepper
- 1 pinch salt
- 1 bay leaf

Directions:
Heat oil in large soup pot over med-high heat. Add onion and bell peppers and cook, stirring occasionally, 3-5 minutes, or until they start to get soft.   Add the garlic and cook 1 minute more. Transfer vegetables to a food processor along with canned tomatoes. Process until smooth. Pour back into soup pot and add tomato sauce, broth and seasoning.   Bring to a boil. Reduce heat and

simmer 15-20 minutes, or until soup starts to thicken and is reduced.   Add the fish and shrimp and cook just until fish is cooked through and shrimp turn pink. Stir in parsley and discard bay leaf before serving.
Nutrition Info: Calories 174 Total Carbs 10g Net Carbs 8g Protein 24g Fat 4g Sugar 6g Fiber 2g

581. Brown Rice & Lentil Salad

Servings: 4   Cooking Time: 10 Minutes
Ingredients:
- 1-cup water
- ½ cup instant brown rice
- 2 tablespoons olive oil
- 2 tablespoons red wine vinegar
- 1-tablespoon Dijon mustard
- 1 tablespoon minced onion
- ½-teaspoon paprika
- Salt and pepper
- 1 (15-ounce) can brown lentils, rinsed and drained
- 1 medium carrot, shredded
- 2 tablespoons fresh chopped parsley

Directions:
Stir together the water and instant brown rice in a medium saucepan.   Bring to a boil then simmer for 10 minutes, covered.   Remove from heat and set aside while you prepare the salad.   Whisk together the olive oil, vinegar, Dijon mustard, onion, paprika, salt, and pepper in a medium bowl.   Toss in the cooked rice, lentils, carrots, and parsley.   Adjust seasoning to taste then stir well and serve warm.
Nutrition Info: Calories 1455Total Fat 4.8gSaturated Fat 0.7gTotal Carbs 8.5gNet Carbs 4.6g Protein 2.1g Sugar 1.7g Fiber 3.9g Sodium 75mg

582. Vegetable Rice Pilaf

Servings: 6   Cooking Time: 25 Minutes
Ingredients:
- 1-tablespoon olive oil
- ½ medium yellow onion, diced
- 1 cup uncooked long-grain brown rice
- 2 cloves minced garlic
- ½ teaspoon dried basil
- Salt and pepper
- 2 cups fat-free chicken broth
- 1 cup frozen mixed veggies

Directions:
Heat the oil in a large skillet over medium heat.   Add the onion and sauté for 3 minutes until translucent. Stir in the rice and cook until lightly toasted.   Add the garlic, basil, salt, and pepper then stir to combine.   Stir in the chicken broth then bring to a boil.   Reduce heat and simmer, covered, for 10 minutes.   Stir in the frozen veggies then cover and cook for another 10 minutes until heated through. Servings hot.
Nutrition Info: Calories 75Total Fat 4.8gSaturated Fat 0.7gTotal Carbs 8.5gNet Carbs 4.6g Protein 2.1g Sugar 1.7g Fiber 3.9g Sodium 7mg

583. Turkey Chili

Servings: 6   Cooking Time: 15 Minutes
Ingredients:

- 1 tablespoon extra-virgin olive oil
- 1 pound lean ground turkey
- 1 large onion, diced
- 3 garlic cloves, minced
- 1 red bell pepper, seeded and diced
- 1 cup chopped celery
- 2 tablespoons chili powder
- 1 tablespoon ground cumin
- 1 (28-ounce) can reduced-salt diced tomatoes
- 1 (15-ounce) can low-sodium kidney beans, drained and rinsed
- 2 cups low-sodium chicken broth
- ½ teaspoon salt
- Shredded cheddar cheese, for serving (optional)

Directions:
In a large pot, heat the oil over medium heat. Add the turkey, onion, and garlic, and cook, stirring regularly, until the turkey is cooked through.   Add the bell pepper, celery, chili powder, and cumin. Stir well and continue to cook for 1 minute.   Add the tomatoes with their liquid, kidney beans, and chicken broth. Bring to a boil, reduce the heat to low, and simmer for 20 minutes. Season with the salt and serve topped with cheese (if using).
Nutrition Info: Calories: 276; Total Fat: 10g; Protein: 23g; Carbohydrates: 27g; Sugars: 7g; Fiber: 8g; Sodium: 556mg

584. Tangy Asparagus Bisque

Servings: 4   Cooking Time: 20 Minutes
Ingredients:
- 2 lbs. fresh asparagus, remove the bottom and cut into small pieces
- 1 yellow onion, diced
- 1 small lemon, zest and juice
- 1 tsp fresh thyme, diced fine
- What you'll need from store cupboard:
- 4 cup low sodium vegetable broth
- 3 tbsp. olive oil
- 3 cloves garlic, diced fine
- Salt & pepper, to taste

Directions:
Heat oil in a large saucepan over med-high heat. Add asparagus and onion and cook, stirring occasionally, until nicely browned, about 5 minutes. Add garlic and cook 1 minute more.   Stir in remaining Ingredients and bring to a boil. Reduce heat, and simmer 12-15 minutes or until asparagus is soft.   Use an immersion blender and process until smooth. Salt and pepper to taste and serve.
Nutrition Info: Calories 169 Total Carbs 17g Net carbs 11g Protein 6g Fat 11g Sugar 7g Fiber 6g

585. Wild Rice And Cranberries Salad

Servings: 6 Cups   Cooking Time: 45 Minutes
Ingredients:
- For the Rice:
- 2½ cups chicken bone broth, vegetable broth, or water
- 2 cups wild rice blend, rinsed
- 1 teaspoon kosher salt

- For the Dressing:
- Juice of 1 medium orange (about ¼ cup)
- 1½ teaspoons grated orange zest
- ¼ cup white wine vinegar
- 1 teaspoon pure maple syrup
- ¼ cup extra-virgin olive oil
- For the Salad:
- ½ cup sliced almonds, toasted
- ¾ cup unsweetened dried cranberries
- Freshly ground black pepper, to taste

Directions:
For the Rice   Pour the broth in a pot, then add the rice and sprinkle with salt. Bring to a boil over medium-high heat.   Reduce the heat to low. Cover the pot, then simmer for 45 minutes.   Turn off the heat and fluff the rice with a fork. Set aside until ready to use.   For the Dressing   When cooking the rice, make the dressing: Combine the ingredients for the dressing in a small bowl. Stir to combine well. Set aside until ready to use.   For the Salad   Put the cooked rice, almonds, and cranberries in a bowl, then sprinkle with black pepper. Add the dressing, then toss to combine well.   Serve immediately.
Nutrition Info:(⅓ Cup)calories: 126   fat: 5.0g   protein: 3.0g   carbs: 18.0g   fiber: 2.0g   sugar: 2.0g   sodium: 120mg

586. No Corn "cornbread"

Servings: 16   Cooking Time: 25 Minutes
Ingredients:
- 4 eggs, room temperature
- 1/3 cup butter, melted
- What you'll need from store cupboard:
- 1 ½ cup almond flour, sifted
- 1/3 cup Splenda
- 1 tsp baking powder

Directions:
Heat oven to 350 degrees. Line an 8-inch baking dish with parchment paper.   In a large bowl, whisk together eggs, butter, and Splenda. Stir in the flour and baking powder until no lumps remain.   Pour batter into prepared dish and smooth the top. Bake 25-30 minutes or until edges are golden brown and it passes the toothpick test.   Let cool 5 minutes before slicing and serving.
Nutrition Info: Calories 121 Total Carbs 6g Net Carbs 5g Protein 3g Fat 9g Sugar 4g Fiber 1g

587. Sugar Free Ketchup

Servings: 28   Cooking Time: 5 Minutes
Ingredients:
- What you'll need from store cupboard
- 12 oz. tomato paste
- 1 ½ cup water
- 1/3 cup white vinegar
- 1 tbsp. salt
- 3 tsp Splenda
- 1 tsp onion powder

Directions:
In a large bowl, combine water, vinegar, Splenda, onion powder, and salt. Whisk in tomato paste until smooth.

Pour into a glass jar with an air tight lid and store in refrigerator until ready to use. Serving size is 2 tablespoons.
Nutrition Info: Calories 15 Total Carbs 3g Protein 0g Fat 0g Sugar 2g Fiber 0g

588. Ritzy Calabaza Squash Soup

Servings: 8   Cooking Time: 45 Minutes
Ingredients:
- 2 pounds (907 g) calabaza squash, peeled and chopped
- 1 large tomato, chopped
- 1 medium onion, chopped
- 1 medium green bell pepper, chopped
- 1 scotch bonnet chili, deseeded and minced
- 8 scallions, chopped
- 3 sprigs fresh thyme
- 1 tablespoon minced ginger root
- 8 cups low-sodium vegetable broth
- Juice of 1 lime
- ¼ cup chopped cilantro
- Salt, to taste
- ¼ cup toasted pepitas

Directions:
Put the calabaza squash, tomato, onion, bell pepper, scotch bonnet, scallions, thyme, and ginger roots in a saucepan, then pour in the vegetable broth.   Bring to a boil over medium-high heat. Reduce the heat to low, then simmer for 45 minutes or until the vegetables are soft. Stir constantly.   Add the lime juice, cilantro, and salt. Pour the soup in a large bowl, then discard the thyme sprigs and garnish with pepitas before serving.
Nutrition Info:calories: 50   fat: 0g   protein: 2.0g   carbs: 12.0g   fiber: 4.0g   sugar: 5.0g   sodium: 20mg

589. All Purpose Beef Marinade

Servings: 8   Cooking Time: 10 Minutes
Ingredients:
- 6 limes zested
- 1 bunch cilantro, diced
- What you'll need from store cupboard:
- ¼ c olive oil
- 6 cloves garlic, diced fine

Directions:
Mix all Ingredients in an airtight container.   Keep refrigerated for up to 3 months or frozen up to 6 months. Serving size is 1 tablespoon.
Nutrition Info: Calories 78 Total Carbs 1g Protein 0g Fat 8g Sugar 0g Fiber 0g

590. Guinness Beef Stew With Cauliflower Mash

Servings: 4   Cooking Time: 8 Hours
Ingredients:
- 2 lb. beef round steak, cut into 1-inch cubes
- 1 large head cauliflower, separated into florets
- 5 sprigs fresh thyme
- 1 medium carrot, cut into 1/2-inch pieces
- 1 stick of celery, cut into 1/2-inch pieces
- 1 cup yellow onion, cut into large pieces

- 2/3 cup Guinness
- 1 tbsp. margarine
- What you'll need from store cupboard:
- 2 cups low sodium beef broth
- 2 tbsp. arrowroot starch
- 1 tbsp. + 1 tsp garlic, diced fine
- 2 tsp olive oil
- Sea salt & pepper to taste

Directions:
Add oil to a large nonstick skillet and heat over med-high heat. Add beef and sear on all sides. Transfer to crock pot. Add thyme, Guinness, carrot, onion, celery, garlic, and broth. Set to low and cook 6-8 hours, or 4-5 on high. One hour before the stew is ready, mix arrowroot with 1 ½ tablespoons water and stir into stew.   For the mash: bring 2 cups water to a boil in a large pot and add cauliflower. Cover and cook 10 -12 minutes, or until cauliflower is soft.   Drain. Add salt, pepper, 1 teaspoon garlic, and margarine. Use an immersion blender and process until it resembles mashed potatoes.   To serve: ladle stew in a bowl and spoon about ¼ cup of the mash on top. Garnish with fresh thyme, parsley, and cracked pepper if desired.
Nutrition Info: Calories 563 Total Carbs 17g Net Carbs 11g Protein 75g Fat 28g Sugar 7g Fiber 6g

591. Maple Mustard Salad Dressing

Servings: 6   Cooking Time: 5 Minutes
Ingredients:
- What you'll need from store cupboard:
- 2 tbsp. balsamic vinegar
- 2 tbsp. olive oil
- 1 tbsp. sugar free maple syrup
- 1 tsp Dijon mustard
- 1/8 tsp sea salt

Directions:
Place all the Ingredients in a jar with a tight fitting lid. Screw on lid and shake to combine. Store in refrigerator until ready to use.
Nutrition Info: Calories 48 Total Carbs 2g Protein 0g Fat 5g Sugar 0g Fiber 0g

592. Cauli-broccoli Tots

Servings: 4   Cooking Time: 10 Minutes
Ingredients:
- 1 cup chopped broccoli florets and stems
- 1 cup chopped cauliflower florets and stems
- ¼ cup diced onion
- 1 large egg
- ¼ cup whole-wheat bread crumbs
- ¼ cup crumbled feta cheese
- ½ teaspoon salt
- ¼ teaspoon freshly ground black pepper

Directions:
Preheat the oven to 400°F. Line a baking sheet with parchment paper.   In a food processor, combine the broccoli, cauliflower, and onion, and pulse until chopped well but still slightly chunky. Or if you don't have a food processor, chop everything on a large cutting board until you have very small pieces. Transfer to a large mixing bowl.   Add the egg, bread crumbs, cheese, salt, and

pepper.   Using your hands, shape small balls, a little smaller than a tablespoon, and carefully place them on the prepared baking sheet.   Bake for 10 minutes, flip carefully, and continue to bake for 10 additional minutes until browned and crisp.
Nutrition Info: Calories: 90; Total Fat: 4g; Protein: 5g; Carbohydrates: 9g; Sugars: 2g; Fiber: 2g; Sodium: 424mg

593. Basic Salsa

Servings: 8   Cooking Time: 1 Hour
Ingredients:
- 8 tomatoes
- 2-3 jalapeno peppers, depending on how spicy you like it
- 2 limes, juiced
- What you'll need from store cupboard:
- 4 cloves garlic
- 1 tbsp. salt
- Nonstick cooking spray

Directions:
Heat oven to broil. Spray a baking sheet with cooking spray.   Place tomatoes, peppers, and garlic on prepared pan and broil 8-10 minutes, turning occasionally, until skin on the vegetables begins to char and peel way.   Let cool. Remove skins.   Place vegetables in a food processor and pulse. Add salt and lime juise and pulse until salsa reaches desired consistency.   Store in a jar with an airtight lid in the refrigerator up to 7 days. Serving size is ¼ cup.
Nutrition Info: Calories   31 Total Carbs 7g Net Carbs 5g Protein 1g Fat 0g Sugar 4g Fiber 2g

594. Cheesy Cauliflower Puree

Servings: 6   Cooking Time: 15 Minutes
Ingredients:
- 2 ½ lbs. cauliflower florets, steamed
- 4 oz. reduced fat sharp cheddar cheese, grated
- 2 tbsp. half-n-half
- 1 tbsp. butter
- What you'll need from store cupboard:
- ½ tsp salt
- ½ tsp pepper

Directions:
Steam the cauliflower until it is fork tender, drain. Add the cauliflower and remaining Ingredients to a food processor. Pulse until almost smooth. Serve warm. You can make it ahead of time and just reheat it as needed also.
Nutrition Info: Calories 145 Total Carbs 10g Net Carbs 5g Protein 9g Fat 9g Sugar 5g Fiber 5g

595. Green Bean Casserole

Servings: 8   Cooking Time: 10 Minutes
Ingredients:
- 1 pound green beans, trimmed, cut into bite-size pieces
- 3 tablespoons extra-virgin olive oil, divided
- 8 ounces brown mushrooms, diced
- 3 garlic cloves, minced
- 1½ tablespoons whole-wheat flour

- 1 cup low-sodium vegetable broth
- 1 cup unsweetened plain almond milk
- ¼ cup almond flour
- 2 tablespoons dried minced onion

Directions:
Preheat the oven to 400°F.   Bring a large pot of water to a boil. Boil the green beans for 3 to 5 minutes until just barely tender but still bright green. Drain and set aside. In a medium skillet, heat 2 tablespoons of oil over medium-high heat. Add the mushrooms and stir. Cook for 3 to 5 minutes until the mushrooms brown and release their liquid. Add the garlic and stir until just fragrant, about 30 seconds.   Add the whole-wheat flour and stir well to combine. Add the broth and simmer for 1 minute.   Reduce the heat to medium low and add the almond milk. Return to a simmer and cook for 5 to 7 minutes until the mixture thickens.   Remove from the heat. Stir in the green beans and transfer to a baking dish. In a small bowl, mix the almond flour, dried minced onion, and remaining 1 tablespoon of olive oil, and stir until combined and crumbly. Crumble over the beans. Bake for 15 to 20 minutes until the liquids are bubbling and the top is browned.

Nutrition Info: Calories: 97; Total Fat: 7g; Protein: 2g; Carbohydrates: 7g; Sugars: 2g; Fiber: 2g; Sodium: 57mg

596. Ceviche

Servings: 4   Cooking Time: 10 Minutes, Plus 4 Hours To Marinate
Ingredients:
- ½ pound fresh skinless, white, ocean fish fillet (halibut, mahi mahi, etc.), diced
- 1 cup freshly squeezed lime juice, divided
- 2 tablespoons chopped fresh cilantro, divided
- 1 serrano pepper, sliced
- 1 garlic clove, crushed
- ¾ teaspoon salt, divided
- ½ red onion, thinly sliced
- 2 tomatoes, diced
- 1 red bell pepper, seeded and diced
- 1 tablespoon extra-virgin olive oil

Directions:
In a large mixing bowl, combine the fish, ¾ cup of lime juice, 1 tablespoon of cilantro, serrano pepper, garlic, and ½ teaspoon of salt. The fish should be covered or nearly covered in lime juice. Cover the bowl and refrigerate for 4 hours.   Sprinkle the remaining ¼ teaspoon of salt over the onion in a small bowl, and let sit for 10 minutes. Drain and rinse well.   In a large bowl, combine the tomatoes, bell pepper, olive oil, remaining ¼ cup of lime juice, and onion. Let rest for at least 10 minutes, or as long as 4 hours, while the fish "cooks."   When the fish is ready, it will be completely white and opaque. At this time, strain the juice, reserving it in another bowl. If desired, remove the serrano pepper and garlic.   Add the vegetables to the fish, and stir gently. Taste, and add some of the reserved lime juice to the ceviche as desired. Serve topped with the remaining 1 tablespoon of cilantro.

Nutrition Info: Calories: 121; Total Fat: 4g; Protein: 12g; Carbohydrates: 11g; Sugars: 5g; Fiber: 2g; Sodium: 405mg

597. Whole Veggie-stuffed Trout

Servings: 2   Cooking Time: 10 Minutes
Ingredients:
- Nonstick cooking spray
- 2 (8-ounce) whole trout fillets, dressed (cleaned but with bones and skin intact)
- 1 tablespoon extra-virgin olive oil
- ¼ teaspoon salt
- ⅛ teaspoon freshly ground black pepper
- ½ red bell pepper, seeded and thinly sliced
- 1 small onion, thinly sliced
- 2 or 3 shiitake mushrooms, sliced
- 1 poblano pepper, seeded and thinly sliced
- 1 lemon, sliced

Directions:
Preheat the oven to 425°F. Spray a baking sheet with nonstick cooking spray.   Rub both trout, inside and out, with the olive oil, then season with the salt and pepper.   In a large bowl, combine the bell pepper, onion, mushrooms, and poblano pepper. Stuff half of this mixture into the cavity of each fish. Top the mixture with 2 or 3 lemon slices inside each fish.   Arrange the fish on the prepared baking sheet side by side and roast for 25 minutes until the fish is cooked through and the vegetables are tender.

Nutrition Info: Calories: 452; Total Fat: 22g; Protein: 49g; Carbohydrates: 14g; Sugars: 5g; Fiber: 3g; Sodium: 357mg

598. Classic Texas Caviar

Servings: 6   Cooking Time: 0 Minutes
Ingredients:
- For the Salad:
- 1 ear fresh corn, kernels removed
- 1 cup cooked lima beans
- 1 cup cooked black-eyed peas
- 1 red bell pepper, chopped
- 2 celery stalks, chopped
- ½ red onion, chopped
- For the Dressing:
- 3 tablespoons apple cider vinegar
- 1 teaspoon paprika
- 2 tablespoons extra-virgin olive oil

Directions:
Combine the corn, beans, peas, bell pepper, celery, and onion in a large bowl. Stir to mix well.   Combine the vinegar, paprika, and olive oil in a small bowl. Stir to combine well.   Pour the dressing into the salad and toss to mix well. Let sit for 20 minutes to infuse before serving.

Nutrition Info:calories: 170   fat: 5.0g   protein: 10.0g   carbs: 29.0g   fiber: 10.0g   sugar: 4.0g   sodium: 20mg

599. Avocado Cilantro Dressing

Servings: 1 Cup   Cooking Time: 0 Minutes
Ingredients:
- 1 large avocado, peeled and pitted
- ½ cup plain Greek yogurt
- ¾ cup fresh cilantro

- 1 tablespoon water
- 2 teaspoons freshly squeezed lime juice
- 1/8 teaspoon garlic powder
- Pinch salt

Directions:
Process the avocado, yogurt, cilantro, water, lime juice, garlic powder, and salt in a blender until creamy and emulsified. Chill for at least 30 minutes in the refrigerator to let the flavors blend.

Nutrition Info:(1/4 Cup)calories: 92   fat: 6.8g protein: 4.1g   carbs: 4.9g   fiber: 2.3g   sugar: 1.0g sodium: 52mg

600. Green Protein Smoothie Recipe

Servings: 2   Cooking Time: 5 Minutes
Ingredients:
- Kale – 1 oz.
- Pineapple – 4 oz.
- Pea protein – 1 Tbsp.
- Water – 1 cup
- Tangerine – 1, peeled
- Avocado – 1/2
- Almonds – 3 Tbsp.
- Ice – 1 cup

Directions:
Except for the almonds, blend everything in the blender. Top with almonds and serve.

Nutrition Info:227Fat: 4Carb: 21g Protein: 7g

Made in the USA
Coppell, TX
12 March 2021